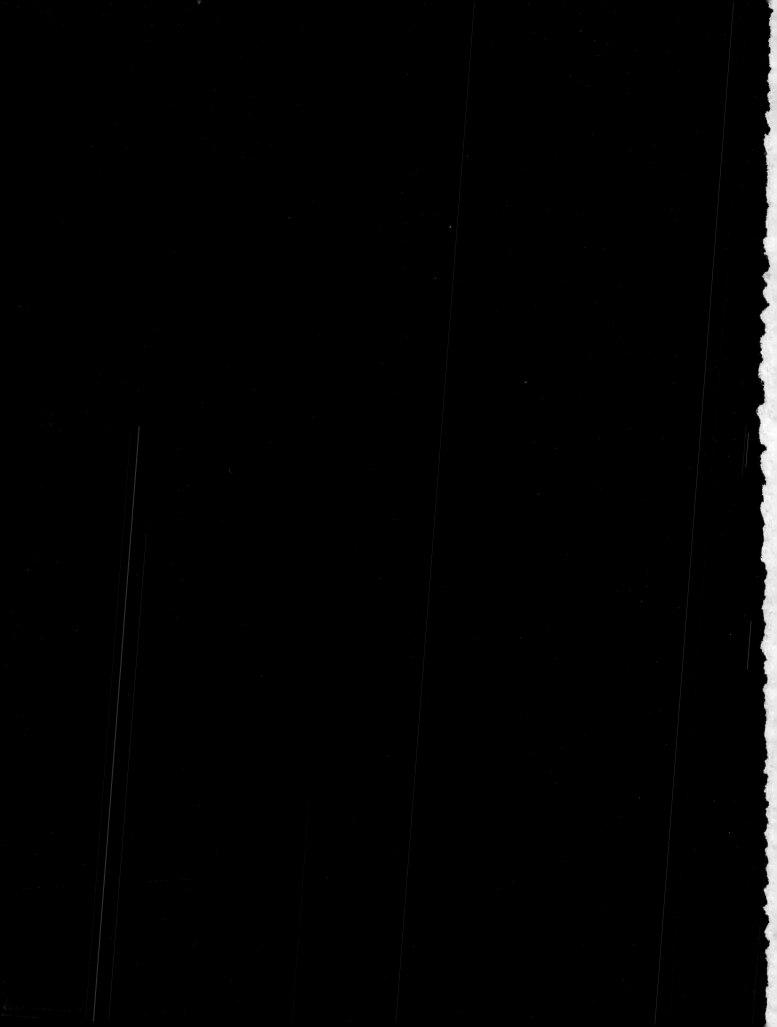

Mastering digital dental photography Wolfgang Bengel

MASTERING
digital dental photography

Wolfgang Bengel

Quintessence Publishing Co, Ltd

London, Berlin, Chicago, Tokyo, Barcelona, Beijing, Istanbul, Milan,
Moscow, Mumbai, Paris, Prague, São Paulo, Seoul, Warsaw

British Library Cataloguing in Publication Data
  Bengel, Wolfgang
  Mastering digital dental photography
  1. Dental photography – Technique 2. Photography – Digital techniques
  I. Title
  617.6'0028
  ISBN-10: 1850971528

© 2006 Quintessence Publishing Co, Ltd
Quintessence Publishing Co, Ltd
Grafton Road, New Malden, Surrey KT3 3AB
United Kingdom
www.quintpub.co.uk

Editor: Kathleen Splieth, Wampen
Layout and Production: Bernd Burkart, Berlin
Printing and Binding: Bosch-Druck GmbH, Landshut

Printed in Germany

ISBN 1-85097-152-8

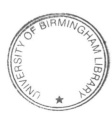

Dedication

To Helmi, Christiane, and Renate

who accompanied our way for many years
with patience, commitment and unlimited loyalty.

Foreword

Photography can be found virtually everywhere in daily life, and it seems that images are being produced everywhere in both personal and professional applications. Bioinformatics, a new field, is speeding ahead, and new applications are being explored at exponential rates as computers and digital tools become mainstream. The actual photomechanical process has become so easy that it might actually be difficult to achieve the quality results one might expect. Practitioners have become a bit spoiled and rarely think about the role and goal of the pictures and are more enamored with the technology and how cool it is.

Photography has experienced an incredible transformation in the last 10 years as digital methods have taken over photographic applications. Originally invented in the late 1830's with silver halide materials, photography's evolution to the 1990's was a long steady continuum of improvements with few, if any, significant departures from methods and materials. Small improvements occurred frequently and were most evident in color photography, but fundamentally used silver halide materials and mostly film. These fundamental principles were grounded in physical and chemical processes.

In specific applications, photography can remember what the mind struggles to and photography can more easily describe what words cannot. Photography, when practiced correctly, can make the invisible visible. Science, and in particular medicine, quickly adopted photography as a tool for the documentation of procedures, disease and treatments. With careful and precise approaches, photography could reproduce reality with a precision that drawing or other illustrative methods could not. It was a powerful way to share conditions and cases that otherwise words struggled to achieve.

As the mid 1990's arrived, digital photography and more specifically digital cameras started to arrive in the marketplace. Although their resolution was low, they created a small buzz and purists argued about their poor picture quality, while innovators were delighted with what might be possible. In the 10 or so years since the Apple Quicktake first appeared in photography stores, digital photography has completely displaced film photography in science and medicine. Digital has achieved in 10 years what took silver halide materials more than 150 years to achieve.

The future is indeed exciting. With CCD and CMOS chips being able to resolve more things than ever using chips that are often 8+ million pixels, applications are being explored daily for imaging situations that otherwise were not possible with film. Display devices, printers, software and a slew of other inventions create a myriad of choices, provide methods, and provide new usages or others that have yet to be considered. Often it is overwhelming and challenging at best to know where to go, how to purchase tools and what are the standards.

The advantages of this new technology do however come with a cost. New technology is very dynamic and standards are being proposed daily for approaches and practices, but are not widely accepted in all industries. It can be frustrating when considering purchasing products for specific applications as the prices are constantly decreasing and improvements are continually made. New software allows things to be measured, changed, shared, and integrated into new communication tools with the click of a mouse. Images now are being animated, used in reports and put onto web sites at exponential rates. These applications are unparalleled in film technologies.

This richly illustrated book by Dr Wolfgang Bengel builds on his initial book investigating *Dental Photography* published in 1984. Excellent practical solutions are shared in very logical manner. Attention to detail is evident upon a quick review of the table of contents. As a practicing dentist and having a long history of using photography, he has produced an excellent book that should serve as a cornerstone of any practitioner of digital photography in a clinical setting.

Professor Michael Peres
Rochester Institute of Technology

Preface and acknowledgements

My last book on dental photography was published in 2002. It dealt with conventional and digital techniques.

When I was asked by the publisher to prepare a 2nd edition, I realized that photography had changed completely.

In the professional world, the transition from conventional silver-halide photography to digital photography was not only underway but nearly completed. I thus decided to write a completely new book concentrating only on digital photography. Of course, the principles of photography have not changed. But in many cases, digital photography has changed the approach to photography.

In my hands-on photography courses, I learned a great deal about problems colleagues have when starting with digital photography and stumbling into the pitfalls of soft- and hardware. Therefore, I have tried to compile a book which is practically oriented. Although the user has to deal with things like image editing programs, archiving programs, and some software problems, digital photography is much easier than the old silver-halide technique. The learning curve in the digital world is much steeper, as there is the great opportunity of immediate image checking. After users have overcome their initial inhibitions about the new technique, they have the chance to explore new worlds of creativity and fascinating possibilities.

I have never yet met a user who returned to conventional photography after he or she had stepped into the digital world.

Writing such a book relies on the help of others. I would like to thank Mrs. Bähr of Olympus, Mr. Scheffer of Nikon, Mr. Hermanns of Canon, and Mr. Bauer of Sigma, as well as Mr. Dieter Baumann and other people not mentioned here. Mr. Hübschen of Kaiser and Mr. Hiesinger of Novoflex supported me with advice on many occasions.

My appreciation goes to my practice staff for their help and patience over many years.

I thank my friend Dr. Steve Chu, New York, for our discussions.

Again, I would like to extend my gratitude to Mr. Haase of Quintessence Publishing for the opportunity of publishing another book. Mr. Burkart was responsible for the production of this work. I would like to thank him especially for his attention to detail and his patience.

At last I have to thank my wife and the whole family for their patience.

Wolfgang Bengel
Bensheim

Contents

Man – Image – Medicine

Man is a visual animal. When our ancestors first attempted to walk erect and our eyes moved from the sides to the front of our skulls, we began to see in three dimensions – not necessarily a disadvantage for a species which swung rapidly from branch to branch through the treetops. At the very latest, when we began to walk on two legs and left the forests to conquer the steppes and the rest of the world, vision became our primary sense. This is still the case today.

Today, now well advanced into the visual age, the image is beginning to replace the word. Images need only to be recognized, but words must be understood. An image always lends authenticity, whereas even the strongest proof cannot wipe off the weaknesses of mere assertions.

Images can inform, and also engender emotions. Images, many of which have since become icons, played a large role in ending the Vietnam War. The image of the Earth taken from space has bolstered the perception of our world as a unified and vulnerable system more than many a politician's speech has been able to do. Lennart Nilsson's images of life in the womb showed us that human beings must be regarded as such from the very beginning, and had a greater impact on the debate about abortions than pronouncements by the Church.

Images create their own credibility, even if they lie. Images can manipulate and deceive. "What do you want to believe, facts or your eyes?" replied a media advisor of former US President Ronald Reagan when asked about the obvious discrepancy between politics and staging. Even 400 years after Copernicus, our planet still does not appear to be revolving, and the sun still appears to set. Media research has found that images linger longer than words, and indeed, their existence is based on it. "A punch in the eye is worth more than three on the ear," is an adage from boxing which also applies to teaching.

Images are perhaps the only remaining way of understanding certain aspects of our highly complex world, albeit by drastically reducing factual relationships sometimes even to the point of narrative fiction. Unfathomable complexity is reduced to simple, perspicuous concepts.

In the meantime, the images we have created, especially televised ones, have long since begun to influence us. As the principal cultural medium, television determines the models, receptivity, and processing of information. Viewed sceptically by the older generation, younger generations grow up which are accustomed to sporadic and distracting perceptions of rapidly changing images replacing one another. While books created a culture of language, even as a mass medium, television images are a mosaic of visual impressions devoid of context, disparate fragments of images held together only by a fictitious correlation. Speeches and intellectual exchanges have been replaced by podium discussions and talk shows in which relaxed debate has been superceded by rapid-fire bons mots.

Imagery, the dominant medium, has also influenced the principles of our media culture even where it is not pre-eminent, such as in this book.

What is true of people in general is especially true in medicine. Images have always been used in this field. When medicine was considered magic, images were too. Images were always created using the prevailing technology. Leonardo da Vinci's anatomical studies are still the pinnacle of artistic expression. The very first photographs also included those for the study of medicine. Medical images today not only portray what we see, but also what is invisible to the naked eye.

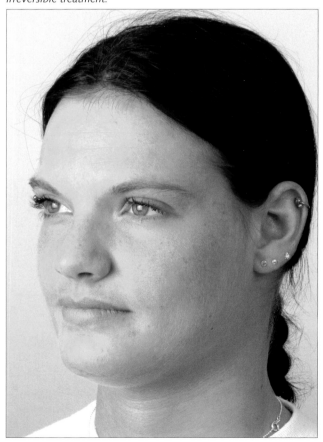

Fig. 0.1 Documentation is the most important application for dental photography. Photography should be done before any irreversible treatment.

Why dental photography?

Dentistry is one of the branches of medicine which has always used photography. There are many reasons for this.

Documentation

The main aim of dental photography is for documentation to supplement treatment. This includes photographs which show the processes and stages of treatment (Fig. 0.1).

As a general rule, images should be made before every irreversible and invasive procedure. This results not only in a stock of interesting dental records, but also provides forensic ones as well. In many instances, disagreements between dentist and patient can also be avoided in this way.

Images should always be made after trauma. This is not only for the dentist's legal protection, but also for the patient's. Dental photography is also useful during treatment and follow-up examination to check for pathological changes in the mucous membranes. Unusual and fleeting results of an examination can be documented to underpin an initial diagnosis. Since stoma-

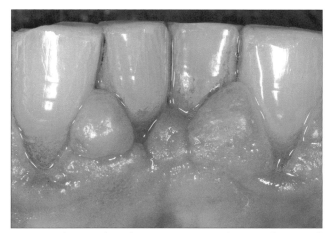

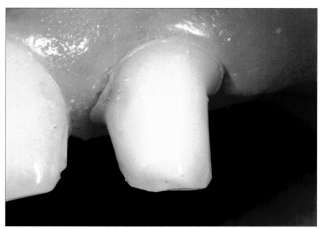

Fig. 0.2   Photography aids in communication between dentist and patient. Preliminary excisions and surgical removal of alterations in the mucous membrane should always be documented preoperatively.

Fig. 0.3   An important consequence of dental photography is the ability to self-check.

tology will be increasingly important in the coming years, these aspects will gain greater significance than before. It should be as natural for anyone interested in stomatology to have a camera at hand at all times as having an X-ray machine has been for decades.

Communication

"One picture is worth a thousand words" is a true and often quoted maxim. Conditions in hard and soft tissue can be quickly and easily photographed, facilitating communications between dentists, doctors, and laboratories. Images give dental technicians important information about structure and color of teeth, allowing them to individually match crowns to adjacent teeth. Even when the choice of color cannot be communicated to the laboratory directly in this way, photography can go a long way toward optimizing dental technicians' work. A pre-operation image sent along with a tissue sample to a pathologist can provide important information and support the diagnosis (Fig. 0.2).

Images also play an important role in patient consultations. The image not only allows the dentist to communicate information to the patient, but gives the patient a far better opportunity to express and articulate his or her wishes and desires.

Self-check

Quality control will become more important to dentists in the coming years. Photography will also gain importance in this context. Even without institutionalized quality control, photography will continue to aid the dentist as a self-check measure. Anyone who has photographed the stages of his or her treatment and then enlarged and projected the results is able to confirm this (Fig. 0.3). Images are also a key element in case presentations as part of training or as part of quality control.

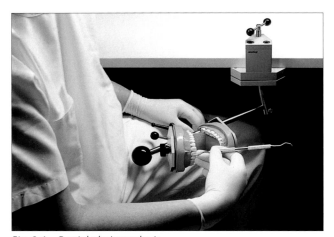

Fig. 0.4   Dental photography is very useful for illustrating the dentist's own lectures and publications.

Illustrations

It is almost inconceivable for lectures and publications on dentistry to be presented without images. These images are taken either for other reasons or specifically for that purpose (Fig. 0.4).

Marketing a practice

The concept of marketing a practice is often misused. Many recommendations by self-appointed "marketing experts" appear all too crass and are quickly seen through by patients. Marketing in the positive sense can allow a patient to directly compare the beginning and the outcome of treatment. Two images, printed side-by-side, are generally sufficient for this and can be given to the patient. Very little text is needed. Patients frequently also show these images to friends and acquaintances: there is probably no better low-key but effective marketing tool than this (Fig. 0.5).

Dres. Beatrix and Wolfgang Bengel
Darmstädter Str. 190a, 64625 Bensheim
Tel.: 06251 – 76095
Fax: 06251 – 76096

Patient: ....

Date: ....

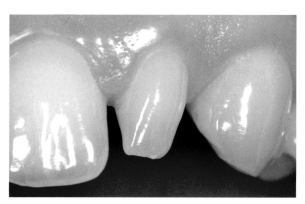

Before treatment

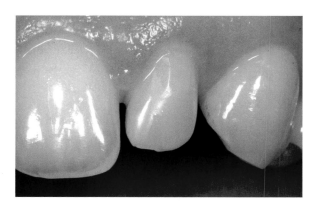

After treatment

Fig. 0.5   The juxtaposition of images taken at the onset and end of treatment not only emphasizes the importance of such work to the patient, but is also an understated yet highly effective marketing tool.

Finally, images also contribute to enjoyment and furtherance of the profession of dentistry, which becomes increasingly important in an advancing career (Fig. 0.6).

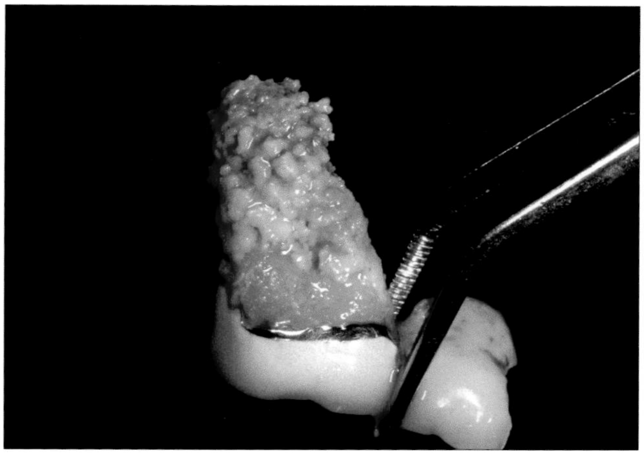

Why digital photography?

Within the last years, photography has changed dramatically. Not in principal: we record images projected by a lens onto a storage medium. The technology of recording the image and storing the information has changed. Silver halide photography (often referred to as conventional photography, although within a short period of time, digital photography will be regarded as conventional) had more than 150 years to develop. Digital photography reached a comparable technical level within a couple of years. It can be expected that this development will proceed.

Fig. 0.6 *Photographing interesting cases or curiosities bolsters interest in dentistry.*

Digital photography is not the technique of the future, it is state of the art.

There are numerous advantages particularly for medical documentation. Some of them are listed here:
- Images are immediately available.
- Exposure can be controlled perfectly right after the image is taken.
- Images are digitized at once: they can be transferred electronically immediately after the shot.
- The learning curve for the beginner is much steeper, as it is a more interactive process.
- The photographer largely is not dependent on costly lighting equipment, at least in object photography.
- Image recording can be adapted to different color temperatures.
- ISO speed of the camera can be adapted for each single shot.
- The photographer is not dependent on a laboratory.
- Although hardware is more expensive, shooting images is less expensive as there are no film or lab costs involved.
- Technical data of every image are recorded automatically, resulting in higher reproducibility.
- Keywords and image captions can be added directly to the image file, facilitating archiving procedures.

There are disadvantages, of course, above all the fact that image preservation makes a pro-active procedure necessary in order to preserve the bits and keep the file formats accessible (see Chapter 14.5).

Many concerns about the "death of photography" were discussed when digital photography was new. A frequently used argument was that digital photography is not valid for medical documentation due to the possible "photographic fakery". Falsification was performed even before photography was invented. Wood engravings were used in the early days of book printing to manipulate images. Metadata added to every image file allow the expert to control image manipulation easily.

Another argument was that "there is no original". Yes, it is true that nobody has seen a digital image up to now. All we can see is the result of a transfer process, by which data have been transformed into an image on a screen or into a print. But who has ever seen a latent image in a film? The influence of film processing on the final image cannot be neglected. If raw files are used, these can be regarded as digital negatives.

Another concern was that digital photographers "don't know what they are doing", as digital technology is rather complicated. This may be true in many cases. But the slogan on which Kodak's world success was based was "You press the button, we do the rest." What is the difference? The advanced photographer should at least know the basics of digital technology in order to understand the procedures and pitfalls of digital imaging. The same is true for silver halide photography.

The main merit of digital photography is that it has aroused huge interest in photography in general. Sales figures of the companies confirm this.

A camera should be part of the standard equipment of every dentist, as images are becoming more and more important. Digital photography has contributed essentially to attaining this goal.

Technical background *Section A*

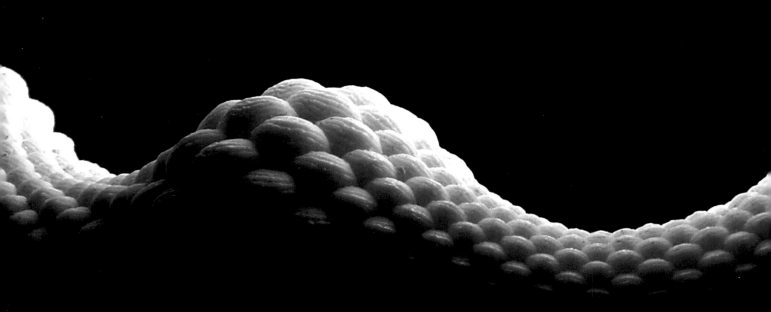

Demands on
the dental photograph

1

Is it justified to publish a book covering only dental photography? This refers to part of medical photography dealing with special photographic procedures applied in dentistry. Are there so many special problems in this field?

In intraoral photography, one of the main problems is the difficult access to the objects to be photographed. These objects are hidden in the oral cavity. This makes illumination a problem. Special equipment is needed to create good images. Another problem is that there are highly reflective areas in the mouth and the objects often show big differences in brightness. This may cause exposure difficulties. As the main purpose of taking photos is documentation, standardization is necessary regarding framing, inclination of the camera, magnification ratio, and illumination. Our objects are tiny. That means we have all the problems of macrophotography: high magnification ratio, shallow depth of field, disturbing perspective distortion, uneven illumination, etc. Even at higher magnification ratios, we need lighting which shows the outline of the object, the surface texture, the color, and even some inner structures of the semitransparent teeth as well.

In portrait photography, standardization is mandatory: framing, camera position, patient position, and illumination should be reproducible.

In object photography we have special problems, too. Objects are small, many of them are highly reflective (polished metal), others have a very low object contrast (e.g., white casts) or are semitransparent. We have to face general problems of macrophotography and we have to use different lighting techniques to get optimum results.

Another field of dentistry where photography is frequently used is surgery. In this field, access to the operating field is difficult and it is not easy to get a clean and dry situation.

The applications mentioned in the introduction of this book result in requirements for images, both in their technical aspects and image composition.

1.1   Technical demands

Technical requirements should present no fundamental problems with the current quality of photographic equipment. These include

- image sharpness
- sufficient depth of field
- suitable reproduction ratios
- correct exposure
- correct illumination, even in the mouth
- correct color rendition
- distortion-free images
- working distance long enough

These requirements are discussed in detail below.

Digital images are described by a file. Therefore, the file format used should be universally readable and the file should have an appropriate file size. That means image resolution/number of pixels should be sufficient to allow high quality images when printed or projected by a beamer.

1.2   Image composition

The requirements for image composition are more difficult to meet and most mistakes are made in this regard. These requirements are not so much creative as technical (e.g., image composition according with the golden section), and cover three specific areas:

- appropriate magnification ratio
- reduction of image contents
- ability to reproduce photographic conditions

One of the most common mistakes made, not necessarily only in dental photography, is having the camera positioned too far away from the subject. The rule of thumb, "Get close to the subject," also applies in this case. A reproduction ratio of 1:2 or greater should be the rule.

Images, which mostly are shown too briefly when used to illustrate lectures, should have a very simple composition in order to allow the viewer to take in their entire contents. Book illustrations are less critical, since the reader can peruse them at his or her leisure. Since it is never clear when a photo is taken what its ultimate use may be, it is best to take it in such a manner that its contents can be perceived quickly. This means reducing the contents, either through an appropriate scale or through selective focusing. Reduced image content is one of the secrets of a "good" or a "beautiful" image, because this image supports visual perception. Visual perception can only work if visual information is reduced dramatically.

Furthermore, it is always possible that a photograph taken almost by chance could become part of a series of illustrations. Thus it is important that the most critical photographic parameters—such as reproduction ratio, camera angle, and center of the photograph—can be reproduced. The goal is not necessarily to be able to precisely recreate these images, but to recreate the conditions under which photographs have been taken, allowing the viewer to quickly analyze images in a series without having to re-orientate him- or herself with each subsequent image because they have been taken from a different perspective.

Object photography also has these requirements. The background is particularly important in this case and should be as uniform as possible in order to avoid a confusing presentation. Images with different colored backgrounds are not only visually disturbing but are also easily recognized as having been pieced together.

Basic components of photography

2

The requirements cited above for a good dental photograph result in those for the camera system itself. In particular these are:

- adequate reproduction ratio
- sufficient working distance
- sufficient depth of field
- even exposure (also within the mouth)
- correct illumination, independent of reflections from subject
- correct color rendition
- easy use
- cost effective

In the following, the main camera system components are discussed with a view toward procuring the best possible equipment to meet the requirements.

The basic components discussed are:

- camera body
- lens
- flash/light

2.1   Camera body

There is no more discussion in the literature that the single lens reflex (SLR) system is most suited to medical photography (Fig. 2.1). This is true for both conventional and digital photography. In principle, it is not necessary to choose the most expensive body in a product range. It makes more sense to spend the money saved on lenses and flash equipment.

Fig. 2.1   Cross section of a modern digital single lens reflex camera (Illustration: Canon).

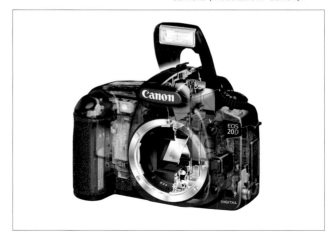

2.1.1   Disadvantages of digital viewfinder cameras

Digital viewfinder cameras offer many sophisticated features. When used for "normal" photography, results are superb. Therefore, many dentists believe that these cameras can be used for medical documentation as well. They often realize after a short time that results are not consistent enough for medical documentation. Some shots are perfect, but there are many images which are far from being acceptable. Hence, digital viewfinder cameras are suitable for medical documentation only to a very limited extent. Some of their properties restrict their use significantly.

Viewfinder parallax
Like conventional rangefinder cameras, digital models have a viewfinder parallax. This means that the image in the viewfinder and that recorded by the sensor are not the same (Fig. 2.2). This can be overcome by using the LCD screen of the camera.

Shutter lag
Most digital viewfinder cameras have a very long shutter lag. This is the time from pressing the shutter release button until the picture is taken. Within this time the image is focused (if autofocus function is switched on), white balance is performed, exposure is metered, and the ISO value is determined. All these functions are time consuming, especially finding the focus, which is performed in viewfinder cameras by using the CCD image.

In clinical photography, pictures are taken "by hand" without using a tripod to stabilize the camera. Therefore, small camera movements cannot be avoided. The result is that the camera is no longer "in focus" when the picture is taken: the image is blurred. The best way to avoid these problems is "pre-focusing" by pressing the shutter release button halfway down. Then the image is framed and the shutter is released.

Fig. 2.2   With a rangefinder camera, the image in the viewfinder and that on the sensor do not correspond at close range (viewfinder parallax).

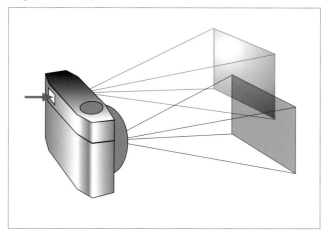

Insufficient viewfinder information
When looking through the viewfinder of a point-and-shoot camera, the information is very limited compared with the information of a SLR viewfinder. Users often look at the LC display (LC = liquid crystal) on the camera back instead of into the viewfinder. Controlling the plane of focus is not possible in this way.

Macro function is not sufficient
Digital viewfinder cameras frequently offer an astonishing macro capability, but only when the zoom lens is in its wide-angle position. Wide-angle position means

short distance to the object. Short working distance means distorted images, which cannot be used for medical documentation.

Flash too far from camera lens

To avoid the "red-eye effect," the built-in camera flash is often located as far as possible from the lens, thus producing difficulties when photographs of the oral cavity are taken from a short distance.

Further disadvantages of digital viewfinder cameras for dental photography sometimes include a low frame rate, rapid battery consumption, and a long time lag between turning on the camera and being able to take the first picture. Therefore, if complete control over the photographic procedure is mandatory, digital SLR cameras (DSLRs) are strongly recommended.

Some digital viewfinder cameras which are useful to a limited extent for dental photography are listed in Chapter 4.

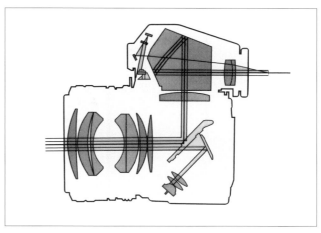

Fig. 2.3   Diagram of a single lens reflex camera.

2.1.2   Single lens reflex cameras (SLR)

The Single Lens Reflex Camera (SLR) is the most versatile type of camera, in which the light passing through the lens is directed by a mirror angled at 45 degrees to the optical axis onto a matte screen (Fig. 2.3). By looking at this matte screen, the photographer is able to frame the picture, and check its sharpness and depth of field. With only a few exceptions, only 35 mm (24 x 36 mm) SLR cameras and digital SLR cameras are used in medical documentation.

Important properties of digital SLR cameras (DSLR)

To make the step from conventional to digital photography easier, manufacturers modified conventional camera bodies so that it is possible to use the old camera equipment—such as lenses and flashes—with the new body. An exception in this respect is the Olympus E-1 system, which was completely redesigned especially for the demands of digital photography, including lenses and flash accessories.

If a DSLR is used for dental photography, it should include the following features.

Fig. 2.4   Exposure is always the product of aperture and exposure time. Short exposure time and large aperture achieve the same result as long exposure time and a large aperture.

Manual exposure/aperture-priority automatic exposure control

Correct exposure of an image is always the result of two factors: aperture and exposure time. A large aperture is coupled with a faster shutter speed and vice versa (Fig. 2.4).

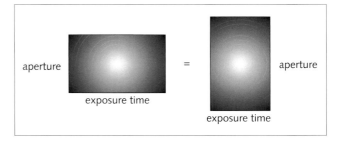

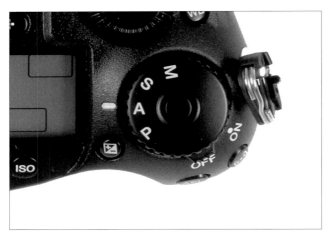

Fig. 2.5 The automatic expo-sure setting of choice for dental photography is aperture priority ("A" symbol) since it allows control of depth of field.

SLRs generally allow the exposure to be selected manually or automatically, in which case various auto-exposure modes can be chosen. The method of choice in this instance should be aperture-priority automatic exposure control, in which the aperture is selected and the appropriate shutter speed determined and set automatically by the camera. To use the aperture-priority mode, set the camera to the symbol "A" for aperture priority (Fig. 2.5). Choosing this exposure mode has the advantage of being able to select the aperture and thus influence the critically important depth of field (see below). Depth of field is determined by the aperture for a given magnification ratio.

Cameras used with TTL (through the lens) metered flashes can be set to manual (M) as well. With a pre-selected aperture (e.g., f 22) and an appropriate shutter speed (e.g., 1/125 s) the flash is set to TTL mode, thus ensuring a proper exposure of the image. This is the method of choice for Canon Digital SLRs.

In addition, the manual mode (M) is important for copy work and for clinical shots taken for color determination.

Fig. 2.6 An interchangeable focusing screen is important for dental photography. Focusing screens with a grid, illustrated in (a) and shown from the lens mount in a camera (b).

Short shutter lag

One of the biggest advantages of SLR cameras compared with digital viewfinder models is the ultra-short shutter lag. The main reason for this is that digital SLR cameras use special detectors for focusing while viewfinder cameras have to use the CCD image. Short shutter lag means better control not only of the time you take the picture but also of image sharpness if you use the autofocus function.

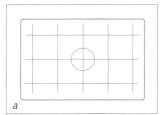

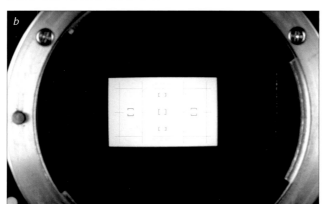

Focusing screens

The focusing screen is part of the focusing system. The mirror projects the image onto the screen; this image is flipped horizontally and vertically by the pentaprism so that it is the right way up and corrected for left-to-right reversal, allowing us to view the image through the viewfinder.

It is advisable to replace the standard focusing screen with a fine matte focusing screen with an engraved grid (Fig. 2.6). The advantage of such a grid screen cannot be overestimated in practical work.

Some cameras offer a feature to switch on a grid screen electronically. This is the case in Nikon-based models such as Nikon D200, D 70s, and Fuji FinePix S3 Prof.

If a digital viewfinder camera is used, grid lines can be painted on the LC display on the camera back or on a protecting foil attached to it (Fig.2.7).

Data back

For conventional cameras, data backs were a very useful aid. They have lost their importance, however, because now every image file gets its own unmistakable number. Beside this, a considerable amount of technical information is added to the file (EXIF file, see below).

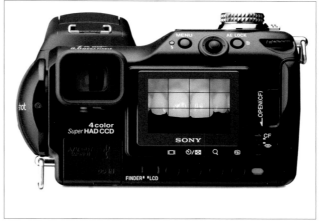

Fig. 2.7 A grid can be painted onto the LC display of viewfinder cameras to improve alignment.

Depth of field preview button

Depth of field is always critical in close-up photography (see below). This can be checked visually in the viewfinder only if the camera has a depth of field preview button. In focusing, the lens aperture is normally fully open to achieve the brightest image in the viewfinder. Pressing the depth of field preview button stops the lens diaphragm down to the aperture which is set (working aperture). Although the image becomes darker, it is possible to visually check the depth of field, an important feature for object photography.

Autofocus function

Modern cameras with the appropriate lenses allow autofocusing. This feature is important in sports and action photography and also for copy work.

However, in clinical photography this autofocus function should be turned off and focusing should be done manually (Fig. 2.8). Since photography in this field is mostly hand-held, it is difficult to avoid a small amount of camera shake. This would mean that the lens motor would continually have to refocus the lens. An even more important reason for switching off the autofocus mode is the fact that the autofocus focusing point is in the center of the viewfinder in most cameras. However, the closest point of the subject is often in the center, too, such as is the case when photographing a set of teeth. If this point is focused on, nearly 50% of the depth of field (that is the area in front of the nearest point) is not used (see below). Thus, it would not be possible to have the entire set of teeth in acceptable focus. For this reason, the autofocus function should be switched off in clinical photography.

Fig. 2.8 In clinical photography the autofocus function of digital SLR cameras should be switched off.

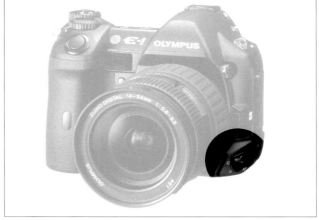

Useful accessories

Most camera systems offer a range of accessories, though only a limited number of these appear suitable for our purposes. These useful accessories, for instance, include dioptric adjustment lenses if this feature is not built in. Another useful accessory is eye cups, which keep out extraneous light and substantially improve the image in the viewfinder. A right-angle finder is very useful when the camera is mounted on a tripod in a very low position or on a copy stand.

Technical details concerning the digital image recording are discussed in Chapter 3 in detail.

2.2   The lens

Dental photography is mostly close-up photography, calling for macro lenses. Zoom lenses with a "macro setting" are not suitable for this purpose, since these can be set only to a reproduction (magnification) ratio of about 1:4.

Fig. 2.9   Close up photography is achieved by increasing the distance from the lens to the film plane/sensor plane. This longer length must be light-tight, for example, by using bellows.

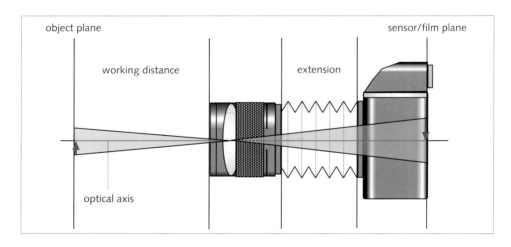

Fig. 2.10   Nikon macro lenses. In front, the old 200-mm medical lens; in the middle, a 105-mm macro lens which achieves a magnification of 1:2; in the back, the newer 105-mm AF macro lens which achieves a magnification of 1:1. Despite the greater magnification, it is physically shorter than the other lenses, since it has floating lens elements. However, this also has a shorter subject-to-camera distance.

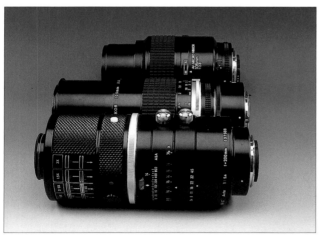

To focus on an object which is closer to the camera than "infinity," the focus setting ring on the lens is turned to increase the distance between the center of the lens and the sensor plane. Most normal lenses are designed to produce a maximum magnification ratio of approximately 1:10 to 1:7. The lens cannot be moved further away from the sensor plane. If the photographer wishes to focus on a subject which is closer, the distance between the lens and the camera must be bridged so as to allow no light leakage (Fig. 2.9). This can be achieved in various ways, for instance by using extension rings, bellows unit, macro tubes, etc. This is easiest with macro lenses, which generally have the means by which the lens can be extended farther than normal. More modern designs permit greater magnification through the use of floating elements. Another advantage of these macro lenses is their ability to compensate for image problems inherent in close-up photography. These lenses are designed and corrected for close-up photography (Fig. 2.10).

Normal lengths of macro lenses are 50 mm, 60 mm, 90 mm, 100 mm, 105 mm, and 200 mm; the 100 or 105 mm lens is best suited to our purpose.

BACKGROUND

Angle of view

The angle that the lens "sees". Normal lenses have an angle of view which roughly corresponds to that of the human eye (about 45 to 55 degrees). Wide-angle lenses have a larger angle of view and telephoto lenses a smaller one (Fig. 2.11).

When a conventional lens is used with a digital camera, the crop factor must be taken into account, as the sensor is usually smaller than the film format 24 x 36 mm. That means that the angle of view is smaller for a digital camera, if its sensor is not a full format sensor.

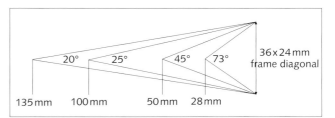

Fig. 2.11   The angle of view of a lens is what it "sees". The diagram shows the angles of view of common lenses. In digital photography, the angle of view is determined also by the sensor size.

Aperture

Opening in the lens which regulates the amount of light. Mostly an iris aperture consisting of overlapping metal blades. Stopping down (closing) the aperture reduces the image brightness and increases the depth of field. The next higher aperture reduces the amount of light by half and the next lower one doubles it. The area of a circle increases with the square of the radius. To double the amount of light (= area of circle), the radius has to be increased by the factor of the root of 2 (about 1.4). This produces the aperture numbers.

Fig. 2.12   The aperture number indicates the number of times the aperture diameter fits in the focal length of the lens. In this case the aperture is f/4.

Lens stop

Reciprocal of the aperture ratio. The lens stop is the ratio of the diameter of the opening (aperture diameter) and the lens focal length lens. F/4, for instance, means that the aperture diameter fits four times in the focal length of the lens (Fig. 2.12). The aperture settings form the "international aperture sequence" of 1, 1.4, 2, 2.8, 4, 5.6, 8, 11, 16, 22, 32, 45.

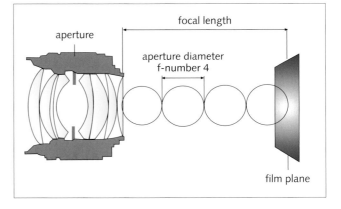

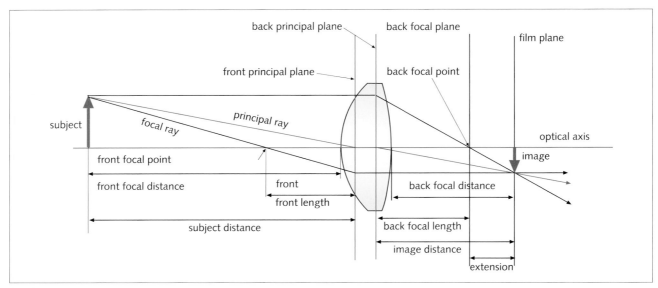

Fig. 2.13
Diagram of key optical terms.

Focal point/focal length

Distance between the focal point to the lens plane (Fig. 2.13). The back focal length, which differs from the front focal length in asymmetrical lenses, is engraved on the front of lenses. In normal lenses, the focal length is approximately equal to the diagonal of the picture frame. In 35-mm cameras with a 24×36mm film format, this is about 43.5mm. Lenses with a shorter focal length are termed wide-angle and those with a longer length telephoto lenses.

Lens speed/relative aperture

The maximum aperture ratio of a lens is called lens speed or relative aperture. This is cited in the ratio of 1:X. A 50-mm lens with an aperture diameter of 27mm thus has a lens speed of 27:50 = 1:1.8. Lenses with extremely wide apertures are not recommended for dental photography as they are not only very expensive, but the image in the viewfinder has a very shallow depth of field. The advantage is their very bright image in the viewfinder. When the shutter release is pressed, this depth of field becomes greater, of course, as focusing is always done with the aperture wide open. When the shutter is pressed, the lens is stopped down to the selected aperture. Nevertheless, a very shallow depth of field in the viewfinder often causes the operator to overlook some details of the subject.

Macro lens

Lenses between 50mm and 200mm which are specially designed for close-up photography (clear color rendition, good resolution, lack of distortion, good field flattening). Today most macro lenses have floating elements which are coupled to the distance setting and allow large reproduction ratios, mostly 1:1, without the use of additional accessories, achieving good image quality. Since these lenses can also be set to "infinity," they can also be used in normal photography.

The lens determines a number of optical and image parameters, and thus it is more important to use a high quality lens than a more costly camera. Unlike in conventional photography, the quality of lenses can only be judged when tested together with an individual camera, as the camera sensor influences image quality as well.

Lenses influence the following parameters:

- image quality (image sharpness, color rendition, contrast)
- magnification
- working distance
  (and by this the lighting angle, when a macro flash is attached)
- depth of field (via aperture setting and magnification)

Image quality

Optical requirements such as image sharpness, color rendition, and contrast should present no problems given the quality of today's lenses. It is not mandatory to use original manufacturers' lenses. Lenses of independent makers differ only in specifications but not in image quality from those of the original manufacturers.

In digital photography image quality is just as much influenced by a number of other factors, e.g., the image sensor and the computer algorithms used for processing image data. Details such as sensor size and type, number and size of pixels, type and quality of sensor filters and many other things are important. Testing the quality of a lens only makes sense when the rating refers to special lens-camera combinations.

Lenses for conventional silver halide photography which are used with digital cameras equipped with 6-8 MPixel chips reach their optical limits, as they have to resolve extremely fine structures of the chips. Increasing the number of the sensor elements without increasing sensor size results in extremely tiny "pixels" (=sensor elements). A further increase of the pixel count would not result in better image quality, as the conventional lenses are not capable of resolving these fine structures. Hence, some manufacturers offer special "digital lenses", especially designed for the demands of high quality digital photography.

Reproduction ratio/magnification ratio

Reproduction ratio is defined as the size of the subject relative to the image on the film. A reproduction ratio of 1:2 means that the subject on the slide or negative would have half its actual size. A reproduction ratio of 2:1 means that the subject would be two times its real size (Fig. 2.14).

In digital photography, film is no longer used. Magnification ratio in digital photography means the ratio of the size of the image projected on the sensor to the object size. The projected image in a digital SLR camera has the same size as the image inside a conventional camera. What differs is sensor size and viewing field. As sensors differ in size and resolution from camera to camera, talking about magnification ratio may thus be confusing.

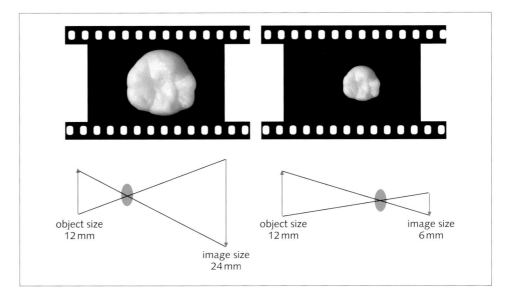

Fig. 2.14   At a magnification of 1:2 the object size (OS) is twice the size of the image. At a magnification of 2:1, the image is twice the size of the object. This is true for conventional and digital cameras containing a sensor which is smaller than the film format.

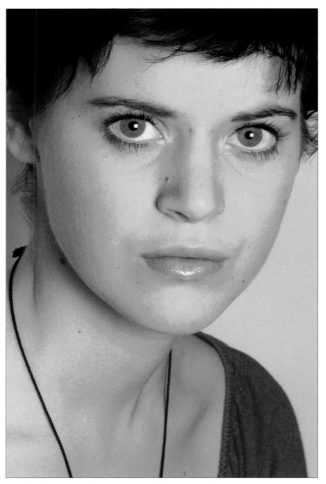

Fig. 2.15   Magnification ratio of about 1:10.

For practical reasons, the magnification ratio may be referred to 35-mm film format. If the frame includes a distance of 36 mm, we speak of a magnification ratio of 1:1. If a full frame includes 18 mm, we are speaking of a magnification ratio of 2:1.

In dental photography the following reproduction ratios are important (approximate):

- 1:10   portrait photography (Fig. 2.15)
- 1:2   image of a set of teeth (Fig. 2.16)
- 1:1.2   whole set of anterior teeth (Fig. 2.17)
- 1:1   anterior teeth with partial canines or pre molars and molars filling the format (Fig. 2.18)
- 2:1   Two maxillary anterior teeth (Fig. 2.19)

Given the same aperture, the depth of field decreases with greater magnification; with the same focal length, the working distance also decreases.

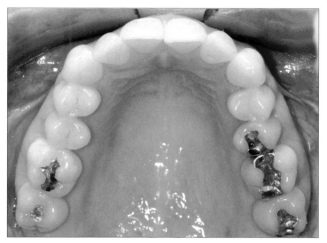

Fig. 2.16   Magnification ratio of 1:2

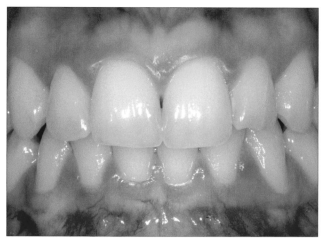

Fig. 2.17   Magnification ratio of 1:1.2

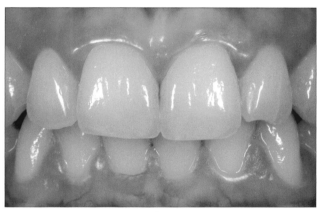

Fig. 2.18   Magnification ratio of 1:1

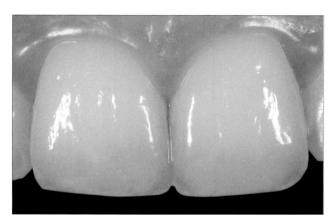

Fig. 2.19   Magnification ratio of 2:1

BACKGROUND

Magnification ratio

Size ratio between the image on the film and the object (Fig. 2.14). A magnification ratio of 1:2 means that in reality the object is twice as large as it is on the film (0.5x magnification). Reproduction ratios in dental photography are usually between 1:10 (portrait photography) and 2:1 (image of two teeth which fill the frame). Macro lenses commonly used today without accessories have reproduction ratios of 1:1. With accessories (extension tubes, auto-macro tubes, bellows units) or optical means (teleconverters, close-up lenses) the maximum reproduction ratio can be further increased.

If a crop factor (see below) has to be taken into account for a digital camera—which is the case in most DSLRs due to the smaller sensor size—the maximum magnification ratio of macro lenses is even larger.

Measurment in horizontal format	magnification ratio
9	4:1
10	3.6:1
11	3.3:1
12	3:1
13	2.8:1
14	2.6:1
15	2.4:1
16	2.3:1
17	2.1:1
18	2:1
19	1.9:1
20	1.8:1
21	1.7:1
22	1.6:1
23	1.5:1
24	1.5:1
25	1.4:1
26	1.4:1
27	1.3:1
28	1.3:1
29	1.2:1
30	1.2:1
31	1.2:1
32–34	1.1:1
35–38	1:1
66–80	1:2

As sensor size is no point of reference and the size of a printed digital image depends on the number of pixels involved and the printing resolution, for practical reasons, the magnification ratio refers to the viewfinder image of a 35-mm SLR camera.

The reproduction ratio can be determined fairly accurately by measuring the image in the viewfinder in millimeters. It should be noted, however, that there are small deviations between the image in the viewfinder and that on the sensor. This can be determined from the camera's technical specifications.

The table allows the reproduction ratio to be determined by measuring the image in the viewfinder (horizontal format).

Focal length multiplier/crop factor

The reproduction ratio is engraved on many lenses and can therefore easily be pre-set. If conventional lenses are used with digital cameras, these engravings are misleading. The reason for that is the fact that most sensors are much smaller than the 35-mm film format for which the lenses were designed (film format 24x36mm, Nikon D70 sensor 15.6 x 23.7mm). That means the image circle generated by the lens has the same dimensions as if used with conventional cameras. The smaller sensor captures only the central part of this circle. This is the same effect as if a lens with longer focal length were used in conventional photography. A so-called focal length multiplier must be taken into account (also called crop factor).

To be able to preset the magnification ratio, which is very helpful in practical work, it is recommended to make one's own engravings for the lens setting of the most often used magnification ratios. This can easily be done within a couple of minutes using a millimeter scale. The lens is set so that the following millimeter ranges fill the frame completely:

- 36-mm range for a "magnification ratio" of 1:1
- 43-mm range for a "magnification ratio" of 1:1.2
- 72-mm range for a "magnification ratio" of 1:2.

One engraving is placed on the top of the fixed part of the lens tube, and the corresponding engravings for the three ratios are placed beside this first mark on the rotatable part of the tube. Otherwise, one has to keep in mind the corresponding values indicated on the lens for the most important magnification ratios (Fig. 2.20 a-c). In this manner, the magnification ratio can be quickly preselected, which speeds up daily work.

Most digital cameras have a crop factor of 1.5 to 1.7. The Olympus E-1 has a crop factor of 2. Using a digital camera also increases the magnification ratio achievable with this lens. To be more precise: the viewfinder image is larger than the viewfinder image of a conventional camera. If a magnification ratio of 1:1 could be achieved with a conventional system, the corresponding ratio is 1.5:1 with a digital camera with crop factor of 1.5. In many cases, therefore, additional equipment to enlarge the magnification is not necessary.

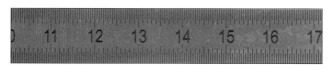

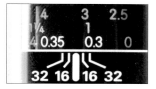

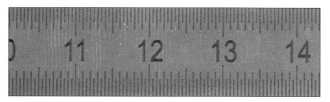

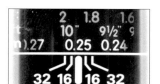

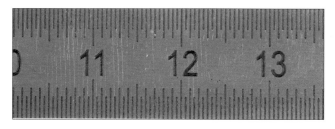

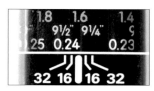

Fig. 2.20a   Magnification ratio of 1:2: 72mm are visible within the frame. Corresponding magnification ratio number of a Nikon lens (orange values).

Fig. 2.20b   Magnification ratio of 1:1.2: 43mm are visible within the frame. Corresponding magnification ratio number of a Nikon lens (orange values).

Fig. 2.20c   Magnification ratio of 1:1: 36mm are visible within the frame. Corresponding magnification ratio number of a Nikon lens (orange values).

If even higher magnifications are required, the use of special accessories is necessary. Teleconverters and close-up lenses are generally used in clinical photography.

Close-up lenses

Close-up lenses act like "spectacles" in front of the camera lens. This means that they reduce the focal length of the lens, thus reducing the subject-to-camera distance. This makes larger images possible.

Close-up lenses have the advantage of being light, easy to use, and for the most part relatively inexpensive. Optically, there is no resulting loss of light.

One disadvantage is that close-up lenses sometimes result in loss of image quality. Thus, it is recommended to use close-up lenses with built-in correction for image quality, such as achromatic lenses corrected for chromatic aberrations. There is also another disadvantage caused by their functional principle. As the focal length of the lens/close-up lens combination is reduced compared to the straight lens, the subject-to-camera distance is also reduced (see below) (Fig. 2.21). If the lens is set to infinity, the focal length of the overall system is equal to that of the close-up lens. Thus it generally makes sense to use close-up lenses only when the basic focal length of the macro lens being used is no less than 100mm. Otherwise, this would present difficulties with lighting and perspective.

Fig. 2.21   A close-up lens reduces the overall length of the optical system. This leads to a shorter working distance. In contrast, a teleconverter (on the right) increases the overall length and thus the working distance.

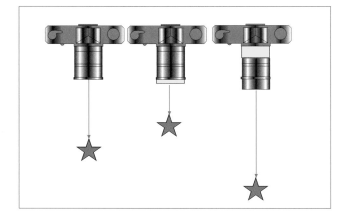

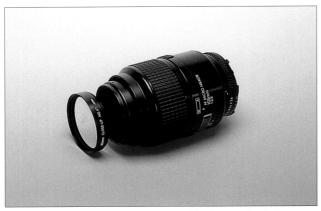

Fig. 2.22 Nikon 105-mm AF-Micro Nikkor lens with 4T close-up lens.

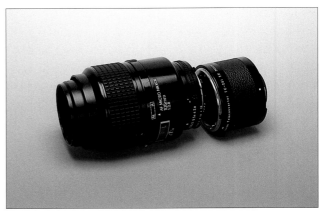

Fig. 2.23 Nikon 105-mm AF-Micro Nikkor with TC 201 teleconverter.

An example of a recommended system is the Nikon 4T close-up lens with the 105-mm Micro AF lens (Fig. 2.22).

Teleconverters

Teleconverters are simple to operate and are therefore frequently used in dental photography. They are a sort of intermediate lens. Fitted between the camera and lens, they increase the lens' focal length (Fig. 2.23). The most frequently used converters are 2x, which double the focal length. Since this does not affect the minimum focusing distance, the result is images in greater magnification. Combining a macro lens with a maximum reproduction ratio of 1:1 plus a 2x teleconverter produces an overall result of 2:1 (the crop factor also has to be taken into account). The ability to set the lens to infinity is retained.

A general disadvantage is that the rays of light travelling from the lens toward the sensor are spread by the converter. This reduces the intensity of light on the sensor surface (Fig. 2.24). A 2x converter loses two f-stops and a 1.4x converter one stop. Teleconverters are thus to be recommended only when the flashgun being used is sufficiently powerful; otherwise, the aperture must be opened up.

Teleconverters reach their limitations with lenses of around 100 mm. Lenses with focal lengths above that, when used with converters, result in too great a focal length and camera-to-subject distance (see below).

Normally, optical quality is not diminished by using teleconverters, since in dental photography, most shots are done with lenses stopped down to f/16 or f/22, thus eliminating most image errors. However, if a lens of a lower quality is used, the faults are intensified by the converter.

Fig. 2.24 The intensity of illumination is inversely proportional to the square of its distance from the light source.

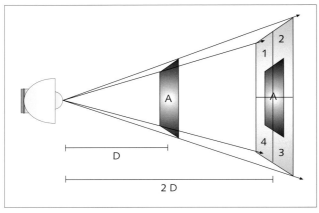

Bellows units

Bellows units allow infinite adjustment of the image distance and thus the magnification. Normal bellows are too clumsy for use in clinical photography. The Novoflex Automatic Bellows are an exception; these are compact and offer direct auto-aperture coupling (Fig. 2.25).

The main advantage of increasing the focal length to achieve greater magnification is that good optical quality is achieved. The disadvantage is the loss of light, since the intensity of illumination is inversely proportional to the square of its distance from the light source. For example, at a reproduction ratio of 1:1, the object width and the image width are equal to double the focal length of the lens. The loss of light is thus two stops.

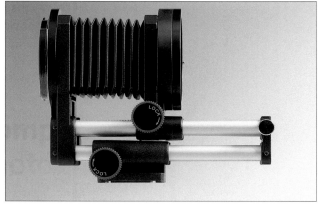

Fig. 2.25   The Novoflex automatic bellows unit is a "portable" solution for dental photography (Photo: Novoflex).

Extension tubes

In dental photography, extension tubes should be used only as a last resort. They increase the distance between the lens and the sensor and thus increase magnification. These are generally sold in sets of three and can be used individually or in combination. The shorter the focal length of the lens, the stronger their effect is; for our purposes, this is not an advantage, since we use longer focal length lenses (Fig. 2.26). Because the light must travel further to reach the sensor, there can be a loss of up to two stops. The subject-to-camera distance is also reduced, although not as much as in using close-up lenses. It is also no longer possible to focus on infinity. The use of extension tubes is not very practical, since it is no longer possible to infinitely vary the magnification.

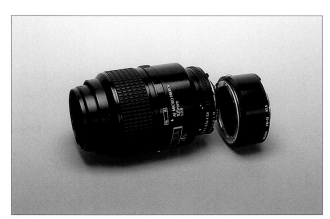

Fig. 2.26   Extension tubes are a compromise solution in dental photography since they do not permit infinite adjustment of the working distance.

Working distance

Working distance is defined as the distance between the subject and the front of the lens. This value is determined by the focal length of the lens and the selected magnification. For a given reproduction ratio, the longer the focal length of the lens, the greater the subject-to-camera distance (Fig. 2.27). At a reproduction ratio of 1:1, the subject-to-camera distance is about double the focal length of the lens in conventional lens design. Lenses with floating elements have a significantly shorter subject-to-camera distance. Working distance must be neither too long nor too short.

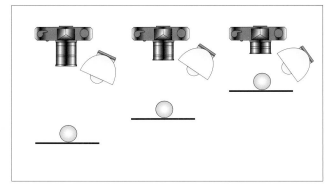

Fig. 2.27   Reducing the working distance means the light comes more from the side. This is problematic for objects in body cavities.

Working distance too long

A subject-to-camera distance which is too long has various disadvantages. The distance between flashgun and subject, for instance, is too great. This means that a high-power flashgun must be used, which can be problematic in the case of macro flashguns. Another disadvantage of a large subject-to-camera distance is that small camera movements have a greater effect on the field of view than with shorter ones. It is difficult or even almost impossible to fill the frame exactly.

Working distance too short

If the subject-to-camera distance is too short, this can lead to hygiene problems when taking pictures. This is to be strictly avoided, particularly in photography during operations. In dental photography, this is merely uncomfortable for the patient if the camera is too close. In intraoral photography in particular, in which the objects are hidden in the mouth, too short a working distance can create problems in lighting if a lateral point flash or a twin flash is used (Fig. 2.28a).

A good rule of thumb for achieving uniform illumination in the mouth is that the working distance should be at least 1.5 times that of the diameter of the ring flash or the distance of the two flash reflectors. Another disadvantage if the working distance is too short is image distortion, which results from an incorrect viewing distance. An eye viewing the subject from the same distance would see the same distorted perspective. The result is that parts of the subject closest to the lens are disproportionally large. In the case of a set of teeth, the incisors would appear larger than they would from a greater distance. A portrait would be completely useless because the patient's nose would appear too large (Fig. 2.28b).

For these reasons, in dental photography, a macro lens with a focal length of about 100 mm has proven most useful. For digital dental photography, lenses with focal lengths of 60 or 100 mm are recommended, as the crop factor must be taken into account (effective focal lengths are about 90 or 150 mm). The difference regarding image perspective is visible but not disturbing (Fig. 2.29-30).

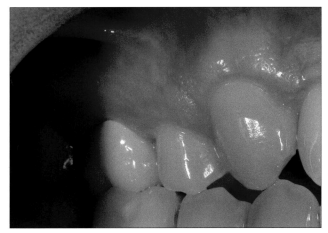

Fig. 2.28a   *Here the working distance was too short for the side lighting, with the resulting shadows in the right molar area.*

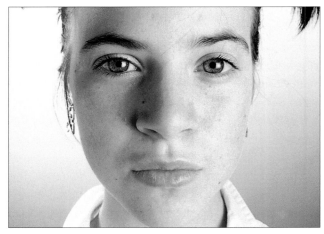

Fig. 2.28b   *The short working distance resulting from using too short a lens leads to obvious distortion in the portrait.*

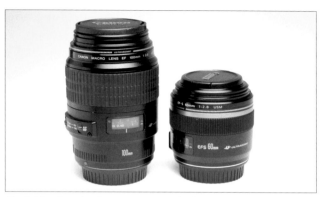

Fig. 2.29   Besides the 100-mm standard lens for dental photography, a 60-mm macro lens can be used as well because the crop factor turns it into a lens with an effective focal length of 90 mm.

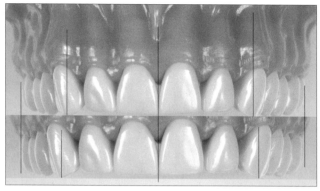

Fig. 2.30   The working distance is responsible for the perspective of the image. The upper image was shot with a 105-mm macro lens, the lower arch of teeth with a 60-mm macro lens. The lower arch is a little bit more distorted when compared with the upper one. That means: Front teeth are a little bit bigger in relation to the whole arch.

Depth of field

When focusing on a tree standing in a meadow, it is obvious that a certain distance in front of and a greater distance behind the tree is still in focus. The distance from the nearest to the furthest point of perceived "sharp" focus in a picture is called depth of field (DOF). (Fig. 2.31). Depth of field depends on the aperture and magnification (Fig. 2.32). It does not depend on the focal length of the lens. A 50-mm lens at a subject distance of 5 m at f8 yields the same depth of field as a 100 mm lens at a subject distance of 10 m. The smaller the aperture (and the higher the aperture number), the greater the depth of field. Depth of field reduces sharply with greater magnification, so that depth of field in the distances involved in dental photography is only millimeters (Table 2.1).

In dental photography, this means that generally photos can be taken only using small apertures. "Standard" apertures should be f/16 or (better) f/22. These require high power flashguns, which is not always the case with ring or macro flashguns. Another option is to increase light sensitivity of the camera (e.g., ISO 200 instead of ISO 100).

It is especially important that depth of field is not sacrificed. It should also be kept in mind that the entire depth of field is both in front of and behind the focusing plane. In normal photography approximately one third of the overall depth of field is in front of this and two thirds behind. In close-up photography with a reproduction ratio of 1:1, this ratio changes, with about 50% of the total depth of field in front of and about

Fig. 2.31   A correctly focused object (A) leads to a sharp image on the film/sensor plane (A"). An object which is closer (B) would be sharp behind the film/sensor plane (B"). The image point of the top of the object is not exactly focused as a point, but as a so-called circle of confusion. If this exceeds a certain size, we perceive the image as being blurred.

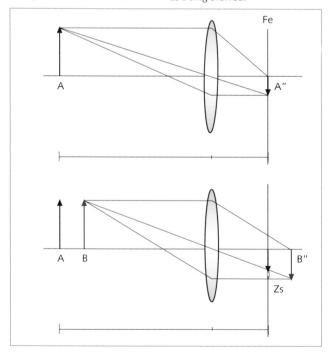

Table 2.1   Depth of field in relation to magnification ratio and aperture. Measurements in millimeters.

Ratio	Aperture						
	5,6	8	11	16	22	32	45
1:10	41	59	81	117	161	234	1260
1:5	11.2	16	22	32	44	64	90
1:2	2.2	3.2	4.4	6.4	8.8	13	18
1:1	0.75	1.07	1.47	2.13	2.9	4.27	6.0
2:1	0.28	0.40	0.55	0.80	1.10	1.60	2.3
3:1	0.17	0.24	0.33	0.47	0.65	0.94	1.33

50% behind the distance focused on. This means that if the closest part of the subject is focused on, 50% of the overall depth of field is in front of the subject and thus not used.

When photographing a set of teeth from the front, the photographer should not focus on the center of the image (contact point of the central incisors), but on the canines (Fig. 2.33). Only in this way can the entire depth of field be used; otherwise it is not possible to keep a set of teeth in sharp focus from front to back.

In object photography, the problem of shallow depth of field can in many instances be overcome by placing the object parallel to the sensor plane. This is possible only to a certain extent in intraoral photography.

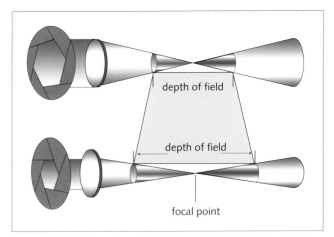

Fig. 2.32   Stopping down the aperture reduces the beam. The diameter of the circles of confusion becomes smaller and the depth of field increases.

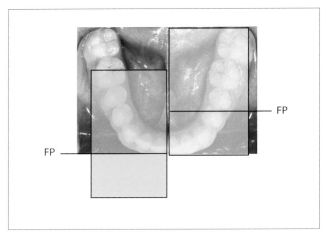

Fig. 2.33   The overall depth of field extends about one third in front of and about two thirds behind the focusing plane (FP). If the closest point in a set of teeth is focused on, the depth of field in front of the focusing point is lost.

BACKGROUND

Hyperfocal distance

If a lens is focused on infinity, the depth of field starts at somewhere in front of the lens and extends to infinity. To be more precise: from that point in front of the lens the scene appears sharp and subjects between the camera and this point are out of focus.

The distance from the camera to this point is referred to as the hyperfocal distance. If the camera is pointed to the end of the hyperfocal distance (where the scene begins to appear sharp), the resulting depth of field starts from halfway from the hyperfocal distance and extends to infinity. By using this technique, depth of field can be used to greater advantage.

Depth of field and digital cameras

There is much confusion about depth of field and digital cameras, resulting partly from failing to take the crop factor into account.

If you use the same lens on a digital SLR camera (with a crop factor 1.6) and a conventional 35-mm film body, and crop the 35-mm image in order to get a comparable field of view, the depth of field is identical. If you use the same lens on a DSLR and a 35-mm film body without cropping the image afterwards, the digital image has a 1.6x shallower depth of field than the 35-mm image would have, because we have different images with different field of views and different magnification ratios.

For an equivalent field of view, the digital camera has 1.6x greater depth of field that a 35-mm camera would have. The 35-mm camera would need a lens with 1.6x the focal length to give the same view.

BACKGROUND

Diffraction

Even if there are very powerful light sources, it does not make sense to close the aperture as far as possible in order to increase depth of field. With decreasing aperture diameter, loss of image sharpness due to light diffraction becomes more and more visible. The depth of field increases, but overall sharpness is reduced.

When light rays pass the lens tube, light is diffracted at edges of mechanical parts (lens margin, diaphragm margin) and is thus deflected from its original direction. If the diaphragm is large, diffracted rays do not meaningfully contribute to the whole image. Loss of quality is negligible. If the diaphragm is small, the proportion of the diffracted and non-diffracted light becomes significant: image quality is reduced. When closing down the aperture, at first image quality (by reducing shortcomings of the lens) and depth of field increase up to a certain point. After this, quality goes down because of the impact of diffraction, causing an overall loss of image sharpness. The aperture at which the best image can be obtained is called the optimum aperture. It should be taken into account in close-up photography.

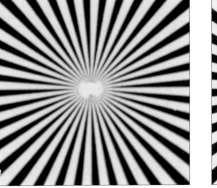
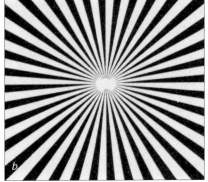
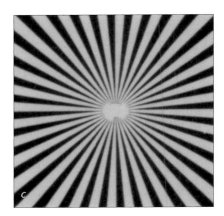

Fig. 2.34   Central part of a test chart photographed with the aperture wide open (f/2.8) (a), stopped down to f/8 (b), and aperture maximally closed to f/45 (c). Image quality at f/8 is the best.

For the same reasons, a standard aperture setting of f16–22 is recommended in dental photography, as this setting is a good compromise between image quality and depth of field. If depth of field is not important, a setting of f8 will give better results in terms of overall sharpness (Fig. 2.34).

Optical zoom – digital zoom

Zoom lenses are not used for clinical dental photography with SLR cameras, but most viewfinder cameras have built-in zoom lenses. There is sometimes confusion about the term optical zoom vs. digital zoom.

A zoom lens is a lens designed so that its focal length can be varied over a certain range. The image is optically magnified and, depending on the lens' setting, will show a larger or smaller field of view (Fig. 2.35ab). With a digital camera, the optical zoom does not change the image size or the resolution. The number of pixels used to describe the image remains constant. In addition to the optical zoom, many digital cameras offer a "digital zoom". This works by capturing only the central portion of the entire image received by the sensor.

Fig. 2.35   View of a zoom lens showing the image with a wide angle setting (a). A longer focal length shows the image with a smaller viewing angle (b).

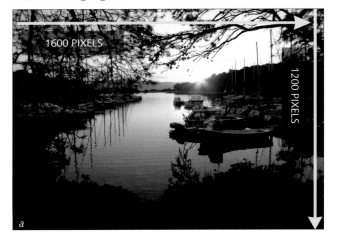
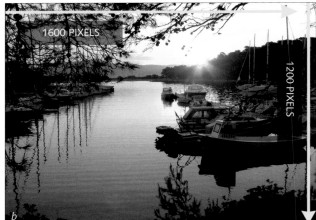

In a real sense, the digital zoom is nothing more than a cropping tool (Fig. 2.36). Cropping can be performed better using an image editing program after the image is taken.

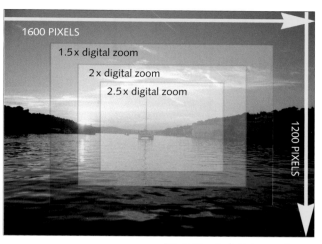

Fig. 2.36 *A digital zoom is a cropping tool, showing only part of the image. The same can be performed using image editing software after the picture is taken.*

2.3   Light and electronic flash

Photography means "writing with light". Therefore, light is the most important factor. Clinical dental photography is undertaken almost exclusively with the aid of flash, unlike in object or portrait photography, where constant lighting can be used optionally.

The undoubted advantages of flash photography are:
- short duration of flash, eliminating the influence of camera shake
- great intensity of light, allowing smaller apertures
- color temperature has the characteristics of daylight, white balance can be pre-set to "flash"
- flashguns are compact, permitting hand-held photography
- little heat, no stress to patient

The main difficulty in using flashguns is proper dosage of light and estimation of the light-shadow distribution of the image, the latter being determined by arrangement and form of the flashguns.

BACKGROUND

Electronic flash

Standard light source for medical photography which provides short-duration, high-power lighting.

Powered by rechargeable power packs or commercial batteries. Can be mains powered for stationary applications.

The flash capacitor is charged with a relatively weak current to several hundred volts via a transformer. The flash tubes are connected to the capacitor. The tubes are filled with xenon. The flash is fired instantaneously via the capacitor. This places a charge of about 10,000 volts on the ignition electrode. The gas in the flash tubes is thus ionized and electrically conductive. In about 1/1000th of a second, the energy of the capacitor is discharged via the flash tubes. The current briefly illuminates the ionized gas. Discharge time depends on the capacitance of the condenser (capacitor).

Simple electronic flashguns always fully discharge the capacitor. Exposure must therefore be regulated via the aperture setting. The guide number of the flashgun gives an indication of this. Modern computer flash and TTL-controlled flashguns limit energy output by shutting off the flash. This is done using a thyristor, which shuts off the power to the flash tubes via a sensor in the flashgun—or, in the case of TTL control in the camera—when there is sufficient light from the flash for correct exposure. This prevents the capacitor from being fully discharged and reduces the time needed to fully recharge the capacitor (recycling time).

TTL flash systems for digital SLR cameras work with a preflash, which is reflected from the object. This preflash is metered and the main flash intensity is adjusted according to the metering result.

When using electronic flash it should be ensured that the correct synch speed is set on the camera; otherwise flash duration will be too short and produce a curtain effect on the film. Since the light from an electronic flash is relatively concentrated and results in a "hard" light, special accessories are used to increase the illuminating surface. These include reflectors, soft boxes, etc., which are particularly useful for portrait and technical photography.

Modern electronic flash units allow several units to be connected which are not only triggered by the camera, but which also permit their output to be controlled. Additional flashguns can be fired via slave units which are triggered by the on-camera flash.

Guide number

Value which indicates the light output of a flashgun. It is based on a film speed of ISO 100 and equals the product of the flashgun-subject distance (in m) and the aperture:

Guide number = distance (m) x aperture

Example: For a flashgun with a guide number of 32 and a subject distance of 4 m, an aperture of f/8 must be set (Fig. 2.37).

At close ranges, calculations with guide numbers are inexact. In order to achieve the correct values, exposure bracketing series are recommended. It is simpler to use TTL controlled flashguns.

If two flashguns with the same output are fired in the same direction (e.g., a twin flash system), the overall guide number is calculated by multiplying the guide number of one flashgun by 1.4.

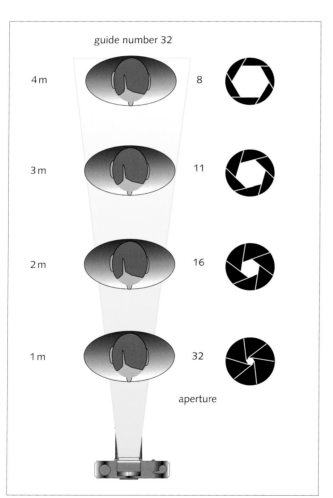

guide number 32

4 m　　　　　8

3 m　　　　　11

2 m　　　　　16

1 m　　　　　32

aperture

Fig. 2.37　The guide number indicates the performance of a flashgun. The required lens aperture is calculated by dividing the guide number into the subject distance (in m).

Dosage of light/flash exposure

When using flashguns, the camera must be set to the correct flash synchronization speed (usually between 1/60s and 1/250s). At the correctly set synchronization speed, the amount of light falling on the film is determined solely by the amount of flash light. There are different ways of determining this amount when using digital cameras:

- manually setting the aperture
- TTL (through the lens) flash metering

Manually setting the aperture

At a specific reproduction ratio and a given lens aperture, the amount of light reflected from an object with normal reflectivity (normal subject) back to the camera is always the same, as the object-camera distance and the amount of light produced by the flash are also always the same. For a particular camera system, the correct aperture can be determined for various reproduction ratios and thus for various subject-to-camera distances. These apertures then have to be set manually before every exposure. With a little bit of experience, it is possible in this straightforward manner to achieve good, reproducible results.

This procedure is necessary if no TTL flash is available for the digital camera. As DSLRs allow an immediate image control, this is no significant disadvantage compared with TTL-metered flashguns.

TTL flash metering

Through the lens flash was originally patented by Minolta, then taken over by Olympus in 1976, and since then offered by every camera manufacturer. TTL means that for flash metering using conventional cameras, only that amount of light is measured which strikes the film through the lens and is reflected from the film surface onto a sensor, generally placed on the camera base (Fig. 2.38).

The advantages of this are obvious. Even in close-up work there is no light parallax. Only that light which was effective for image exposure is measured. Thus, it is possible to control the aperture (and consequently the depth of field) and use light-absorbing accessories such as polarizing filters or bellows units without the danger of incorrect exposure. This type of flash photography has taken the guesswork out of close-up photography. It is also possible to control several flash units through a TTL unit. Naturally, TTL flash also has disadvantages.

Since the camera does not "know" what it is photographing, a mid-range exposure is selected corresponding to a medium gray level (Fig. 2.39). If the subject has very bright highlights, the exposure in the rest of the image is reduced so that the overall exposure is equal to that of a subject with medium reflectivity. Thus, for ex-

Fig. 2.38 With TTL flash metering, the light reflected from the subject passes through the lens to the film; part of this light is reflected by the film surface and strikes a sensor in the base of the camera. The sensor measures the amount of light, transfers the data to the camera's computer, which cuts off the TTL flash when sufficient light has struck the film plane. This "real" TTL flash metering is not possible with digital cameras as the sensor surface has a completely different reflectivity compared with film. Digital TTL flash systems use a preflash instead.

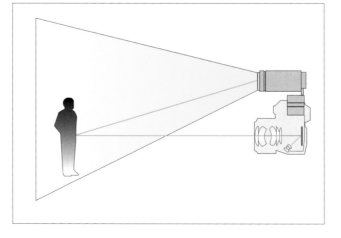

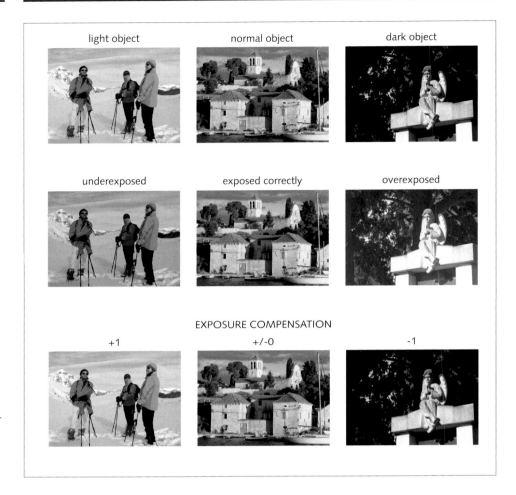

Fig. 2.39   If the brightness of
an image is much higher or lower than a "normal" image with
medium brightness values, an
exposure compensation is necessary in order to get a proper
exposure.

ample, reflections from metal operating instruments can cause such underexposure
that the image is unusable. If the image is almost completely filled with white teeth,
the image can likewise be too dark.

This must be taken into consideration and can be corrected by using the so-called
exposure compensation (in this case, a plus correction) on the exposure setting of
the camera (Fig. 2.40 a–c). The amount of correction depends on the surface and
the brightness of the white objects.

In intraoral photography, in which there are always white surfaces from teeth, it
generally pays to set the aperture to +2/3 of a stop. When teeth fill the entire content of the frame (e.g., a photo of the two central incisors in a reproduction ratio of
2:1) an exposure correction of at least one aperture is required.

Conversely, the same sort of approach must be taken with subjects which are
darker than average. The amount of light must be reduced to prevent the object being overexposed (Fig. 2.41 a–c).

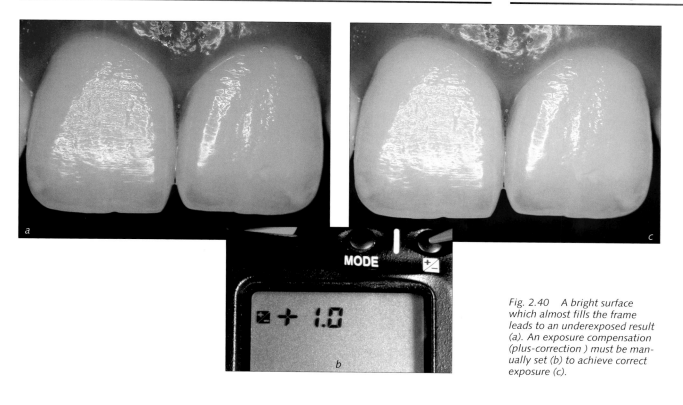

Fig. 2.40 *A bright surface which almost fills the frame leads to an underexposed result (a). An exposure compensation (plus-correction) must be manually set (b) to achieve correct exposure (c).*

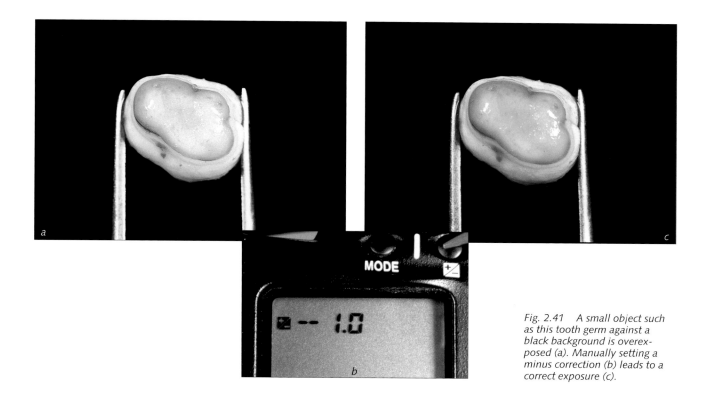

Fig. 2.41 *A small object such as this tooth germ against a black background is overexposed (a). Manually setting a minus correction (b) leads to a correct exposure (c).*

TTL flash metering with digital SLR cameras

As the reflectivity of an electronic sensor is completely different from reflectivity of a film surface (mainly due to the micro lenses), TTL metering for DSLRs had to be modified. Instead of an internal metering of the reflected parts of light, digital cameras use a preflash, which is fired just before the "main" flash. In a split second, the camera determines correct exposure on the basis of the reflected light metering of the preflash falling onto the outer surface of the shutter and adjusts the amount of light necessary for the suitable exposure with the second flash. In addition, data concerning the camera-to-object distance are taken into account. Unlike in conventional photography, where the light reflected from the film surface was metered (shutter open), in digital SLR cameras, the light falling on the shutter surface is metered and the flash is adjusted for the last time when the shutter is still closed. TTL flash metering for conventional cameras means metering the light and controlling the flash during exposure. In digital SLR photography, it means metering the light and adjusting the flash before the exposure.

These advanced TTL flash metering systems are called eTTL or eTTL II (here color temperature of the flash is also metered) by Canon, iTTL by Nikon, sTTL by Sigma, and by Minolta ADI.

Lighting – effects of light

In addition to light dosage problems, lighting the subject and assessment of light and shadow distribution present further principal problems of flash photography. These can be assessed through the viewfinder when constant lighting is used, but not with flash due to its short duration. The lighting effect is dependent on the form of the flash reflectors and their arrangement. There are a number of types available for flash photography.

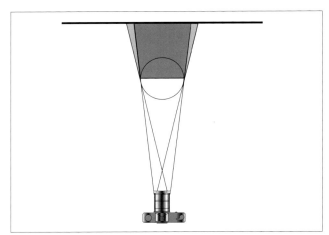

Fig. 2.42   The light from a ring flash surrounds the optical axis. This results in a ring-shaped shadow zone surrounding the subject and a flat, shadowless image of the subject.

Ring flash, sector flash

Ring flashes are widely used in taking images in body cavities, and thus also in the mouth. These types also include sector flashes, in which two to four individual flash tubes are arranged around the lens (Fig. 2.42). In the case of a genuine ring flash, one flash tube surrounds the lens. Sector flashes with four flash reflectors and ring flashes do not differ appreciably in terms of lighting effect. In both of these types, the light practically surrounds the optical axis. The main advantage of this arrangement is that relatively inaccessible objects deep in the oral cavity can be evenly lit, even when ring light is partially obscured by the lips or cheeks (Fig. 2.43). Inexperienced photographers, too, are thus able to produce correctly exposed and illuminated images in inaccessible areas. Another advantage of this type of front illumination is natural color rendition. However, ring flashes have the disadvantage of producing an image almost without shadows. Images tend to look flat and frequently not very brilliant because the shadows, which are necessary to create a three-dimensional effect, are lacking (Fig. 2.44 a,b). This does not substantially affect images taken in the mouth, since light is always partially obscured here anyway, and the characteristics of the ring flash are not evident. For this reason, images taken with ring flash can generally only be distinguished through direct comparison with images taken with side lighting.

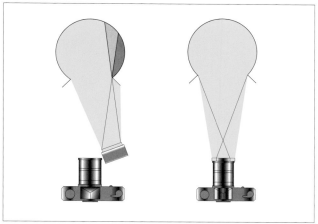

Fig. 2.43   Ring flashes are ideal for illumination of body cavities. If it is not closely enough placed to the lens, illumination by a point flash may result in shadows.

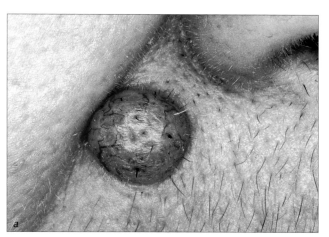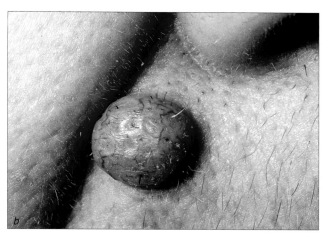

Fig. 2.44   Using a ring flash results in correct color rendition, but a flat representation of the naevus. Sidelighting results in better depth and plasticity (b).

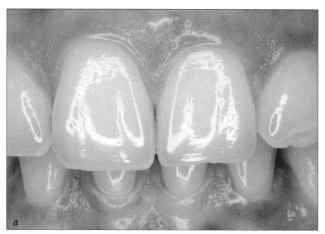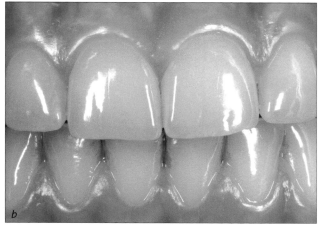

Fig. 2.45   Image of front teeth taken with a ring flash: Lack of shadow and plasticity, disturbing reflections on tooth surfaces (a). Better results with a bilateral flash (b).

The quality of the image can be improved by putting a finger over parts of the ring flash or an individual flash tube, or, if possible, turning them off separately. Modern macro flashes with two lateral single flashes make it possible to reduce the light output of one side. This can be done electronically (e.g., Canon or Sigma) or by moving an built-in diffuser over one side (e.g., Nikon SB-29s). Using asymmetric lighting, the image gains plasticity and depth (Fig. 2.45 a,b).

In general, ring flashes are relatively low powered. When used with teleconverters or other extension accessories, it may therefore be necessary to increase the camera's ISO value.

Point flash

A point light source from the side produces a directional light with strong shadows which aids in the three dimensional appearance of the final image. Macro flash units with bilateral flash tubes provide the option of switching off one tube completely and only using the other tube.

If a twin flash is used with swivelling single flashes, one of these can be turned completely away. This can be necessary for lateral shots to avoid unwanted shadows cast by the second flash.

Depending on the part of the mouth which is to be photographed, the position of the side lighting has to be altered before each exposure. This requires some experience. Overall, front views require the flash to be located at the 12:00 o'clock position; for side lighting, the positions are at 3:00 and 9:00 o'clock. With very short subject-to-camera distances the flash must be located very close to the optical axis to avoid disturbing shadows. For this purpose, a rotatable side flash unit which is mounted close to the lens would be suitable.

Combinations

To compensate for the disadvantages of ring and side flash, or to combine their advantages, several flash units can be combined.

The use of ring and side flash together is not prevalent. Lester Dine (USA) offers a flash unit with both point and ring flash. The flashes can only be used alternatively.

More often, twin flash systems are used with two flash units to be mounted to the left and right of the lens (Fig. 2.46 a,b). The resulting light is intense enough to allow the lens to be stopped down quite far, having a positive effect on depth of field. This set-up achieves illumination even deep in the oral cavity, while at the same time yielding greater plasticity of the image. However, in order to achieve the best possible results, the direction of the flash heads has to be checked and adjusted before each exposure, depending on the subject-to-camera distance. The output from one of the two flash tubes can be reduced by using a diffuser. The use of dual flashes also requires some experience on the part of the operator, if uniformly good results are to be achieved.

Summary: the deeper the object is in the oral cavity and the greater the magnification ratio, the more suitable a ring flash is. Side flash should be used for images

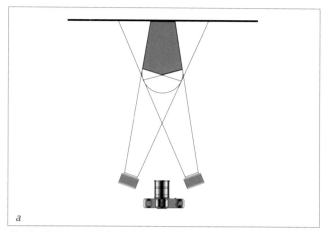 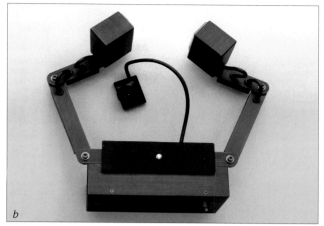

Fig. 2.46   Using a bilateral flash (a) provides high light output and even illumination. An example of such a flash bracket system is the BINZ flash, a handmade high-end system.

taken outside the mouth. Ring flash should be avoided for object or portrait photographs. The use of a bilateral flash system is optimum, but requires a certain amount of experience on the part of the user. Moreover, they are heavier and clumsier to use than ring flashes.

A disadvantage of many macro flash units is their low output. This is indicated by their guide number. A low guide number, such as 8, can mean that higher ISO values (e.g., ISO 200) must be used in order to achieve small enough apertures.

General characteristics of light
Light has certain properties that should be borne in mind when taking pictures.

Light intensity
Finding the proper exposure is always a question of the right aperture in combination with the right shutter speed. Opening the aperture by one stop and shortening shutter speed by one step will lead to the same exposure (Bunsen-Roscoe reciprocity law). Vice versa, shutter speed can be longer and the aperture one stop smaller. It always depends on the intention. If a large depth of field is the aim, the aperture must be closed. If the object moves, a short shutter speed is necessary and the aperture has to be opened wider. Sometimes we reach the limits of these possible combinations. Then we have to use additional light, e.g., electronic flash, or we have to put the camera on the tripod to prevent the camera shaking. In digital photography, we have one more option: we can select a higher ISO value. If this is not exaggerated, image quality will not suffer too much from increase of noise.

Color temperature
A white sheet of paper illuminated by sunlight appears to us as white. This is also the case if we use tungsten light. The reason for this is that our brain is able to fool us

(white adaptation). From an evolutionary point of view this makes sense, as it is an advantage to be able to recognize a poisonous mushroom by its color, independent from the time of the day or the weather.

In conventional silver halide photography, two types of film were used: daylight film and tungsten film. Each of them was sensitized for a certain color temperature of light. But there are more than just two color temperatures. Color temperature of light depends on the mixture of colors it contains.

The term color temperature is borrowed from physics. A so-called black body radiates light when it is heated. The color of this light depends on the temperature. First it will glow dark red, then orange and yellow and then it turns white and blue-white. The hotter the body becomes, the more the color moves from red to blue, and the higher the color temperature will be. Color temperature is metered in degrees Kelvin (K). In this context, our language is a little bit confusing. When talking about "warmer" colors, we mean colors with a tendency to yellow or red, which have a lower color temperature. If we talk about "cooler" colors, we are referring to more bluish colors with a higher color temperature (Fig. 2.47 a–d).

Fig. 2.47   Different light sources show different color temperatures: candle light (a), halogen light (b), blue LED light (c), blue sky in the mountains (d).

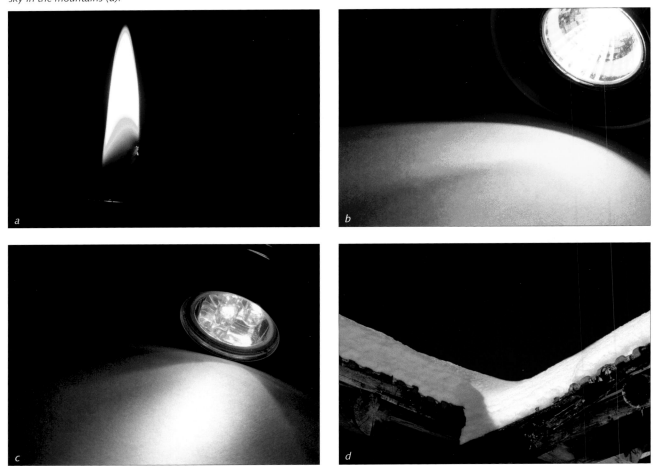

The table on the right shows some light sources and their typical color temperatures.

Unlike our eyes, a digital camera can distinguish color temperature. The result should be an image with colors that look as they were, or how we perceived them when viewed in daylight.

A digital SLR camera offers different modes to adapt it to different color temperatures.

Light source	°Kelvin
Candle	1000-1500
Sunrise/sunset	2000-3500
Household light bulb	2500-3000
Photo flood lights	3000
Halogen bulb	3200
Fluorescent light	4200
Daylight, electronic flash	5000-5500
Bright sunshine, clear sky	6000
Sky slightly overcast	7000
Hazy sky	8000
Open shade at clear sky	8000-9000

Automatic white balance adjustment (AWB)

Works very well in most "normal" situations, for example, during summer vacation when different shots are taken under changing conditions. In these cases, it should be tried first. AWB should be avoided in situations where we have a predominant color. The system "expects"an average distribution of hue, which are combined to produce a neutral gray or white. The automatic function evaluates the overall field of view, and tries to average the present light values with respect to hue in order to eliminate any overall color bias. If there is a color bias (e.g., red mucosa or a blue-stained microscopic specimen), the summed pixel response is not similar to the "expected" overall average and the white balance adjustment will not produce accurate color rendition. Hence, it is not recommended for dental photography. As we always use electronic flash in clinical photography, we should use the preset flash white balance setting first, which may need some fine-tuning.

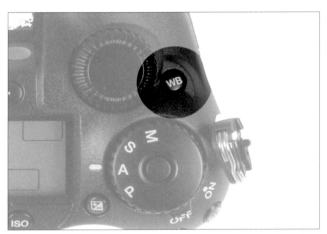

Fig. 2.48   Setting the white balance means adapting to the different color temperatures, one of the major advantages of digital photography.

White balance settings ("presets")

Every camera offers different white balance settings for certain illumination conditions, such as flash, fluorescent, tungsten, cloudy, shade, and sun (Fig. 2.48). By preselecting one of these settings, the cameras' white balance system is set to a certain color temperature so that colors appear the way they would look if shot in daylight (Fig. 16.11). Besides these fixed values, good cameras offer the possibility to "fine-tune" color temperature by 100-K steps in both directions (Fig. 2.49).

In dental photography, the flash setting is recommended, as we normally use electronic flash. If the automatic white balance were selected, the outcome would be more variable.

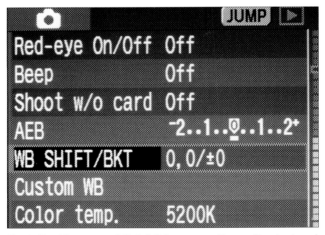

Fig. 2.49   The menu of digital SLR cameras allows a fine-tuning of white balance.

Manual white balance

When working under mixed lighting conditions, the "manual" white balance could be the best way. The procedure differs in detail from one camera to the next (for details, see the respective camera handbook). In principle, the camera is aimed at a white or gray neutral background (white or gray paper, gray card) illuminated in the same way as the following shot. The white object fills the field of view. White balance adjustment is initiated by switch settings or selection in an operation menu (depending upon the specific camera). By this, the camera is "told" that the object is neutral and the camera makes appropriate sensor adjustments to render the target white.

Adjustment by reference to a defined white object is performed under the same lighting conditions employed during acquisition of the image. This method can provide very accurate color balance calibration. If the illumination situation changes, the procedure must be repeated.

This method can be employed by experienced photographers to achieve a desired esthetic effect rather than perfect color rendition, for example, to obtain cooler or warmer colors. For this purpose, bluish or reddish white balance reference cards are available. If the intention is to capture warmer colors (e.g., for portrait photography), a reference card with a light blue color can be used.

More sophisticated cameras allow "white balance bracketing": one shot is taken at the preselected color settings, two more images are generated by the camera, one more blue, the other more red.

If the RAW file format is selected, no white balance setting is used. The ideal white balance can be found later, when converting the image with visual control on the screen.

There are two more important characteristics of light which are only mentioned briefly here, but are discussed later in more detail.

Direction of light

If the light comes parallel to the optical axis (as is the case when using a ring flash), illumination will be very flat, not giving the image plasticity. For portrait work and object photography, shadowless light should be avoided.

If the light comes "from below", the image can be irritating. We are used to seeing light emanate from above (as sun light). From this experience during our evolution, we have learned to deduce from a certain distribution of shadows and illuminated parts that an object has a concavity or a convexity. If light comes from the "wrong" direction, this can be misleading. Therefore, the main light should always come from above (Fig. 2.50–2.51).

Surface of the light source

If the light source used is small in comparison to the object, illumination appears to be "hard". A large light source gives softer light.

A portrait shot under blue sky is always contrasty. Better portraits are obtained under a sky which is at least partly overcast, because the clouds function as a diffuser or reflector, making the light source larger and the light softer. Therefore, in object

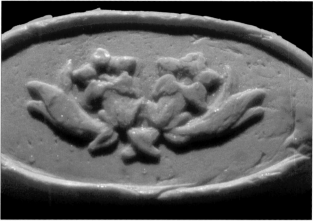

Fig. 2.51   If the object is turned 180 degrees the convexity appears as a concavity.

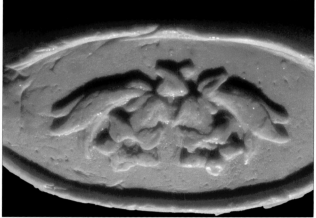

Fig. 2.50   If the light comes from above, a convexity appears as a convexity.

photography, the light source should always be relatively large in comparison with the object itself. A soft-box or diffuser should be used.

BACKGROUND

Exposure measurement

To find the proper exposure, light intensity has to be measured. This can be done more or less automatically by using the bulit-in light meters or with a separate hand-held meter.

There are two methods of measuring light: incident reading and reflected light reading. To take an incident reading, the hand-held meter is pointed in the direction of the camera. The measuring angle is increased through the use of a translucent dome over the light-receiving element. One variant of this way of measurement is flash metering using a flash meter. In taking a reflected light reading, the light reflected by the subject is measured. Camera light meters have different types of measurement depending on the ratio of the sensor surface to the size of the field being measured:

- averaged metering (Fig. 2.52 a)
- selective metering
- spot metering (Fig. 2.52 b)
- matrix metering (

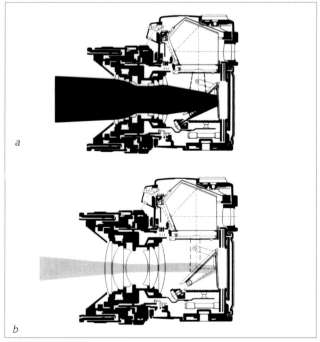

Fig. 2.52   In averaged metering, the illumination from the entire image is measured (a); in spot metering (b), only one point in the center of the image (1-2 degrees) is measured.

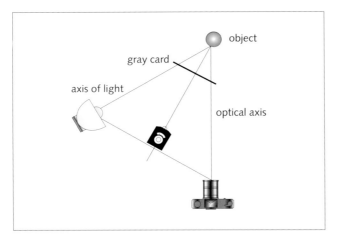

Fig. 2.53   Using a gray card to determine exposure leads to better exposures in many instances. With side lighting, the gray card is placed between the optical axis of the camera and the axis of the light.

With averaged metering, the overall brightness of the subject is measured. With selective metering, the most important part of the image is measured. Most SLRs have center-weighted averaged metering. This means that although the overall light intensity is measured, the center is given greater prominence (e.g., 80%). Modern light meters use a matrix; certain parts of the image are given greater prominence in determining the exposure. Spot metering covers an extremely small angle (e.g., 1 degree).

In many instances it makes sense to take a substitute reading, for example, when the subject cannot be directly measured because it cannot be reached, or when a subject varies substantially from an average reading (bright crowns filling the image frame, portrait of a dark-skinned person), or the subject is high contrast. The photographer's own hand can be used for a substitute reading. In many instances, for example, in technical photography and copy work, the use of a gray card makes sense. This is a piece of cardboard or sheet of plastic which reflects about 18% ("normal" object). This means that 18% of the light is reflected back from the surface. All meters are calibrated to this medium gray value. The gray card is held as close as possible to the object in a front view, in the direction of the camera, and with side lighting, positioned between the axis of the light and the optical axis (Fig. 2.53). If metering is done with the camera's own light meter, the camera is set to "manual" (manual light reading) and an aperture/shutter speed combination is selected which achieves the correct exposure. Thereafter, the gray card is removed and the image is taken using the values set.

Controlling exposure

One of the key advantages of digital photography is the possibility of checking the proper exposure directly after the shot, not by looking at the LCD image on the camera back, but by checking the histogram. This is discussed more in detail in Chapter 7.4.3.

Built-in light meters of modern cameras adjust the exposure in a way that a standard 18% gray reference card is rendered as a midtone. Modern cameras read multiple areas of a scene and average out the readings, hopefully resulting in the best compromise exposure for that scene.

Digital cameras offer a histogram function. A histogram is a bar graph showing the distribution of all tonal values in the photograph. This graph can be superimposed on the reviewed image or displayed separately. The horizontal axis represents the tonal values, beginning with the dark tones on the left and ending with the bright ones on the right. If the distribution of tones is shifted to the left, the image is underexposed or it is a low-key image with numerous dark tones. If the distribution is shifted to the right, we have an overexposed image or a high-key image. By checking this histogram after each exposure, perfectly exposed images should be the result. Therefore, the histogram is sometimes referred to as the 21st century light meter.

Digital technique

3

Within the last few years, digital photography has replaced the conventional technique in nearly all photographic applications. Especially in the field of medical documentation, digital photography has major advantages compared with the old silver halide photography. The main advantages are:

- images are immediately available
- no lab is necessary
- images are available in a digitized form

In the beginning poor image quality was a disadvantage of the new technique, but today there are digital high quality camera systems in use with high resolution and excellent image quality.

3.1   Image capture

In digital cameras, an electronic component—in the position where conventional cameras have the film pressure plate—converts the light falling on it into an electrical signal. These components are solid-state sensors, typically charge-coupled device (CCD) or complementary metal oxide semiconductor (CMOS, pronounced C-moss) photodiode detectors. The image capturing process can be broken down into individual steps to make it more understandable. In reality, these individual processes occur in parallel and simultaneously:

- rastering the image into pixels
- determination of pixel brightness
- conversion of analog to digital
- adding information about color

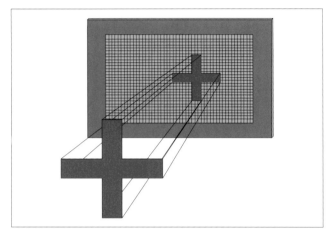

Fig. 3.1 The image projected onto the CCD/CMOS chip is rastered into millions of pixels.

3.1.1   Rastering the image into pixels

First, the image is converted into individual pixels. The greater the number of these, the higher the resolution of the image and the sharper it appears to us. Good digital cameras raster an image into about 6 to 8 million pixels (picture elements = pixels) or more (Fig. 3.1). The rastering is done by the CCD/CMOS chip, which comprises about the same number of single CCD/CMOS elements (about 6 to 8 million). The image is projected by the optical system onto the CCD/CMOS chip. Each single element can convert the light striking it into an electrical current. Thus, in the first approximation, the number of CCD/CMOS elements determines the image quality: the greater the number of CCD/CMOS elements, the better the image quality, comparable to a mosaic.

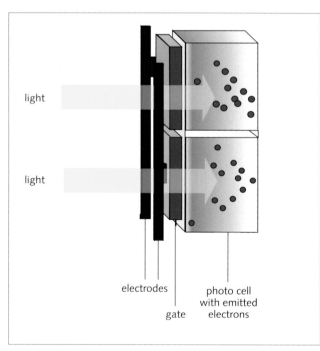

Fig. 3.2 The photo cell emits electrical signals in relation to the amount of light striking it.

light

light

electrodes

gate

photo cell with emitted electrons

3.1.2   Determination of pixel brightness

A CCD element consists of an electrode grid and a silicon layer. The energy of the light falling on the CCD element releases electrons in the silicon layer which are bundled by a current on the gate. The brighter the light signal, the more electrons are released (Fig. 3.2). Each CCD element thus produces a signal which is proportional to the amount of the light reflected off the object and which strikes the single photo element. This weak electrical signal is first produced as an analog current voltage. The brightness of a pixel can therefore be expressed as the strength of the current which can be measured when this pixel is accessed.

Voltage levels are useless to a computer; the analog voltage value has to be converted into computer-readable, digitized form. This is performed by the analog-digital converter.

3.1.3   Analog-digital converter

An analog-digital converter converts the infinitely variable voltage value into a limited number of discrete digital values (Fig. 3.3). In the simplest case, this means current = yes = 1, no current = no = 0. Such a converter can distinguish only between black and white. For text recognition or line drawings, this alone would already be sufficient. If it is necessary to enter images with gray scales into the computer, detectors must be used which can distinguish these minimal differences in brightness. An important criterion for the quality of such digitizers is the number of brightness values they can distinguish.

In addition to resolution, which is determined by the number of pixels and is used to describe the so-called pixel resolution or—better—"structural resolution," there is also a grayscale or color resolution, which describes the ability to discriminate grayscale or color. In addition to the quality of the lenses or sensors, an important factor is the analog-digital converter. Its resolution is expressed in bits (bit depth).

A computer stores numerical values as a series of zeros or ones. The smallest unit of information which a computer can process is called a bit (bit = binary digit). A bit has either a value of 0 or 1. If four bits are used to code a numerical value, 16 different values can be clearly represented.

0000	0001	0010	0011
0100	0101	0110	0111
1000	1001	1010	1011
1100	1101	1110	1111

These can represent, for example, the numbers 0 to 15, gray levels, or other values.

A byte equals 8 bits. A byte can represent 256 (= 2^8) different sequences of zeros and ones. These can be the numbers of 0 to 255, 256 characters, or, for example, 256 gray levels. A kilobyte (kB) equals 1024 such units of information. A megabyte is equal to 1024 x 1024 or 1,048,576 bytes. A digitizer with a 4-bit resolution can thus convert the analog signals produced by the photo sensor into 16 digital values, allowing 16 gray levels to be distinguished.

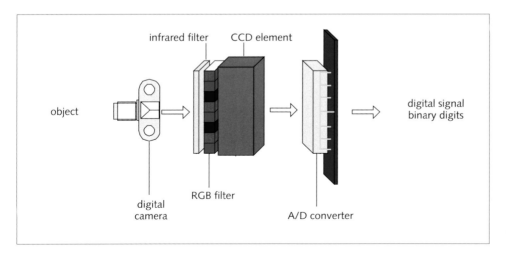

Fig. 3.3   Functional diagram of digital photography: rastering of image, conversion into electrical signals, and subsequent digitization.

Resolution in bits	Numbers	Gray levels
4	0–15	16
5	0–31	32
6	0–63	64
8	0–255	256

The left table shows the relationship between resolution in bits and grayscale resolution

The better the resolution of the analog-digital converter, the greater the number of gray levels which can be distinguished.

How many gray levels are needed to convert a halftone into a computerized form without significant loss of quality?

Aside from the scientific assessment of the image, the human eye is the yardstick, which can distinguish a resolution of about 2 % difference in grayscale. That means about 64 gray levels can be distinguished. Thus, a 6-bit resolution is sufficient in principle, but to compensate for any possible errors, an 8-bit resolution is often used. With 8 bits, 256 shades of gray can be created. Advanced cameras have even higher resolutions offering more data for certain image editing procedures.

At this point, the image consists of about 6 to 8 million pixels which vary in brightness from one another. Now color must be added.

3.1.4   Color information

A color image has information about color as well as brightness. The individual light-sensing elements of CCD or CMOS detectors are only able to measure the intensity (brightness) of light. Different wavelengths (colors) cannot be registered, as the photodiodes are colorblind.

To record color information, a trick is used. The CCD/CMOS elements achieve their color sensitivity by passing the incident light through miniature polymeric thin-film filters that are placed in a mosaic pattern over each pixel of the array. The most common filter arrangement is an ordered mosaic array of red, green, and blue colored filters that repeats an G-R-G-B pattern over the entire sensor. This arrangement, termed a Bayer filter pattern, incorporates 50 % green, 25 % red, and 25 % blue filter elements (Fig. 3.4). The additional green sensor pixels allow the imaging device to more closely approximate the color response of the human visual system. The human eye can differentiate differences in brightness of green light better than of red or blue light. In addition, the green information also provides the signal for luminance (brightness).

These small filters do what color filters always do: they let light of their own color through and block the light of the complementary color. This means that the CCD element with a red filter only measures the brightness of the red part of the light, the neighboring "blue CCD element" only the blue portion, etc.

The image data file of a 6 megabyte chip at this point is 6 million bytes. Each byte contains information about the position, brightness, and color information about a basic color of the particular pixel.

Fig. 3.4   A mosaic filter allows only its own color through, so that each CCD/CMOS element only registers the brightness information of "its" color.

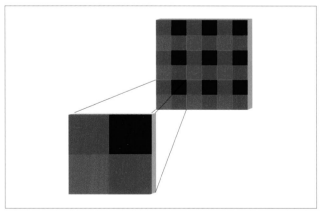

The missing color information of the individual pixels (e.g., the brightness of the green and blue portion of a "red CCD element") is added by the computer through interpolation of the neighboring pixel values, thus increasing the amount of data. The image data file, which was 6 megabytes, is now suddenly 18 megabytes. The electronic image loses brilliance and sharpness through this process of interpolation and must therefore be subsequently enhanced, for instance, through electronic sharpening. It must be kept in mind that only the color information is interpolated, and not the physical resolution. Correspondingly, a pixel is defined as the smallest unit of a digital image containing the full color information.

As we saw before, each pixel has a color depth of 8 bits for each of the basic colors R, G, and B. That means every pixel has 256 possible values for each of its red, green, or blue components (in the RGB model). Therefore it has a 24-bit color depth, also called "true color". When the 3 components are combined there are 256 x 256 x 256 = 16,777,216 possible colors.

The term color depth is defined as the number of bits per pixel available for storage of color information.

$$N_{colors} = 2^{\,color\ depth}$$

Normally, images are stored and displayed on a monitor with a color depth of 24 bits.

The relation between file size in bytes (uncompressed file format such as TIFF) and number of pixels can be estimated according to a rule of thumb:

Number of bytes = number of pixels x 1 (black and white)

Number of bytes = number of pixels x 3 (color)

If you take a normal 24-bit picture stored in RGB mode and transfer it into CMYK mode (CMYK = cyan, magenta, yellow, and key color black) before printing, file size is increased by one third and color depth is now 32 bits. But this has nothing to do with the real, existing colors. In theory, we should have 2^{32} colors (about 4 billion). As the CMYK color space is smaller than the RGB color space, the number of CMYK colors is smaller than the existing RGB colors.

True color with more than 16 million colors is more than sufficient for printing and for displaying colors on computer monitors. Why do some scanners offer more than 24-bit color depth? There are scanners which allow 48-bit color depth (2^{48} colors!). That means instead of 8 bits to represent a single color, 12 or 16 bits are used. A 16-bit image can handle 65,536 discrete levels of information instead of the 256 levels that an 8-bit image can. This can make sense if a high-end image editing procedure follows, using a program that can handle 48-bit images. The main advantage of a high-bit image is that by using the Levels or Curves to compress or stretch the data (see Chapter 17) you have more data to work with. A low-bit image leaves gaps (toothcomb effect) and these gaps manifest themselves as jumps in color or brightness levels of the final image, which is termed posterization.

The heart of the camera, the CCD/ CMOS chip, thus predominantly determines the image quality, and also the price of the camera. The current developmental trend for digital cameras is the appearance of new models at least every six months; these differ from the previous models in particular in that the CCD chip offers yet another million pixels.

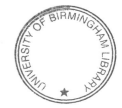

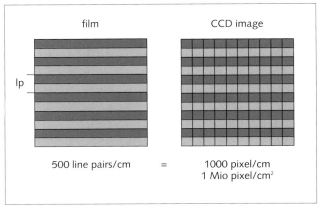

film   CCD image

lp

500 line pairs/cm   =   1000 pixel/cm
                        1 Mio pixel/cm²

Fig. 3.5   The resolution of film translated into electronic terms. A resolution of 500 line pairs per cm corresponds to a resolution of 1000 pixels/cm. This results in a resolution of over 8.6 million pixels for the overall area of a 35-mm slide or negative. This corresponds to more than a 20-MB data volume per individual image.

An alternative to the conventional CCD sensors is CMOS (=complementary metal oxide semiconductor) technology, used in many cameras (see Chapter 4).

The "gold standard" in terms of resolution continues to be 35-mm film. A good 35-mm image has more than 500 line pairs (Lp) per cm (Fig. 3.5). Translated into the language of digital technology, a line pair corresponds to two pixels. Hence, 500 Lp correspond to 1000 pixels per cm or 1 million pixels per cm². With a total area of about 8.6 cm² per slide, this means about 8.6 million pixels per image. This produces more than 20 MB of data per slide. In comparing image quality, digital cameras have as a yardstick this resolution of current 35-mm slides or negatives. Another opinion is that a 12 MPixel SLR camera produces results close to good 100 ISO 35-mm slides. Therefore, we can conclude that a digital SLR camera with a resolution between 8 and 12 MPixels will give us results comparable with good slide films.

3.2   New developments in sensor technology

In principle, the transformation of light hitting the sensor elements into an electric signal proceeds in nearly the same manner in all sensor types. As these components are the heart of every digital camera, some properties of the sensors and newer developments are discussed more in detail.

Designation	Aspect ratio	Width (mm)	Height (mm)
1/3.6"	4:3	4.0	3.0
1/3.2"	4:3	4.5	3.4
1/3"	4:3	4.8	3.6
1/2.7"	4:3	5.3	4.0
1/2"	4:3	6.4	4.8
1/1.8"	4:3	7.2	5.3
2/3"	4:3	8.8	6.6
1"	4:3	12.8	9.6
4/3"	4:3	18.0	13.5
Sigma SD 10	3:2	20.7	13.8
Canon EOS 300D,10D	3:2	22,7	15.1
Nikon D1, D70, D100	3:2	23.7	15.6
Canon 1D MkII	3:2	28.7	19.1
Canon EOS 1Ds	3:2	36.0	24.0
Kodak DSC-14n	3:2	36.0	24.0

Sensor size/number of pixels

With increasing size of the sensors, manufacturing costs increase disproportionately. According to a rule of the thumb, doubling the sensor size increases the costs of production eight times.

Up to now, a higher sensor resolution has been achieved by placing more single sensor elements on the chip, not by increasing sensor size. Most of the digital SLR cameras (DSLR) have sensors which have the dimensions of the APS film format. Consumer cameras have sensors which are far smaller (see table below).

The designation of the sensor is based on specifications for old TV tubes used in the 1950s. One of the mysteries of digital technology is why these designations are used for modern digital sensors, as the "sizes" don't really relate in any consistent way to the actual physical size of the sensor.

The following table shows some typical sensor sizes. For costs reasons, "full format sensors", which have the size of 35-mm film (24 x 36 mm) are used only in a few DSLRs. These cameras are not the first choice for dental photography as they are much too expensive.

As the table above shows, there are big differences in sensor size (Fig. 3.6). A very popular sensor in consumer cameras is the "1/1.8" sensor", which is about 23 times smaller than 35-mm film and nearly 10 times smaller than the typical sensor used in DSLR cameras. The same is true for the single "pixels" of a CMOS sensor. A single sensor element of the chip built in the Canon EOS-1D is 12 times larger than a single sensor element on the chip of Canons G2 consumer camera.

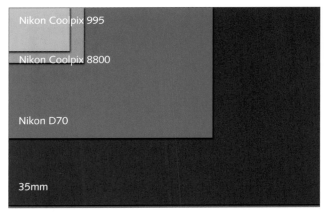

Fig. 3.6   Sensor size of different cameras in relation to 35-mm film format.

The consequence is that the tiny consumer sensors are less light sensitive than the SLR sensors. The problem that smaller sensors are less light sensitive can be overcome by amplifying the output signal. But this causes another problem: amplifying the signal means amplifying the noise as well. The image shows a significant loss of quality. Therefore, most consumer digicams cannot operate above ISO 400, while DSLRs can be "pushed" up to ISO 3200 with noisy but acceptable results.

BACKGROUND

Image noise

"Noise" is defined as an electrical or acoustic activity that can disturb communication. When listening to a radio station which is not set perfectly, you cannot improve the quality by amplifying the signal, which means increasing the volume. The result would be that the noise is amplified as well.

Noise in digital images can be compared with film grain, caused by excessive clumping together of silver particles in the film emulsion, visible on large format prints or used intentionally for artistic reasons. Digital noise appears like multi-colored TV "snow", particularly visible in shadow areas, skin tones and in solid sky or other even-colored areas.

There are different sources of noise in digital images:
- A certain level of internal "electronic" noise is normal for every CCD or CMOS sensor. If ISO speed of the camera is increased, the output signal of the sensor is amplified, together with the noise, which then becomes visible.
- During long exposure times, the imaging device becomes heated up, causing pixels to saturate and appear as noise.
- During long exposure times, some pixels become saturated and may cause noise in surrounding pixels.
- Pixel interpolation can cause noise.

- The more pixels that are arranged on tiny sensors, the noisier the image becomes, due to the signal amplification of the less light sensitive pixels and because of a pixel-to-pixel contamination. Therefore, an 8 MPixel viewfinder camera with a small sensor generates far more noise than an 8 MPixel SLR camera with a bigger sensor.
- Noise can be intensified by JPEG compression and by sharpening an image.

Visible noise in images is divided into "luminance" (brightness) noise and "chroma" (color noise). Luminance noise results in grainy-looking images, visible on screens, but not when printed. Chroma noise is characterized by random blue and red pixels.

Reducing noise is possible, but there is always a decision necessary: how much image softness and color damage can be accepted in order to reduce noise?

Solutions
- If noise becomes an issue, the built-in noise reduction features should be used.
- Cameras with larger sensors (SLR camera) show significantly less noise.
- Editing programs offer noise reduction features.
- Special software (e.g., Neat Image) can be applied to reduce noise.

Functionality of the sensor is also different. Small sensors can read the data in real time using a scheme called "interline transfer". These sensors give a live image on the camera's LCD screen, and no mechanical shutter is necessary for exposure control.

The more expensive sensors of digital SLRs use a "full frame" scheme to read the data from the sensor (in this context, "full frame" refers to the design, not to the size). That means they need a mechanical shutter for exposure control and cannot generate a live image on the LCD screen, nor can they record video. The advantage of this type of sensor is that the whole pixel area can be used to capture light, while interline transfer CCDs use part of each pixel to store charge, causing a higher noise level.

Therefore, comparing two cameras only on the basis of their pixel numbers makes no more sense than comparing a sports car and a truck simply because they have similar horsepower.

BACKGROUND

The lens of the camera generates a round image according to its image circle. This image is projected on the CCD or CMOS chip in the back of the camera.

The number of the single photo sensors integrated in the chip is called the total pixel number or physical pixels. Not all are used to capture the image.

Picture pixels/image pixels

The picture pixels, also called image pixels, are used to capture the image. They can be used as indicators for the sensor resolution. Other pixels are not used to capture the image, but to process the image, or they are not used at all, because the image circle is larger than the sensor. These plus the image pixels make up the total pixels (Fig. 3.7).

If the image circle is much smaller than the sensor diameter, there will be a big difference between total pixels and image pixels, as many pixels will be wasted (Fig. 3.8). The opposite can also be true: the image circle is much larger than the sensor. This is the case when conventional lenses are used with DSLRs. The picture area of the sensor does not cover the full 35-mm format (Fig. 3.9).

The ratio of picture pixel area diagonal to the diagonal of 35-mm film determines the so called "focal length multiplier". The focal length of a lens must be multiplied by this factor to find the "effective focal length" when used with a DSLR camera (Fig. 3.10).

Effective pixels

The number of the effective pixels includes the image pixels plus the pixels used to calibrate the black by a zero reading from masked pixels not exposed to light. To complete the confusion: the definition of the PIMA (Photographic and Imaging Manufacturers Association) for image pixels is the same as the Japan Camera Industry Association's definition of effective pixels.

Recorded pixels

Cameras allow storage of the images in different sizes. By doing this, the number of recorded pixels is changed.

Output pixels

Sometimes the recorded image has to be cropped to fit standard dimensions (XGA, SVGA etc.) or to fit certain aspect ratios (4:3, 16:9, 2:3). In these circumstances, the number of the recorded pixels differs from the number of the output pixels.

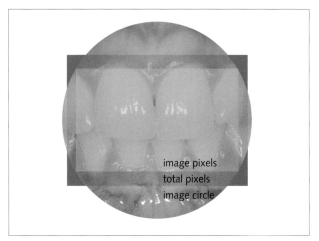

Fig. 3.7   Not all pixels are used to capture the image.

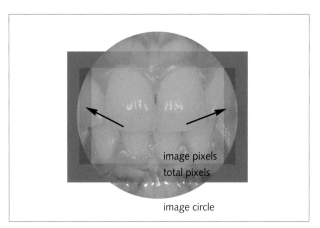

Fig. 3.8   Sometimes pixels are wasted.

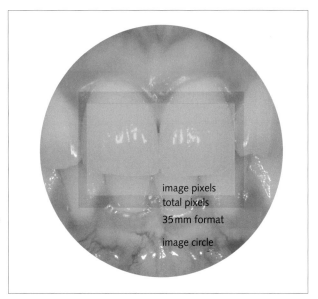

Fig. 3.9   When using conventional lenses, the image circle is much larger than sensor size.

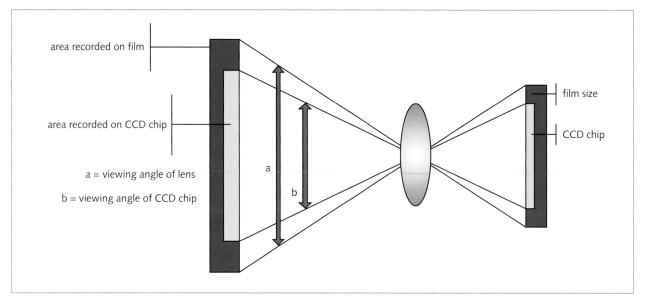

Fig. 3.10   Since CCD chips are presently smaller than 35-mm format, only the middle portion of the image in the viewfinder is taken. This can be compared to using a telephoto lens instead of a normal lens. Thus, this is referred to as conversion factor (or crop factor), with which the lens has to be multiplied in order to compare this to 35mm format.

In most cameras, sensors are used which are much smaller than the 35-mm format. A side effect of this is the so-called lens factor (also called crop factor), which is about 1.5 to 1.7 for most DSLRs. The focal length of the lens has to be multiplied by this factor in order to find the effective focal length (Fig. 3.10). For example, a 100-mm lens used in combination with a Nikon D1X (lens factor 1.5) has an effective focal length of 150mm.

This is not a major problem for dental photography, as we use telemacro lenses with longer focal length. It can, however, be a problem in the wide angle range. To achieve a wide angle image, one must use a lens with a very short focal length.

SuperCCD

The development and further improvements of the "SuperCCD" by the Fujifilm company show how sensor technology is undergoing an evolutionary process (Fig. 3.11 a-d).

In conventional chips, the individual CCD elements are arranged in a rectangular pattern (Fig. 3.11 b). In the SuperCCD chip (Fuji), the individual cells are rotated by 45 degrees and are also octagonal (Fig. 3.11 c). The result is interpolated pixel data surpassing the data of the physically existent pixel. The advantages are better resolution of the chip in horizontal and vertical directions, greater light sensitivity, and better contrast. The first digital SLR to use the SuperCCD chip was the Fuji FinePix S1.

In the meantime, there is a SuperCCD Chip of the next generation on the market (SuperCCD SR; SR = sensitivity range). Here, large high sensitivity S sensors are used together with low sensitivity R sensors (Fig. 3.11 d), improving the dynamic range (more details in shadows and highlights, richer tonality, improved skin tones). On the chip of the FinePix S3 Prof. (SuperCCD SRII) 6.17 million S pixels are arranged beside 6.17 million R pixels. R and S sensors are separated (fourth generation of the

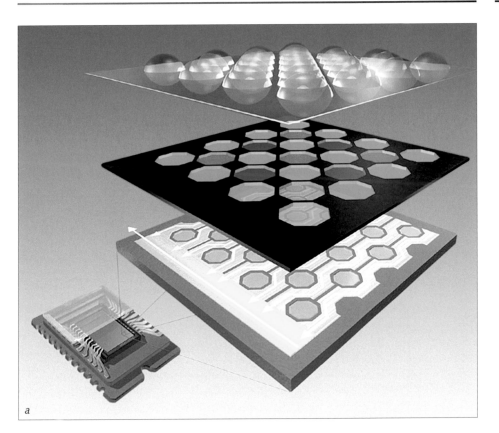

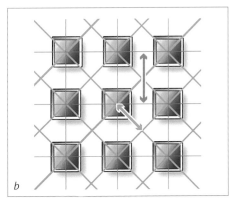

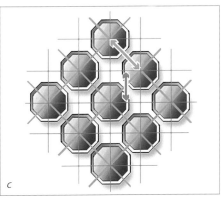

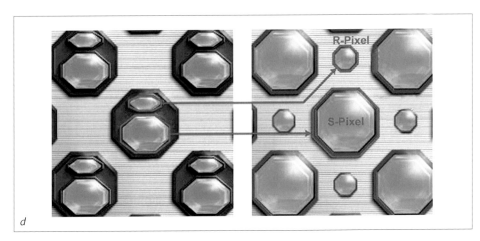

Fig. 3.11   The Super CCD technology is aimed at improving image quality. Components of the chip in principle (a). Unlike conventional rectangular CCD elements (b), the light sensitive sensors on the SuperCCD are octagonal (c). The next generation doubled the number of pixels (d) and the last generation moved the R-pixel into the space between the S-pixels. (Illustration: Fujifilm)

SuperCCD sensor). The data of both sensor types are combined and result in images showing details in both dark and light areas, without losing contrast.

The evolution of this SuperCCD sensor is only an example. Similar improvements have been made by all manufacturers. One has to keep in mind that film technology had more than 150 years to reach its current level. Sensor technology has just started this process.

CMOS technology

CMOS (complementary metal oxide semiconductor) technology is an alternative to conventional CCD chips. In principle, a CMOS sensor works similar to a CCD. Unlike a CCD, a CMOS chip consists of millions of single photodiodes, each of them with its own underlying A/D converter. Processing of the electronic signal is there-

Fig. 3.12   Structure of CCD and CMOS sensors in principle.

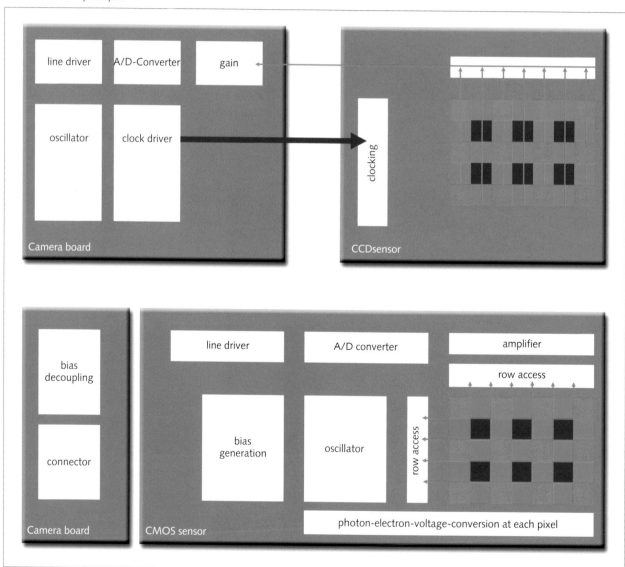

fore faster and less energy consuming (Fig. 3.12). The production of such CMOS chips is far less complicated and thus significantly less expensive than that of the complicated CCD chips.

Some differences are shown in the following table:

Properties	CCD	CMOS
Pixel signal	Electron packet	Voltage
Chip signal	Voltage (analogue)	Bits (digital)
Signal out of camera	Bits (digital)	Bits (digital)
Fill factor	High	Moderate
System noise	Low	Moderate to high
System complexity	High	Low
Sensor complexity	Low	High
Responsivity	Moderate	Slightly better
Dynamic range	High	moderate
Uniformity	High	Low to moderate
Speed	Moderate to high	Higher
Clocking	Higher voltage	Low-voltage

The first DSLR with a CMOS sensor was the Canon EOS D30. The subsequent camera models (D60, 10D, 20D) have CMOS sensors as well. The full-format sensors of Kodak and Canon are also CMOS-type sensors. At the beginning, CMOS-type sensors produced images with higher noise and poor image quality. These disadvantages have since been eliminated.

The sensor of the Sigma SD 10 is also a CMOS-type sensor (Foveon X3 sensor). But this component employs a completely different technique.

Foveon X3 sensor

A completely new approach to sensor technology was taken by the Foveon company: the X3 sensor. In these sensors, every single pixel captures the whole color information of red, green, and blue light. This is possible as the sensor does not use a mosaic filter (capturing only part of the color and constructing the color by interpolation), but has three layers of pixel sensors, one on top of the other. This can be compared with the principle of conventional film. The layers of the X3 sensors are embedded in silicon to take advantage of the fact that red, green, and blue light penetrate silicon to different depths (Fig. 3.13).

The advantage of the X3 sensor is that the time-consuming and complex interpolation performed by conventional CCD or CMOS sensors is not necessary for reconstructing missing information. The result: sharper images, better color reproduction and saturation, and no artefacts such as moire.

This new type of sensor was first used in the Sigma SLR camera SD 9.

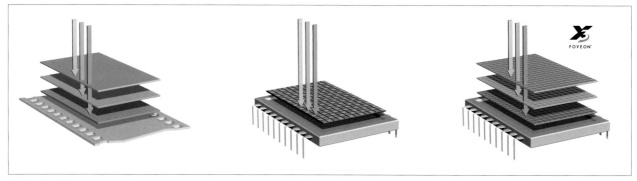

Fig. 3.13   X3 sensors record colors as film does. No Bayer pattern filter is used, therefore no interpolation is necessary to generate data.

3.3   Current trends and developments to improve image quality

The development of digital photography has been characterized by constantly increasing resolution of the cameras and consequently also image quality. There are different ways to reach the goal:

- increasing sensor resolution
- increasing lens resolution
- combinations

Increasing sensor resolution

In the recent past, a given digital camera model has been replaced nearly every six months by its successor version with 1 million pixels more. Today this development has reached a certain plateau or has at least slowed down. Currently, most high-end cameras in the semiprofessional and professional field have 5 to 8 megapixels or more.

	D70	D2X
	6 MP	12 MP
Pixel dimensions	2000 x 3008	2848 x 4288
Print size at 300 dpi in cm	16.25 x 25	23,75 x 35,75

When discussing the pixel count and image size, one must bear in mind that increasing the pixel number by 100% results in an increase in image size of only 50%, because the dimensions of the image increase by only 50%, as the left example shows. In other words: You must quadruple megapixel count to double resolution (horizontally or vertically). A twelve MP sensor of today has only twice the resolution of a three MP sensor of yesterday.

The increase in image dimensions going from a 6 MP camera to an 8 MP camera results in an image only 16% larger. The step from 8 MP to 12 MP results in an image only 25% larger. Pixel numbers which are very impressive at first glance shrink in importance when the real effect is evident.

In order to obtain a higher resolution, there are different possibilities of arranging more single photo elements on a CCD chip:

- increasing the size of the chip
- decreasing the size of the single photodiode on the chip

Up to now, the actual size of the CCD sensor has hardly changed. This is due to the very costly production of the sensors. These are produced from silicon wafers which are coated in various steps. A certain number of CCD sensors can be produced from a wafer. If larger sensors are to be produced, fewer of these can be gained from one silicon wafer. The fewer the sensors produced from a wafer, the higher the rejection rate due to impurities which can occur even in spite of clean-room conditions. Thus, the costs rise almost exponentially if larger chips are produced. A chip twice the size costs eight times more to produce. For this reason, manufacturers seek a compromise between quality and cost.

The current trend of putting more and more CCD elements ("pixels") on almost the same size chip necessarily means that the pixel size and the space between pixels are being reduced. This requires the use of higher performance lenses in order not to negate the advantages of the larger number of pixels by bad optical quality.

The resolution of a lens, like that of a film, is measured in line pairs/mm. Very high quality 35-mm lenses are able to achieve 70 to 100 Lp/mm. Most lenses used for conventional photography do not reach this quality level. A resolution of 70 Lp/mm means that the lens can render a maximum of 140 pixels per mm. This corresponds to a pixel distance of 0.007 mm (7 μm). Modern digital viewfinder cameras have 1/1.8" or 2/3" CCD chips with approximately 5 to 8 million CCD elements. This results in a "pixel distance" of 4 μm or less. In other words, upward of 250 CCD elements are found on a length of 1 mm. To keep these separate requires a high quality lens which can resolve at least 125 Lp/mm.

This is exactly the reason why digital cameras which use conventional lenses constructed for silver halide photography have a resolution of about 6 MPixels. The quality of the lens is the limiting factor. In other words, it does not make sense to arrange more photodiodes on a small chip as long as the resolution of the lens is not improved as well. Otherwise, the full potential of the sensor cannot be exploited. Therefore, some manufacturers decided to construct special lenses for digital photography with higher resolution and smaller image circle, especially adapted to the chip size. Nikon offers newly developed lenses for the DSLR cameras with smaller image circle diameter which cannot be used with conventional SLR cameras. Olympus offers high-end lenses for the E-1 system, and Tamron and Sigma have developed especially designed "digital" lenses.

Besides this, a smaller CCD element also has the disadvantage of being less light sensitive than a larger one. This is compensated for by slightly increasing the amplification of the sensor signals. This not only increases the light sensitivity, but also the background noise, which in turn adversely affects the image quality, analogous to turning up the volume on a radio set for a distant station.

These considerations make it evident that increasing the number of pixels per CCD/CMOS chip sooner or later reaches its limits. CCD/CMOS chips with a larger surface and the same size elements would be one way to improve image quality. Despite the fact that production of full-frame sensors is far more costly, Canon and Kodak decided to go this way with their full-frame sensors (24×36mm) in order to increase image quality.

Full-frame sensors

A full-frame sensor (24×36mm) has two main advantages: more single photodiodes can be arranged on its surface, and conventional lenses can be used without the loss of wide-angle capability. According to this, the Canon EOS 5D has a resolution of 12.8 MPixels and Kodak DCS Pro 14n about 14 MPixels.

Yet there is no light without shadow. Full-frame sensors also have disadvantages. If conventional lenses are used in digital photography, only the light passing the center of the lens hits the center of the chip perpendicularly. The light beams reaching the corners of the chip hit the single sensor elements at a very steep angle of incidence. This means that because the image circle of the lens is utilized completely, we are confronted with problems of image sharpness (as we had in the marginal areas in conventional photography, too).

This is not as critical for silver halide film as it is for electronic sensors, as film has very good stability and sensitivity against lightbeams over a broad range of angle between beam and film plane. In the same situation, electronic sensors are very intolerant and can show visible loss of quality, partly due to the decreasing amount of light reaching the corners of the chip (cornershading).

One reason for this is the construction of such a sensor. The depth of the light-sensitive sensor area is only 2 to 10μm (the light-sensitive area of a film has a depth of 20 to 25μm). The complete chip is a sandwich consisting of the light-sensitive CCD or CMOS sensor, covered by a protecting glass and a filter (infrared or anti-aliasing filter). Furthermore, we find the colored mosaic filter and some chips have special micro lenses to channel the light beams on to the CCD surface. This construction must have an influence on image quality.

Especially when using a full-frame sensor, these deficiencies have to be compensated by extremely sophisticated position-dependant signal processing in order to increase sharpness and brightness in the corners of the image. Therefore, the sensor sensitivity has to increase from image center to corner. A side effect of this is an increase of noise and loss of dynamic range from center to corner.

It seems that full-frame sensors present a number of problems at the moment, which have to be overcome by sophisticated technical means.

Full-frame sensors may be suitable for wide-angle photographers. For medical photography, this is not a major issue, as in most cases telephoto macro lenses are used.

In terms of image quality, interdependence between lens construction and chip construction has a side effect which is worth mentioning. When a lens for conventional photography was tested, the result was independent of the quality of the camera used for the test. When a lens for digital photography is tested, the type and the construction of the image sensor are crucial for the testing result of the lens. Therefore, only camera-related test results of lenses are relevant for digital photography.

Combination of improved lenses and improved chip

As we have seen, enlarging the chip size and increasing the number of single photodiodes are technological dead ends, as long as the old lenses for conventional photography are used. A good approach seems to be to change both the lenses and camera sensor. This is the option Olympus chose for its 4/3 system. Here, lenses designed especially for digital purposes channel the light more accurately to the 4/3-type image sensor, giving excellent image results from edge to edge. With this completely new construction, the lens mount diameter and the sensor size and distance could be harmonized perfectly (Fig. 3.14). Aside from that, a FT-CCD (Frame Transfer CCD) is used. Unlike many so-called Interline CCD sensors, which use a lot of chip surface for electronic pathways on which image data can travel, the FT-CCD is a "Progressive Scan Sensor". This type of sensor utilizes nearly the whole chip surface for gathering image information. The result: better image resolution, higher dynamic range, and lower noise.

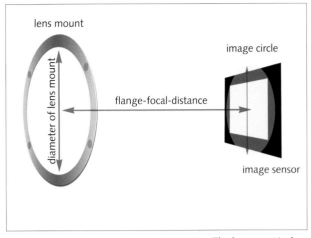

Fig. 3.14 The lens mount of the E-1 system is larger than the lens mount used before for conventional SLR cameras.

Summary

To distill out the most salient points:

1. Using digital cameras with conventional lenses will not give optimum results, especially when zoom lenses are used.
2. Lens resolution in the margin areas is often not sufficient to match sensor resolution. This is especially true for full-format sensors and wide-angle zoom lenses.
3. These are minor problems when good telephoto macro lenses are used, as this is the case in dental photography.
4. Results of lens tests should be camera related.

In order to obtain optimum results, all other factors influencing image quality should be respected:

- Use of a lens hood to prevent flare
- Clean lens surfaces (front and back)
- Proper illumination
- Aperture not closed maximally to prevent diffraction effects
- Use of a tripod, if possible (not for intraoral, clinical routine work)

3.4   Signal processing and in-camera storage

Aside from the CCD/CMOS chip, other electronic components determine the quality of the various cameras.

Image data are first stored in RAM (random access memory) and then in the camera's internal storage. Their capacity and processing speed determine the rate at which pictures can be taken in succession. Generally, amateur cameras allow two or three pictures to be taken in a row before the camera's computer has to process them. Top grade professional cameras can shoot up to 8 or 9 images per second and up to 40 consecutive JPEG or 25 RAW (NEF) full-resolution (2,464 x 1,632 pixels) images in high speed burst mode. Naturally, this requires far more sophisticated electronics than are necessary in amateur cameras.

There are also differences in data formats. Professional cameras allow the user to select the storage format. Most allow images to be stored simply in JPEG format with various compression levels, in which image data, and thus image quality, are lost. Deterioration of the image is only visible, if compression is performed at a low quality level and/or the image is saved repeatedly in such a "lossy" file format.

Other cameras allow storage in TIFF mode without compression or in RAW format, or RAW/JPEG combination making subsequent use of transfer/conversion software necessary.

The next step is the image data transfer from the RAM into a removable storage medium.

The most common storage media are:

- CompactFlash cards
- IBM microdrives

*Fig. 3.15
Structure of a compact flash card.*

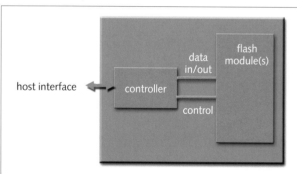

CompactFlash cards

CompactFlash cards are robust and fast. Currently, they have a maximum capacity of 8 GB (Fig. 3.15 and 3.16). They can be downloaded into the PC by integrated card readers or by simple USB card readers or PC card adapters. CompactFlash cards are the most common storage medium for professional digital cameras.

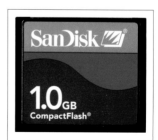

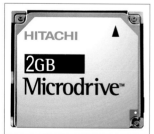

Microdrive

The Microdrive is a miniature hard drive which has a CompactFlash interface. It can be used in any system which accepts CompactFlash cards type II. Although this storage medium weighs only 16 g, it can store up to 4 GB. Its disadvantage is that it contains a rotating microdrive. If it falls or is dropped, there is the danger of data loss (Fig. 3.17).

Fig. 3.16   CF cards have a huge capacity for data storage.

Fig. 3.17   Microdrives contain a rotating hard drive disk.

SD Card

The SD Card (SD = Secure Digital) is a stamp-sized flash memory card, which weighs approximately 2 g. The SD Card can be used in a variety of digital products. The main advantages are small size, low battery consumption, and a user-selectable mechanical write-protect switch on the exterior card casing. Its storage capacity goes up to 1 MB (Fig. 3.18).

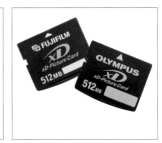

Fig. 3.18   sD cards have the size of a stamp and are used more and more for cameras.

Fig. 3.19   xD picture cards are tiny media with enormous capacity.

MMC

MultiMedia Cards (MMC) are closely related to SD cards. The SD card uses more pins. You can use a MMC in a device that is equipped with a SD card slot, but you cannot do the opposite. SD cards will not work in an MMC-only device.

Fig. 3.20   Memory Stick (Sony) with adapter.

xD-Picture Card

The xD-Picture card provides a high capacity in one of the smallest memory formats available today. It is used in Olympus and Fuji cameras. Featuring rapid data transfer speeds, it is ultra compact with capacities ranging from 64 MB to 1 GB (Fig. 3.19).

Memory Stick

The Memory Stick is a storage format which is currently found only in Sony cameras. The Memory Stick Pro type has a capacity of up to 2 MB. It is also used for DVD-quality video in real time (Fig. 3.20).

SmartMedia card

SmartMedia cards have the advantage of being small, fast, and light, thus being well suited to small amateur cameras. They are not used for DSLRs.

For dental office purposes, it is recommended to use two fast CompactFlash cards with medium capacity (256 or 512 MB) instead of one with ultra high capacity. This forces the user to transfer the image data to the computer regularly.

The table below shows the approximate number of shots per memory card for various digital camera pixel counts using high quality JPEGs for storage.

	3 MP	4 MP	5 MP	6 MP
128 MB memory	116	87	70	58
256 MB memory	232	174	140	116
512 MB memory	464	348	280	232

	Capacity	Size (mm)	Transfer rate: writing	Transfer rate: reading	Compatibility
CompactFlash I/II card	4 GB	36.4 x 42.8 x 3.3 / 36.4 x 42.8 x 5	8-16 MB/s	6-16 MB/s	CF I → CF II slot
MicroDrive	4 GB	36.4 x 42.8 x 5	6 MB	4.2 MB	MD → CF
IISecure Digital card (SD)	1 GB	32 x 24 x 2.1	12.5 MB/s	12.5 MB/s	—
MultiMedia card (MM)	512 MB	32 x 24 x 1.4	2.5 MB/s	2.5 MB/s	MM → SDslot
xD-Picture Card	1 GB	20 x 25 x 1.7	5 MB/s	3 MB/s	xD → CF II (adapter)
Memory Stick	128 MB	50 x 21.5 x 2.8	2.5 MB/s	1.8 MB/s	MS → MS
(Pro)	2 GB		20 MB/s	20 MB/s	Pro-Slot
SmartMedia Card	128 MB	45 x 37 x 0.76	0.8 MB/s	2.1 MB/s	—

Important features of storage media

3.5   Image data file formats

Image data files are stored in different file formats by the camera, which must be pre-selected. The most important file format types for digital photography are:

- JPEG
- TIFF
- RAW

3.5.1   JPEG

Nearly all digital SLR cameras offer the JPEG format (JPEG = Joint Photographic Expert Group; file extension .jpg) as an option, normally at different quality levels. The advantage of the JPEG format is that images can be reproduced very well by relatively small image files. Today, JPEG is the most widespread image format. It is recommended for routine use also in dental photography, as it represents the best compromise between image quality and file volume.

It has to be taken into account that JPEG uses a "lossy" compression mode. In principle, groups (8 x 8 pixels) of equally colored pixels are combined, which are afterwards represented by one single pixel. Thus, an image containing expanses of blue sky or red mucosa can be compressed very effectively. The degree of compression—and by this image quality—can be selected by adjusting the camera, or later when using an image editing program. Photoshop, for example, offers 13 quality levels (0 to 12). For routine work, a maximum quality setting is recommended to avoid image deterioration. Then the lost image information cannot be detected by the naked eye.

JPEG files should not be opened, edited, or saved repeatedly, as image information is lost with every cycle, and image quality deteriorates visibly. Data loss does not happen when the image is opened or saved, but when it is closed again. For extended editing procedures in different sessions, the use of "non-lossy" file formats, such as TIFF or PSD, is recommended.

To avoid image degradation, the following procedure is recommended:
- Open a JPEG.
- Save the file with a new name.
- Work on it.

Following these steps, the original will not be degraded.

In many situations, a JPEG file directly from the camera can produce very high quality prints. Nevertheless, a JPEG file has undergone many manipulations by the camera (linear conversion, matrix conversion, white balance, contrast, saturation, and a potentially destructive compression). If you use a camera able to shoot images as RAW files in a 12-bit mode (84,096 tonal values) and then save the file as a JPEG, the software converts it to 8-bit mode with only 256 tonal values. The rest of the data is thrown away and lost forever.

The secret to using JPEG files is: set a proper white balance and make a proper exposure. If you are using the auto white balance, color may be not consistent from one file to the next, so set a custom white balance or use a gray card in the first image.

There are cameras on the market which have a color bias in JPEG mode, e.g., a higher saturation in the reds. This can be corrected in Photoshop or by using the RAW mode.

Reasons to use JPEG format:
- Files are smaller; they need less space on storage media in camera and computer.
- Smaller files can be handled more easily (image editing, online transmission).
- In many situations, image quality is more than sufficient (routine shots in daily practice, family pictures etc.).
- In the daily routine of a dental practice, there is no time for post-processing the files.
- No technical skill is necessary to extract the maximum image quality, in contrast to shooting RAW files.

3.5.2   TIFF

The TIFF format (TIFF = Tagged Image File Format, file extension .tif) is also a universal image file format, which can be read without problem nearly everywhere. It is used also in the preprint work, where it is a standard for embedding high resolution pixel images in layout documents. The great advantage of TIFF is that it can be opened and saved over and over again without quality loss.

Some image editing programs offer a non-lossy compression method, the LZW (Lempel-Ziv-Welch) procedure.

TIFF should be used if images are undergoing a complex editing procedure, especially when performed in different sessions. Image files which are used for printing purposes should be stored in TIFF as well. If the camera offers a TIFF option, it can be selected if memory volume does not play an important role.

The following table shows different file sizes after compression using different quality levels:

Compression	No	TIFF (LZW)	JPEG (Q12)	JPEG (Q5)	JPEG (Q0)
Size in MB	17.6	9.8	3.8	0.45	0.20
% of original	100	56	21	2.5	1.1

3.4.3   RAW

Professional digital SLR cameras offer the option of storing the image in a TIFF and/or JPEG format and, in addition or alternatively, as a RAW file. Depending on the company, these RAW file extensions are named differently: CRW/CR2 = Canon, NEF = Nikon, RAF = Fuji, MRW = Minolta, ORF = Olympus.

The Sigma SD 10 has a special status, as it is the only digital SLR offering only a RAW file type for internal image storage. It can be expected that future Sigma cameras will offer a TIFF or JPEG option as well, just to satisfy the needs of the camera users.

The RAW format offers unadulterated digital image data, a "digital negative". Such a RAW file can be compared with a latent image contained in an exposed but undeveloped film. The key advantage of shooting RAW files is that the photographer is able to extract the maximum possible image quality afterwards (Fig. 3.21).

To transfer RAW data to the PC and to edit the images, specific software of the individual manufacturer is necessary. Professional image editing software programs such as Photoshop CS can also read, open, and edit RAW files. Updates of these RAW converters are available as new camera models are released.

RAW files are stored uncompressed in the camera, but their volume is significantly smaller than a TIFF file.

Every digital camera shoots in raw mode, but if you select the JPEG format, you let the camera apply the built-in conversion program. Therefore, a good option is saving both RAW and JPEG files simultaneously, which is possible with most cameras. Then you have the advantage of a ready-to-use image for routine applications, and in addition the image data for advanced post processing.

It is recommended to select the option RAW file in the camera menu, if every single image is edited afterwards individually. RAW files are not the option for routine shots in the busy dental practice. RAW is the format of choice if maximum quality images are the goal and if the photographer has the skill to post-process every single image individually. Furthermore, RAW data offer an additional option for the future. Future image editing programs may offer improved post-processing methods, resulting in even better images. Therefore, archiving RAW files is strongly recommended. No photographer in conventional photography would dream of throwing away the slides or negatives in order to keep the prints only.

Fig. 3.21   Function of a RAW converter in principle.

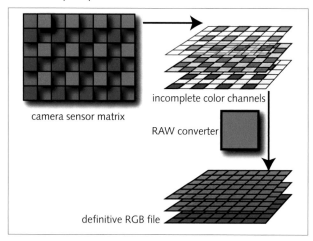

camera sensor matrix

incomplete color channels

RAW converter

definitive RGB file

Reasons to use the RAW file format

- Maximum image quality is possible by post-processing.
- Fine tuning of white balance is possible without image degradation.
- Algorithms of high-end image editing software may be more sophisticated than those used in digital cameras.
- Contrast and saturation can be adapted more individually.
- A 12-bit file offers a broader range of tonal values, which is particularly important, when opening up shadows. Less or no posterization effects will be visible.

BACKGROUND

TIFF

Tagged Image File Format, industry standard, all color depths, non-lossy compression.

Can be read and used nearly everywhere.

Disadvantage: image file volume is rather large.

JPEG

Joint Photographic Expert Group, all color depths, lossy compression. Different quality levels can be preselected (in Photoshop 13 different levels, ranging from 0 to 12).

Excellent for storage of images, less suitable for black and white drawings or image-text combinations.

BMP

The "Bitmap" format was developed by Microsoft for the Windows PC operating system. The format can be read by any Windows-based PC. The other operating systems cannot read BMP files. Therefore, BMP format is not appropriate for professional use.

GIF

The Graphic Interchange Format was developed to display symbols and small drawings with small file sizes. It is mainly used to distribute images over the Internet. As different image parts or images can be stored within one file, which can be displayed in a predetermined sequence, GIF files can be used for small animations. It is not suitable for photographic images, as only 256 colors can be represented. Because data compression is protected by patents, many image editing programs cannot handle compressed GIF data.

PNG

The Portable Network Graphic Format was developed because of the licence problems with GIF. The compression is lossless and results in very small image files. It is a disadvantage that not all editing programs support PNG files. Especially old browsers cannot read this file type.

DNG

The Digital Negative Format was developed by the Adobe company as a universal format for camera RAW data. Adobe offers a free DNG converter, transferring most RAW data of numerous cameras. The intention is to use a public format, which will still be in use years later, making sure that digital photographs can be stored in their original format for future generations.

Format	Color depth	Color mode	Compression	Further data
TIFF (.tif)	any	all	LZW, lossless	alpha channels, paths
JPEG (.jpg)	up to 24 bit	RGB, CMYK, gray levels	lossy	paths
BMP (.bmp)	any	RGB, gray levels, indicated colors	RLE (similar to LZW)	alpha channels
GIF (.gif)	8 bit	indicated colors, gray levels	LZW, lossless	absolute transparence animations
PNG (.png)	8, 24, or 32 Bit	indicated colors, RGB	lossless	at 32 Bit alpha channels

Fig. 3.22 Data transfer can be done by cable or by the storage media.

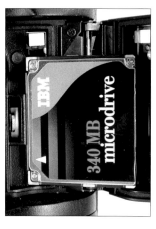

3.6   PC connection – Transferring the images

Aside from special applications, it is more sensible and practical to use the camera as stand-alone and not interfaced via cable with the computer.

At the very latest, when the camera's own storage medium is full, the images have to be downloaded into a computer. There are various means of doing this. Data transfer can be done with or without a cable, or via the camera's own storage medium (Fig. 3.22).

Image transfer via a cable can be performed very fast using a USB 2.0 cable or via the fast IEEE 1394 FireWire interface. The transfer process can be automated so far that it starts after a mouse click in the moment the camera is connected to the PC. In the near future, data transfer using a W-LAN interface may play a more important role than today.

Aside from using a cable, the best method of data transfer is to use the camera's own internal memory cards. Modern personal computers offer integrated card readers where the memory cards can be inserted directly. Another option is to use an external USB card reader or a memory card adapter which can be inserted into the PC card slot of a notebook. Then the memory cards are accessed like a hard drive. This is the fastest way to get the images into the computer and a way which does not misuse the camera as a memory card reader. Special software is not necessary for image transfer.

3.7   Camera set-up

Even if every camera offers different features and has its own set-up modalities, there are some things which most have in common.

There are two main concepts of operating and setting up the camera:
- Adjustments can be done directly using switches and buttons
- Adjustments can be performed over the menu of the camera

The more professional camera models have more buttons and switches for the most important settings, which greatly facilitates handling. You work with buttons in one of two ways: some buttons must be pressed one or several times to switch modes; others must be pressed down while turning a dial.

Normally, all functions that can be reached with the buttons can also be reached over the menu.

Basic set-up of the camera

The following settings usually can be performed using buttons on the camera body.

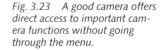

Fig. 3.23   A good camera offers direct access to important camera functions without going through the menu.

Exposure mode: There are different exposure modes which can be selected (Fig. 3.23).

Manual mode ("M"): shutter speed and aperture are set manually.

Aperture priority mode ("A"): the aperture is preset, the shutter speed is set by the camera automatically.

Shutter priority mode ("S"): the shutter is preset, the aperture is set by the camera.

Program mode ("P"): shutter and aperture are set by the camera.

In dental photography, the aperture priority mode ("A") or the manual mode ("M") can be used.

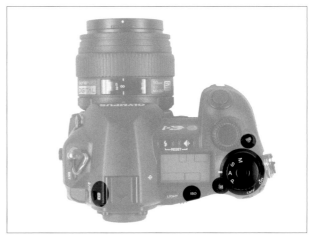

Aperture priority mode

The advantage of this mode is that we can control the critical depth of field by presetting the aperture. This works as long as there is a TTL metered flash, because in flash photography, the camera does not set the shutter speed but the flash duration to control the amount of light falling on the sensor.

Examples of systems which should be used in the "A" mode are: Olympus E-1, Nikon D70s (in combination with Sigma flash EM-140).

Selecting an aperture value is normally done using a wheel on the camera back or top; apertures are not set at the lens as previously in conventional photography.

The "standard" aperture value for dental photography is f/22.

Exposure time (when using a flash it is the synchronization time) is normally set automatically, when flash is turned on.

Manual mode

Another possibility is to preset exposure time (synchronization time) and the aperture.

If the camera system offers the feature of TTL flash metering, the amount of light falling on the sensor is controlled by the TTL metering system (examples: Canon EOS 20D, Digital Rebel XT, Nikon D70s in combination with the Sigma macro flash EM-140). If not, the flash has to be used manually and the correct exposure has to be found by setting the appropriate aperture (example: Nikon D70s in combination with the Nikon SB-29s).

Exposure time (synchronization time, when using a flash) is usually selected by using a wheel on the camera back or top. The time can be between 1/60 and 1/250s, depending on the camera.

ISO-value/light sensitivity

Digital cameras allow preselection of an ISO value for each shot (in conventional photography, you had to put a new roll of film into your camera). Usually the lowest speed is the camera's native ISO speed, which is typically noise free. Setting a higher ISO value does not mean that your camera sensor becomes more sensitive to light; it only means that the output signal of your sensor is amplified a little bit more than before. This also amplifies the noise, which can deteriorate image quality. Therefore, leave the ISO value on the lowest possible value.

Exposure metering characteristics

Good cameras offer different ways to meter exposure: spot metering, center-weighted metering, and matrix metering. For dental photography, center-weighted or matrix metering are the best.

Exposure compensation

Even highly sophisticated cameras do not "know" which type of object you are aiming at with your camera, whether it is a very bright object, or very dark, or has a medium gray level. In dentistry, we often have an image with white teeth in it. Therefore it can be recommended to put the exposure compensation to +2/3 stops. This exposure compensation only makes sense if you are not working in the manual mode.

Autofocus

It should be switched off, in order not to waste depth of field. There is a button at the camera and at the lens, which has to be set to manual focusing mode.

White balance

Our brain has the capacity to adapt to color temperatures. A white sheet of paper is white in our perception, no matter which color temperature the illumination has (at least after a couple of seconds). A digital camera records the color temperature of the illumination as it is. Daylight appears neutral, tungsten lighting has a more or less strong tendency to yellow-red, halogen bulbs give a somewhat greenish lighting.

One of the big advantages of digital cameras is that we can adapt them to the lighting in terms of color temperature. There is usually an automatic white balance function which determines color temperature after pressing the shutter release button and sets the white balance according to the result.

In dental photography, we usually work with electronic flash lighting. To obtain repeatable results, we should preset white balance to "flash photography" (flash symbol). This will give constant results for color reproduction.

In addition, good DSLRs offer the possibility of "fine tuning" the setting in small steps to improve color reproduction. The procedure of fine tuning differs from model to model. A very easy method is offered for the EOS 20D by Canon. In the camera menu, the feature "White Balance Correction" is selected. A color matrix is displayed on the LCD representing the basic colors. Within this matrix, a cursor can be moved towards the desired color using a tiny joystick on the camera back.

Settings using the camera menu

Although there are differences from one camera model to the next, the following items can usually be set using the menu (Fig. 3.24).

Language: must be set to your native language.

Acoustic signals/beep: may be helpful for the beginner, but after a short time they are disturbing and should be switched off.

TV mode: Every digital camera can be connected to a TV monitor. The setting depends on the country where you live. PAL is the right setting for Europe, NTSC for the United States.

Memory card: It is recommended to format the memory card in the camera before it is used for the first time. Then you are certain to get the maximum storage capacity. Formatting the cards should be done in the camera, not on the computer. Otherwise, there is a risk that the card will be unreadable in the camera.

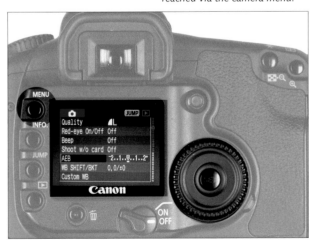

Fig. 3.24   Functions which have to be changed rarely can be reached via the camera menu.

Resolution/quality/image size: Normally, the maximum optical resolution (without interpolation) should be selected, as it is always possible to reduce but not enlarge the image.

Data file format: There are different file formats which can be selected. Some professional cameras allow the storage of two different formats at a time. RAW format should be selected if the picture is converted manually afterwards and the intention is to obtain the highest quality possible. JPEG format is recommended for routine operations. A JPEG setting is recommended with highest quality (meaning lowest compression). TIFF format can be recommended, if storage space is not important. For special purposes, two formats at a time can be selected, e.g., RAW plus JPEG.

Image sharpening: Most cameras allow preselecting a degree of sharpening the image. It is usually preferable to do this with image editing software. Therefore, leave this function at zero.

Contrast: The same is true for image contrast.

Color saturation: Neither should color saturation be enhanced by the camera.

Color space: Professional cameras allow the preselection of different color spaces, in most cases Adobe RGB and sRGB. The choice depends on the purpose of the images. The sRGB space is better for displaying the images on monitors. The Adobe RGB is the larger color space. By recording images in the Adobe RGB color space, the greatest range of colors possible is recorded. Therefore, it should be preferred in most cases. For dental photography, it is not critical which space is selected, because the main colors—which are important here—are represented in both spaces.

Review time: Cameras allow a short review of the image after it is taken. A review time between 8 and 10 s is appropriate for most cases.

Histogram/Superimposed display: Many cameras offer the option of displaying a histogram superimposed on the review image after every shot. Cameras should be set for a 10-second review. With the histogram, exposure can be checked perfectly (see also Chapter 7.4.3): leave ON.

Auto rotate: Advanced cameras "know" which camera position—landscape or portrait—was used. They rotate the image automatically, if necessary. A helpful and time saving feature to leave ON.

Auto power off: To save batteries, the time after which a camera is switched off automatically can be selected within a wide range. Two to 5 minutes are appropriate.

File numbering: Image files are numbered automatically. A "continuous mode" should be selected. Otherwise the camera starts again with "1" after each session, with the result that there may be many image files with the same file name.

Noise reduction: Not important in our context: turn OFF.

ISO expansion: only important in special situations (e.g., available light photography): OFF.

Mirror lockup: only for macro photography using a tripod to prevent camera shake. For clinical photography: OFF.

Shutter curtain synchronization: The flash can be synchronized with the first or the second shutter curtain. For clinical photography: 1st curtain.

4

Camera systems suitable for dental photography

The market has been flooded with digital cameras for years. Today, more than 1100 different cameras are on the market, most of them digital. Hence, it is not possible to present a complete and up-to-date survey of the market in a book, as the technical development cycles of these products are extremely short, and there is a delay between finishing the manuscript and publishing the book. With this in mind and without striving for completeness, I will concentrate on cameras which can be used effectively for dental photography.

Digital cameras can be divided into three groups: amateur, semiprofessional, and professional. Obviously, in dental photography, only semiprofessional and professional cameras should be used.

4.1   Semiprofessional cameras

Semiprofessional cameras include advanced viewfinder cameras and single lens reflex (SLR) cameras without interchangeable lenses. There are some disadvantages and limitations when these cameras are used for dental photography. In most cases, the flash position is not ideal for cavity photography, as the distance between the flash and the front lens is too great. Some cameras offer a "macro" function that is not sufficient or that is only available in the wide-angle position of the zoom lens. The wide-angle position necessitates a short working distance, which results in distorted images. To use these cameras for dental photography, modifications of the lighting system were developed, often in combination with a macro lens. I have outlined some examples of semiprofessional cameras.

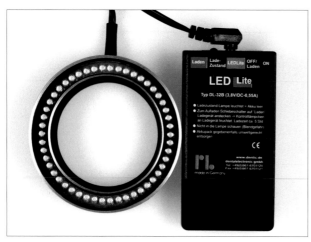

Fig. 4.1 The LEDLite system was the first lighting system on the market using LED technology.

LED RingLite®
(Dentalelectronic GmbH, Weiden, Germany)

The LED RingLite is a lighting system that uses light-emitting diodes (LEDs) on a ring, which is mounted on the camera in combination with a macro lens (Fig. 4.1). It is available for a variety of digital camera systems. An advantage of such ring light systems is that they provide a bright viewing field for framing, as the LEDs are a constant light source. Disadvantages are that the light output is only moderate and the aperture cannot be closed completely; therefore, the depth of field is limited. Some systems show a "light hole" in the center of the picture if the working distance is too short. The color temperature is "white", but does not correspond exactly with daylight.

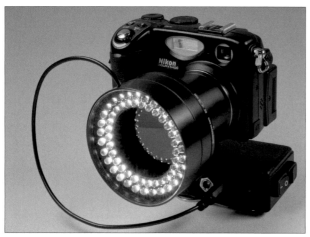

Fig. 4.2 The Doctorseye system offers a broad variety of LED lighting equipment.

Doctorseyes Lighting System (www.doctorseyes.com)

Another LED-based lighting system is the so-called Doctorseyes system. For a variety of digital cameras, there are LED ring lights with different numbers of single LEDs. The power supply is provided by a rechargeable battery, mounted under the cameras (Fig. 4.2).

In addition to the ring light, a macro lens and an adapter are necessary, depending on the camera model. Various intraoral photographic mirrors can also be mounted under the LED ring.

The doctorseyes lighting system is rather bright. Its color temperature is about 7000 K.

The mains adapter can be used to recharge the batteries and as a 220 V plug.

The advanced rechargeable battery is not only bigger and has a higher capacity, but it offers a two-step switch as well, allowing two different brightness levels. Newer developments allow side lighting, giving the images more plasticity.

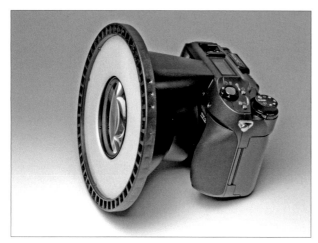

Fig. 4.3
The MedicalD system uses the built-in flash for illumination.

Medical-D System
(DentalPrestige SA, Yverdon, Switzerland)

Medical-D is a modified Olympus Camedia 7070 with a flash diffusor and macro lens. It is simple to use and provides even and soft illumination. A distance guide helps to find the proper working distance of 12 cm. The magnification ratio can be adjusted using the camera's zoom lever (Fig. 4.3).

Kodak DX7590 Dental Digital Camera Kit (Kodak Company)

The Kodak DX 7590 is a five-megapixel viewfinder camera combined with a macro lens and an integrated ringflash. A detachable distance guide helps one find the right working distance for the different magnification ratios. The camera is simple to use. A docking station allows image transfer to the personal computer. A "dental positioning grid" is placed on the LCD screen to facilitate aligning.

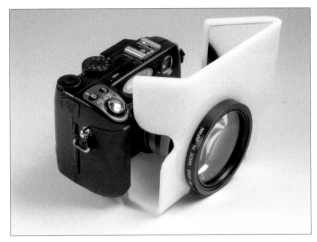

Fig. 4.4
Flash diffuser from PTJ International with the Nikon Coolpix 5400.

PTJ® Diffusor Systems (PTJ International France; PhotoMed International, Van Nuys, CA, USA)

The French company PTJ International offers diffusor systems that are combined with macro lenses for different cameras. These diffusors overcome the problem of a "wrong" flash position when used for dental photography. These diffusors can be the right solution if you already have a camera and want to use this camera in the dental office without spending much more money (Figs 4.4 and 4.5)

The PTJ homepage gives up-to-date information on which camera can be combined with such a diffuser system (www.photo-dentaire.com).

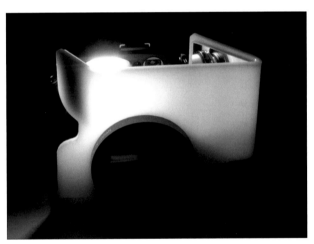

Fig. 4.5   Flash diffuser from PTJ gives a broad and soft illumination.

Minolta Dimage® 7, 7i Hi, A1, A2

The Minolta Dimage 7i and the following camera models are advanced 5- to 8-MPixel digital cameras without interchangeable lenses. The interesting feature for dental purposes is that the Minolta macro flash can be combined with the Dimage camera. Alternatively, a PTJ Diffusor can be used.

If magnification is not sufficient, a close-up lens can be attached to the camera.

The latest models feature an anti-shake system. Studio flash equipment can be connected to the camera (Fig. 4.6).

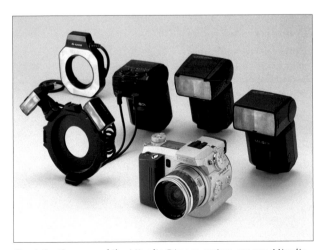

Fig. 4.6   Cameras of the Minolta Dimage system can use Minolta macro flashes.

Limitations of semiprofessional cameras

Although many dentists may be satisfied with the results obtained with these cameras, there are, of course, limitations. The most important is that these cameras do not allow perfect image control, since in most cases, the liquid crystal display (LCD) screen has to be used as a viewfinder. As a result, there is no control over the position of the focusing plane and, therefore, the depth of field. Very often, one has to rely on the autofocus function.

Some cameras have a rather long lag time, which makes focusing difficult when working in the close-up range without stabilizing the camera with a tripod. The lighting of these systems is not variable and cannot be adapted to the situation. A major disadvantage is that not all cameras of this group allow manual exposure and flash mode.

Important features a semiprofessional camera should offer are an external flash shoe, short lag time, screw mount for a close-up lens, manual exposure mode, and proper magnification ratio even in the telephoto position of the zoom lens.

A simple way to optimize a semiprofessional camera is by painting grid lines on the LCD screen. This helps to align the camera according to the anatomic axes and planes of the patient (Fig. 2.7). In order to protect the LCD surface before painting on the lines, you can cover the surface with a self-adhering vinyl-protector material (Kaiser Fototechnik, Buchen, Germany; Kinetronics Company, Sarasota, USA).

There is no doubt in the professional world that these cameras are always a "second choice" for professional routine use in dentistry, although it is possible to achieve good results. If predictable professional results are the aim, digital SLR cameras should be used, although they are more bulky, more expensive, and probably seem to be more complicated at the beginning. After a short time, even an inexperienced user will see that daily work with these cameras is not as complicated as it first appeared.

If a user of a conventional SLR camera switches over to the digital world, the purchase of a digital SLR camera is strongly recommended. Otherwise, he or she will not be happy with the results or the photographic procedure.

4.2   Professional digital cameras

Digital SLR cameras with interchangeable lenses belong to this group. These are rec-ommended if professional results are expected, if perfect image control is essential, and if a user of a conventional SLR camera begins to work with digital photography. These digital SLR cameras are mainly based on conventional bodies, which means that interchangeable lenses and flash equipment of the same brand can be used for digital photography as well.

As prices are dropping constantly and have nearly reached the price level of ad-vanced viewfinder cameras, digital SLR cameras are the first choice for professional photographic documentation.

4.2.1   Nikon based digital SLR cameras

Nikon D50

The Nikon D50 is a 6.2 MPixel camera based on the N80 body. It is the cheapest digital SLR from Nikon. It pro-vides good color rendition, especially neutral skin tones, and connects to a personal computer by means of a USB cable (Fig. 4.7). The camera has a sensor of 23.7 x 15.6 mm (crop factor 1.5) and an SD Memory Card as storage medium.

Unlike the D70 s, grid lines cannot be activated elec-tronically.

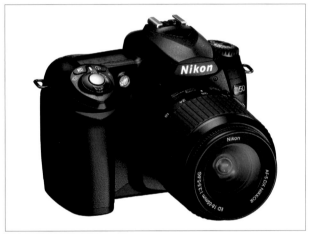

Fig. 4.7   Nikon D50 as an example of a low cost DSLR camera.

System components

Lens: 105 mm AF Micro-Nikkor/60 mm AF Micro-Nikkor. Alternatively: SIGMA Makro 105 mm F 2.8 EX DG or other Nikon compatible macro lenses from other man-ufacturers.

Flash: Nikon SB-29 s

Flash must be used in manual mode, as it currently does not provide iTTL flash metering. As an alternative, the new Sigma macro flash EM 140 DG can be used with iTTL metering. Other alternatives: Novoflex ring flash or twin flash (manual mode).

Camera settings (with SB-29s)

- Exposure mode: M
- Shutter speed: 1/125 s
- Aperture: depends on magnification ratio, a reasonable starting point is f32, when SB-29s is set to M/4. Display control of the image is recommended.
- Lens: lens is bolted, aperture is set on the camera
- SB-29s Flash: manual mode ¼ light output (M1/4)

Camera settings (with Sigma EM 140 DG)

- Exposure mode: A
- Shutter speed: 1/125 s
- Aperture: f22
- Lens: lens is bolted, aperture is set on the camera
- Sigma flash EM 140 DG: TTL

Nikon D70 (s)

Highly rated digital 6.1-MPixel SLR camera made by Nikon. It offers the Nikon F mount and therefore is compatible with most Nikkor lenses (Fig. 4.8).

Microdrive or Compact flash card as storage media.

System components

- Body: Nikon D70(s)
- Lens: 105 mm AF Micro-Nikkor 1:2.8 D. Lens is locked, aperture is set on the camera. This lens is preferred if a long working distance is necessary, e.g., when using a twin flash.

  An alternative is the Nikon AF Micro Nikkor 60 mm 1:2.8 D. Taking the crop factor into account, an effective focal length of about 90 mm results.

  The following table compares the working distances for both lenses for different magnification ratios. Magnification ratio refers to 35-mm film format, where a 1:1 full frame includes 36 mm , a ratio of 1:1.2 includes about 43 mm, and a magnification ratio of 1:2 includes 72 mm.

  Alternatively: SIGMA Makro 105 mm F 2.8 EX DG or other Nikon-compatible macro lenses from other manufacturers.

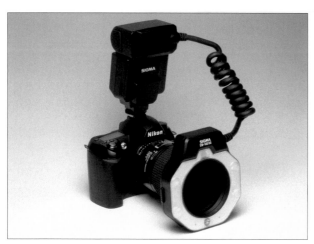

Fig. 4.8   Nikon D70 and D70s are high-end DSLR in a price range for amateurs.

MR	60 mm	105 mm
1:1	10.5	18.5
1:1.2	12	21.2
1:2	19	33.6

- Flash: R1 Wireless Close-Up Speedlight System (see below, Nikon D200) Nikon SB-29 s (Fig. 4.9). Flash must be used in manual mode, as the combination D70-SB-29s does not allow iTTL flash metering. As an alternative, the new Sigma macro flash EM 140 DG can be used, which offers iTTL metering and is compatible with D 70s.

  Other alternatives: Novoflex ring flash or twin flash (manual mode).

Camera settings

1. Nikon D70 (s) used with Nikon SB-29s

There are two possibilities to attach the SB-29s to the AF Micro Nikkor 105 mm lens: the 52 mm adapter ring can be fixed at the screw mount near the front lens or the 62 mm adapter ring can be fixed at the rear screw mount of the fixed part of the lens. The second possibility is recommended as the distance between flash and patient or object is a little bit larger, thus facilitating close-ups, especially important when shooting lateral mirror views of the premolars and molars. A third position of the flash is possible by attaching it to the power unit on top of the camera.

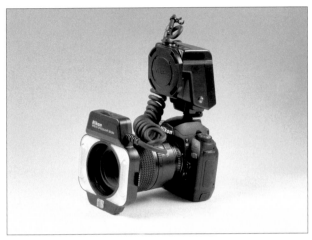

Fig. 4.9   Nikon D70 in combination with Nikon macro flash SB-29s.

As the D70 (s) is very light sensitive (ISO 200), the light output of the flash has to be reduced to M1/4 or M1/32. The following table gives information about the aperture to be set depending on the magnification ratio (MR) and light output reduction. The aperture indicated in the top camera window is the so-called effective aperture, which depends also on the magnification ratio. The SB-29s is attached in the rear position. The camera is in the manual mode (M), exposure time is 1/125.

Magnification ratio	Aperture for M1/4	Aperture for M1/32
1:2	f/29	f/13
1:1	f/40	f/18
1,56:1 (maximum lens extension)	f/57	f/25

The aperture values must be regarded as starting points. A display check of the image and the histogram is recommended after each single shot. The table above shows that aperture setting and light output reduction also depend on the object to be photographed.

If a photo of the whole dentition has to be taken, a large depth of field is necessary which extends from the central incisors to the second molars. In this case, flash light must be reduced to M1/4 in order to use the aperture f/29, which allows sufficient depth of field. Depth of field is not such a problem if only the front teeth need to be photographed, since they are more or less line up in the same plane. In this case, light output can be reduced to M1/32, in order to be able to use the aperture f/18. When depth of field is not an issue, image quality with f/18 is better than the quality of f/40 shots, because diffraction has an influence on image quality.

For those who do not want to keep both variables in mind (aperture setting and light output reduction), the M1/4 reduction is recommended.

2. Nikon D70 (s) used with Sigma EM 140 DG (Nikon)

Flash is set to TTL BL by pressing the MODE button below the flash display. When the camera is switched on, "d" appears on the flash LCD.

Two exposure modes can be used: M and A.

MANUAL mode ("M"):

- Exposure time is set to 1/125 s.
- Aperture is set to f/29.
- Exposure is controlled by the flash light output within a wide range of aperture settings.

APERTURE PRIORITY Mode ("A"):

- Exposure time is set automatically to 1/60 s, when flash is switched on.
- Aperture is set to f/22.
- Exposure is controlled by the flash light output within a wide range of aperture settings.

3. Nikon D70 (s) with Nikon R1 Close-up Speedlight System: see below: Nikon D200

Special features: viewfinder with grid lines can be switched on electronically via the camera menu (individual function 08).

Nikon D200

Advanced DSLR camera with a 10.2 MP CCD sensor (23,6 x 15,8 mm) with 3,872 x 2,592 pixels. Crop factor 1.5 (Fig. 4.10).

Lightweight magnesium alloy body, large LCD monitor. Light sensitivity from ISO 100 to 1600. Grid-screen can be switched on electronically.

System components
See D70 (s)

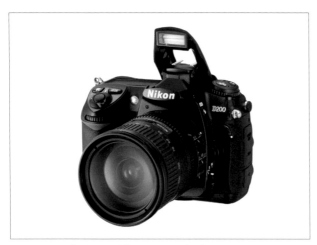

Fig. 4.10   Nikon D200 (Illustration: Nikon).

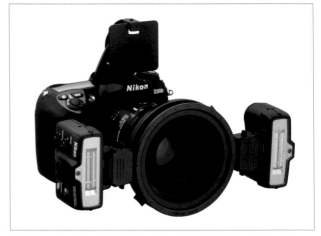

Fig. 4.11   Nikon D200 with the new macroflash (Illustration: Nikon).

R1 Wireless Close-Up Speedlight System

For dental photography the R1 Wireless Close-Up Speeedlight System is very interesting, which came with the Nikon D200 (Fig. 4.11).

This macro flash system works with Nikon i-TTL SLRs with built-in Speedlights
with Commander mode including D200, D70S and D70. The built-in flash of these
cameras serves as system's Master controller. Two or more SB-R200 Speedlights can
be used. Up to four of them can be attached to the SX-1 Master Attachment Ring.
If the ring is taken off the camera, up to eight Speedlights can be used.

Flash compensation or ratio control for special lighting effects is possible. The SB-
800 and/or SB-600 Speedlights can be combined and controlled for additional creative lighting effects or for object or portrait photography.

The system includes not only different adapter rings, but also color filters, Speedlight stands, and extreme close-up adapters.

Fuji FinePix S3 Pro (Fujifilm Company)

The Fujifilm FinePix S3 Prof is based on the N80 Nikon body. Compared with the
D70(s), the S3 offers a higher resolution (Super CCD SR II sensor) and a faster cable
connection (Firewire) with the PC.

System components

- Lens: 105 mm AF Micro-Nikkor.
- Alternatives: SIGMA Makro 105 mm F 2,8 EX DG or other Nikon-compatible
  macro lenses from other manufacturers.
- Flash: Nikon SB-29 s.
  Flash cannot be used in TTL mode. Only in M mode.
  Alternatively, the new Sigma macro flash EM 140 DG can be used.
- Other alternatives: Novoflex ring flash or twin flash (manual mode).

Camera settings

- Exposure mode: M; Shutter speed: 1/125 s.
- Aperture: f32, depending on the magnification ratio.
- Lens: lens is locked, aperture is set on the camera.
- Flash settings: M1/4.
- Special features: Viewfinder with grid lines can be switched on electronically.

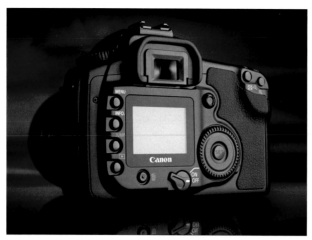

Fig. 4.12   *The Canon EOS 20D is a high-end DSLR camera (Illustration: Canon).*

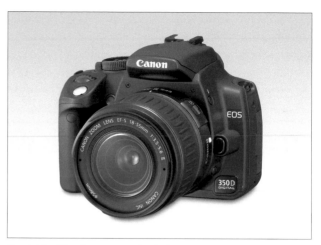

Fig. 4.13   *The Canon Digital Rebel XT (in Europe 350D) nearly has the same functionality as the EOS 20D. (Illustration: Canon).*

4.2.2   Canon-based digital SLR cameras

Canon EOS 20D

The Canon EOS 20D is an advanced 8.3-MPixel camera with a CMOS sensor. For dental photography a ring flash and a twin flash with eTTL II metering can be used. USB 2.0 connection to the PC. Solid but light magnesium alloy body. (Fig. 4.12).

The Canon EOS 20D is a digital SLR with many interesting features. The only disadvantage is that there is no interchangeable grid screen available, nor a grid screen which can be switched on via the camera menu. A cheaper alternative is the Canon EOS Digital Rebel XT.

Canon Digital Rebel XT

Digital SLR camera, similar to EOS 20D, but with a cheaper amateur body (Fig. 4.13). Contains 8-MPixel CMOS sensor. Sensor dimensions 22.2 x 14.8 mm, crop factor 1.6x. USB 2.0 cable connection. Compatible with more than 50 Canon lenses. E-TTL II flash metering system.

System components for EOS 20D and Digital Rebel XT
- Body: EOS 20 D or Digital Rebel XT
- Lens: Canon EF 100/2.8 USM Makro. Aperture ring on the lens is locked. This lens is preferred if a long working distance is necessary, e.g., when using the twin flash. An alternative is the Canon Macro lens EF-S 60 mm f/2.8 USM. Taking the crop factor into account, an effective focal length of 90 mm results.

MR	60 mm	100 mm
1:1	12.5	20.2
1:1.2	14.3	23.7
1:2	22.5	36.5

The table compares the working distances for both lenses for different magnification ratios. Magnification ratio refers to 35-mm film format, where a 1:1 full frame includes 36 mm, a ratio of 1:1.2 includes about 43 mm, and a magnification ratio of 1:2 includes 72 mm.

The EF-S 60mm lens can only be used with cameras containing a "non-full-frame" sensor. In cameras with full-frames sensors the lens interferes with the mirror.

- Alternatively, the SIGMA Makro 105mm F 2.8 EX DG can be used or other Canon-compatible macro lenses from other manufacturers.
- Flash: Canon Macro Ring Lite MR-14EX and/or Macro Twin Lite MT-24EX. Both are eTTL II metered. The more powerful twin flash has a cooler light; images tend to be a little bit more bluish, which can be compensated. As an alternative, the Sigma flash EM 140 DG can be used (Canon compatible). Further flash systems: Novoflex ring flash or twin flash.

Settings for EOS 20D and Digital Rebel XT with Canon flash lights
There are two possibilities for dental photography: Manual (M) mode and Av mode.

Manual (M) mode (recommended)
- Exposure mode: M.
- Shutter speed: 1/125–1/200s.
- Aperture: f22 (has to be set on the camera using the wheel on the camera back). Other aperture settings are possible within a wide range, depending on the depth of field necessary.
- Flash: eTTL II mode is selected.
- The amount of light reaching the camera sensor is controlled by the eTTL II-metered flash.

Av mode (aperture priority mode)
- Alternatively, the camera (only Canon 20D) can be set to "Av" instead of M. In this case, the flash sync speed has to be fixed to 1/200s, which can be done in the menu (custom function 03).
- Aperture: f/22. Other aperture settings are possible within a wide range, depending on the depth of field necessary.
- Flash: eTTL II mode.

EOS 5D
At the moment the smallest and cheapest full-frame DSLR camera on the market. Due to the relatively "moderate" price, the camera is mentioned in this context.

EF lenses can be used without taking a conversion factor into account. 12.8 Megapixel CMOS sensor (4,368×2,912 pixels). Light magnesium-alloy body.

Due to the full-frame sensor the 60mm macro lens cannot be used. The first reason is that the focal length is too short (no conversion factor). The second reason is that the lens would interfere with the bigger mirror, probably causing damage.

The 100mm macro lens is the lens of choice (see above). The camera features the Canon E-TTL II flash metering system.

The Canon Data Verification DVK-E2 is an option for the EOS 5D (and EOS 20D). Like its predecessor, this kit can verify whether or not a photo is an untouched original.

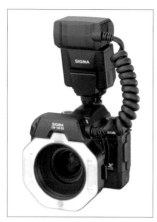

Fig. 4.14   The Sigma SD10 with macro flash. This flash is also available for Nikon, Canon and Minolta cameras.

4.2.3   Sigma SD10

Based on the conventional Sigma SA-9 body, the Sigma SD10 contains a Foveon X3 sensor with 3.5 MPixel resolution (Fig. 4.14). Since every photodiode receives the whole color information, the Sigma company talks about "10.2 Million color sensors" (2268 × 1512 × 3). The X3 image data file has a size of about 6 MB. After conversion into a TIFF file, the TIFF data file has more than 19 MB. If the software option "double size" is used, the file size has more than 78 MB.

Unlike other cameras, the SD 10 only generates RAW data files. These files must be transferred to the computer using the Sigma software and then can be transformed to TIFF or JPEG files using the very useful conversion software. At first sight this seems to be a little bit complicated, but the idea behind it is to avoid destroying the advantages of the X3 sensor results by using a "lossy" file format like JPEG, and to be able to convert the images individually. The Sigma software allows individual correction of sharpness, color, saturation, brightness etc. in three modes. The X3F mode stores the original settings of the image at point of capture. In the auto adjustment mode, the software analyzes and automatically makes adjustments of RAW data. The custom mode allows the photographer to make individual adjustments to exposure, contrast, shadow, highlight, sharpness, and saturation.

Changes made by the software can be attached to the RAW data file. This enables the user to cancel all changes at a later date.

A special highlight of the conversion software is the "fill light" function, which improves image quality by adding extra light to shadow regions, without changing highlight details. A similar function is part of the Photoshop CS version (Shadow/ Highlight Filter). A special feature of the camera is the dust protector. Most digital SLR cameras are typically vulnerable to dust entering the body, especially when the lens is dismounted for changing. Dust and dirt entering through the lens mount of a digital camera can create serious defects in image quality. The dust protector of the SIGMA SD10 prevents dust from entering and adhering to the image sensor.

The Electronic Flash Macro EM-140 DG is a multifunctional flash that controls the light with latest TTL exposure systems. It is fully dedicated with new TTL flash control systems of all popular camera manufacturers: Sigma STTL, Canon sTTL, Nikon iTTL, Minolta ADI, Pentax pTTL. Dual flash tubes can fire simultaneously or separately. Guide number is 14 (ISO 100). Seven power levels from 1/1 to 1/64 can be preselected.

System components

- Body: Sigma SD10.
- Lens: SIGMA Macro lens 105 mm F2.8 EX DG (recommended).
  Alternatively, the 50 mm F2.8 EX DG macro can be used. Due to the crop factor, results in an acceptable focal length.
- Flash: Sigma Macro flash EM 140 DG (Sigma STTL).

Settings

Camera settings

- Exposure mode: A.
- Shutter speed: 1/125 s.
- Aperture: f22.

Flash: TTL

If other flashes are used, camera must be set to the Manual mode: "M".

Lens: aperture ring is blocked.

4.2.4   Pentax *ist D

Compact digital SLR camera system with a 23.5 x 15.7 mm CCD sensor (3008 x 2008 pixels). The camera is compatible with existing Pentax 35-mm format lenses and accessories. Although very light, the camera is extremely rigid, as it has a stainless steel body. It offers all the functions an advanced SLR should have today.

Recommended equipment for dental photography:
- SMC P-FA 100 mm F2.8 Macro, AF-140 C Ring Flash.

4.2.5   Olympus E-1/E-500

The 4/3 system was created by Olympus and Kodak as an open system. The Olympus E-1 camera is the first digital SLR camera with interchangeable lenses developed particularly for digital photography. An especially designed sensor (5 MPixel, 18 x 13.5 mm) and lenses promise high quality images, overcoming the limitations of conventional lenses used in digital SLR cameras (Figs 4.15, 4.16). A ring and a twin flash (both TTL metered) are available. A cheaper alternative is the E-500 body, containing a sensor with 8 MPixels.

The diameter of the lens mount is designed to be approximately twice as large as that of the image circle. This gives higher flexibility of lens and sensor design. Thanks to this lens mount design and the telecentric design of the lenses, most light can strike the image sensor from nearly straight ahead, ensuring clear colors and sharp details even at the periphery of the images.

The 4/3 system is a very interesting development. For dental photography, the only drawback is the short working distance, posing problems if the twin flash is used. Due to the short working distance, pictures have a high plasticity.

System components
- Body: Olympus E-1, E-500.
- Lens: ED 50 mm, f2 macro. Due to the sensor size, a crop factor of 2 results, thus giving an effective focal length of 100 mm.

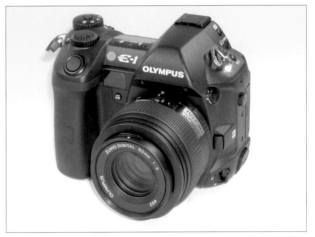

Fig. 4.15   The Olympus E-1 is a professional camera of the newly created 4:3 system.

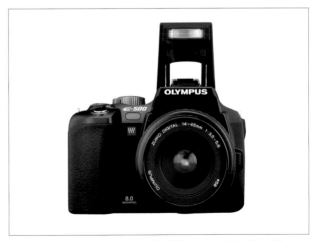

Fig. 4.16   The Olympus E-500, the little sister of the E-1 with higher sensor resolution.

If the twin flash FS-STF22 is used, the additional use of the EC-14 teleconverter is recommended to enlarge working distance, as the distance of the two flash reflectors is rather large.

There are no lenses from other manufacturers available at the moment.

- Flash: Ring Flash FS-SRF11 and/or Twin Flash FS-STF22. For both, the Macro-Flash Controller FS-FC1 is necessary. Both flashes offer TTL-metering.

Settings
Body
- Exposure mode: aperture priority mode ("A").
- Shutter speed: 1/125 s.
- Aperture: f 22 (set on the body).
Flash: TTL mode.
Special features:
- Interchangeable viewfinder screen with net grid is recommended (FS-2; only for E-1).
- Angle viewfinder is recommended for special purposes (e.g., copy work).

4.2.6   Konica – Minolta system

After the fusion with Konica, Minolta is back with a real digital SLR camera, compatible with lenses designed for the Minolta lens mount (Fig. 4.17).

System components
- Body: Dynax 7D, 5D.
- Lens: AF-Macro 2.8/100 mm. Alternatively: SIGMA Macro 105 mm F2.8 EX DG or Minolta compatible macro lenses from other manufacturers.
- Flash: Macro ringflash R-1200 and/or Macro Twinflash 2400. As an alternative, the new Sigma ringflash EM 140 DG can be used (ADI TTL-flash, compatible with Minolta).

Fig. 4.17   The Minolta 7D, the first Minolta SLR camera with interchangeable lenses.

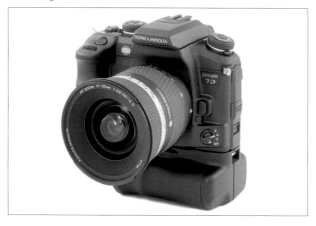

Settings
Body:
- Exposure mode: aperture priority ("A").
- Shutter speed: 1/125 s.
- Aperture: f 22.

Lens: aperture ring is blocked.
Flash: R-1200 or twin flash 2400 in TTL-mode.
Special features: An anti-shake device is integrated in the camera body. For dental photography, this is not very important, as flash is always used.

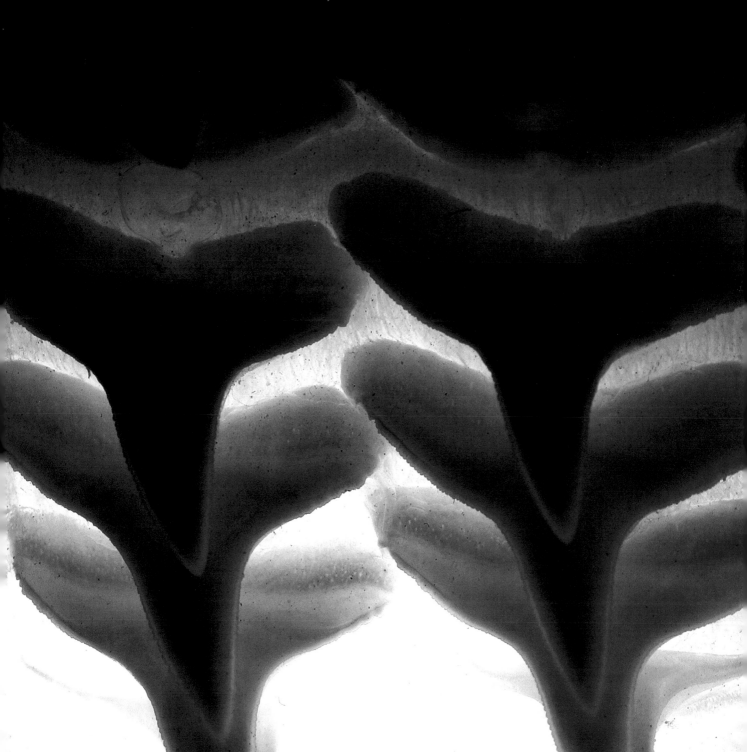

Perioral and intraoral photography

5

The chief focus of dental photography is, of course, the mouth and the perioral region. Its purpose is to document the status and changes in the teeth, mucous membranes of the mouth, and the perioral region under conditions which can be reproduced. The main problems are the inaccessibility of oral structures, lighting within the mouth, framing the image, and achieving conditions which can be reproduced.

The reproduction ratio required for this type of work is between 1:3 (perioral region) and 2:1 (central maxillary incisors filling the frame, individual molar).

The following points are of interest:
- Aids to intraoral photography.
- Visualization.
- Standard views.
- Photography of segmental views of teeth.

5.1   Accessories for intraoral photography

In addition to the camera equipment, a number of aids for intraoral photography are necessary. They enable subjects which are hidden behind lips, cheeks or the tongue, or which are not accessible for a direct view due to their position, to be made visible and photographed.

5.1.1   Lip and cheek retractors

Good intraoral images are not possible without the use of lip retractors. Opening the oral cavity with the use of retractors is not only necessary in order to access the zone to be photographed, but also to achieve optimum illumination.

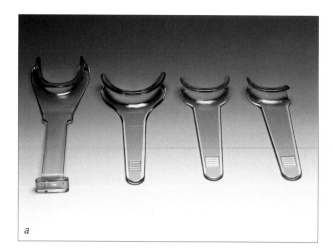

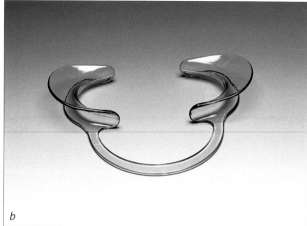

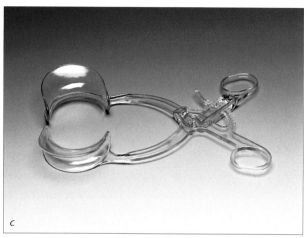

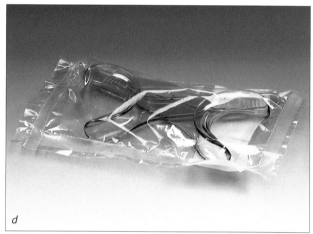

Fig. 5.1   Retractors are available in many forms and made of different materials. The most useful are individual retractors made of plastic. It is sensible to modify individual lip and cheek holders by trimming one of the curved ends (a) right retractor. (b) and (c) are self-expanding retractors which are used if not enough assistants are available to help. Plastic retractors can be chemically sterilized and prepacked hygienically (d).

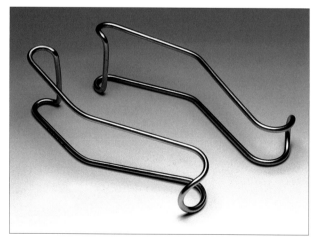

Fig. 5.2
Metal retractors can be easily sterilized in an autoclave.

The most commonly used lip holders are those made of clear plastic; these are available in a variety of sizes (Fig. 5.1). They are the most comfortable for the patient and, if photographed, do not interfere with the image, since they allow the underlying structures to shine through. They also have the advantage that their size and shape can be altered.

It is recommended that one or two pairs be modified by separating a handle or cutting off one end. This allows mirror photography to be done more easily. Retractors made of wire are also in use, which have a larger or smaller bend at either end (Fig. 5.2). The disadvantage here is that the center of the lips is not held and that the highly polished metal can cause reflections.

Making the surface more matte (blasted with aluminum oxide) can reduce the amount of reflections. Such wire retractors are recommended for photography with a long buccal mirror since the mirror can be inserted more easily between the upper and lower bends of the wire than when using plastic lip holders. Self-expanding wire retractors are also in use and available in a variety of sizes.

Lip retractors made of metal (not wire) are not recommended, since the reflections from them cannot be controlled and spoil the image. They can also cause incorrect exposures when using TTL flash, because the flash sensor can be "fooled" by the strong reflections. These metal retractors are also difficult to modify.

Lip holders are generally used in pairs. As a rule, the largest lip holder possible should be used to open the mouth as wide as possible. The size depends not only on the size of the oral cavity, but also on the tone of the lips. Creme should be applied to dry and cracked lips beforehand to avoid lesions. The lip holder is moistened, inserted over the lower lip and carefully turned into the corner of the mouth. In so doing, no pressure should be exerted on the gingiva. See Chapter 5.3 and 5.4 for handling of lip retractors in various photographic situations.

5.1.2 Dental photo mirrors

Intraoral mirrors permit the indirect photography of areas of the mouth which are not directly accessible and, if correctly placed, alleviate the problem of depth of field (Fig. 5.3 a,b).

There are two types of photographic mirrors. Metal mirrors are less expensive, robust, and can easily be sterilized in an autoclave. Optically, they are inferior to glass mirrors, especially on the edges. Metal-film plated glass mirrors are more fragile and expensive, but yield far more brilliant mirror images and are therefore to be preferred (Figs 5.4 to 5.7). A set of coated mirrors is commercially available, consisting of two palatal mirrors in varying sizes and a buccal mirror (Manufacturer: Evaporated Metal Films Corp.; PTJ International France). This set permits overall views of the maxilla and mandible and buccal and oral partial views. This type of

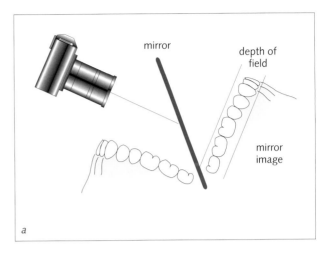

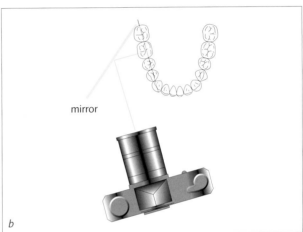

Fig. 5.3   *The use of photo mirrors alleviates the problem of depth of field and makes areas of the mouth accessible which are not directly visible (a). Thus, a vertical view of the posterior teeth is possible (b).*

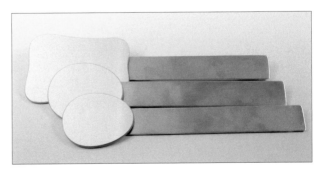

Fig. 5.4
Different types of handle mirrors from PTJ International France.

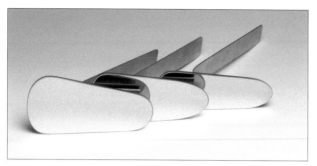

Fig. 5.5   Surface coated lateral glass mirror from PTJ International France with a stainless handle, which works as a retractor.

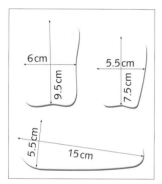

Fig. 5.6   Set of photo mirrors of plated glass, consisting of a buccal mirror and two different size occlusal mirrors.

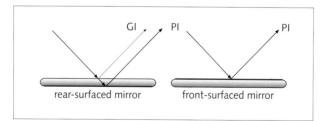

Fig. 5.7   Glass mirrors with glued-on handles (Filtrop company) can facilitate intraoral photography in many cases.

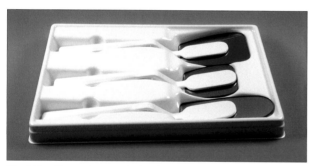

Fig. 5.8   Rear-surfaced mirrors provide a primary image (PI) from the back reflective surface, but also a secondary image from reflection off the front glass surface ("ghost image" = GI). Such mirrors are inexpensive, but not suitable for our purposes.

intraoral mirror is available with and without stainless handles. The handle of the buccal mirror functions as a built-in retractor.

A set of mirrors developed in Professor Rateitschak's Department of Periodontology (Basel, Switzerland) is also commercially available. These are coated glass mirrors with a plastic handle affixed to the back in the manner of a cake knife. The plastic handles make them easier to manipulate (Manufacturer: Filtrop, Liechtenstein) (Fig. 5.7).

Rear-surfaced glass mirrors produce a double image, depending on the angle of the mirror and the thickness of the glass. The main mirror image is produced by the back of the mirror, and the secondary mirror image is produced by the glass surface. This often makes the image appear to have camera shake (Fig. 5.8). Thus, they are not recommended for our purposes.

Coated glass mirrors should be cleaned and disinfected carefully to avoid damaging the delicate metal coating. Soap and water or alcohol are suitable for cleaning before chemical sterilization.

Some points must be kept in mind in order to achieve good images using mirrors.

- If possible, the image should be framed so that only the mirror image of the teeth is captured. The image can then be reversed and then resembles a photograph which was taken directly. Structures or edges of the mirror should be hardly or not at all visible.
- The fingers holding the mirror should be as far to the front as possible so that they do not appear in the photograph. Mirrors with handles are an advantage.
- Fogging on the mirror's surface can be prevented if an assistant warms the mirror first or directs air at it. Anti-condensation liquids can also be used.
- The patient is instructed to breathe in through the mouth and out through the nose during photography.

For suggestions on use of the mirrors for the various standard views, see below.

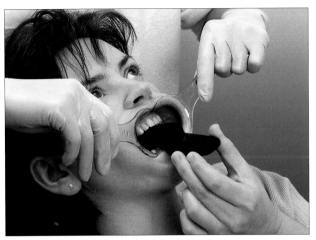

Fig. 5.9 *A black plexiglass background produced in the practice is held in back of the teeth to "isolate" these.*

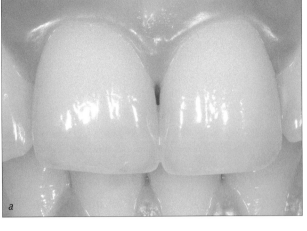

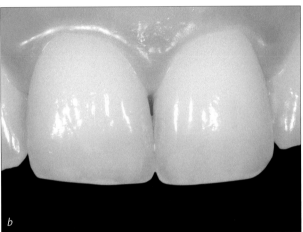

Fig. 5.10 *Isolating the teeth (b) can improve image quality compared to not isolated teeth (a).*

5.1.3 Black background/contrasters

In images, particularly those taken of the front teeth, structures in the back are often disturbing. This can be rectified by placing a black background made in the dental practice in back of the teeth (Fig. 5.9). Black plexiglass is most suitable for this purpose (available from do-it-yourself or hobby stores). This should be cut to size and rubbed with fine sandpaper to achieve a matte surface. Black cardboard or black plastic are also suitable, although less so for use near the posterior teeth. The black background makes the front teeth appear in isolation (Fig. 5.10 a,b). The image is improved because attention of the viewer is focused on the teeth to be shown. A black background is particularly recommended if the translucent regions of the teeth are to be shown. Black backgrounds are commercially available as "contrasters" (PTJ International France, PhotoMed International, Fig. 5.11) or BlackGround (Anaxdent).

5.1.4 Other accessory equipment for intraoral photography

In many photographs, the tongue must be restrained. This can be done using a plastic or glass spatula or the handle of a cheek holder. Disposable plastic spoons are also suitable; these can be used to hold back the lips of children.

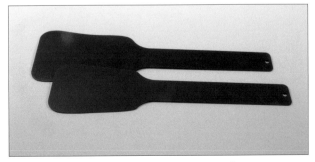

Fig. 5.11 *Metal contraster from PTJ International.*

Dental mirrors should be used for mirror photography only as an exception, and even then only if front coated mirrors are used.

For the most part, the metal holder around the glass is disturbing in the image. However, they are very suitable for holding the tongue or lips, especially when photographing lesions in the lip area. Making the metal surface matte reduces the reflections from the polished metal surfaces if the manufacturer has not already done this. In many instances, the lips or cheeks can be held back with fingers (gloves). This should be done in such a way that the fingers do not appear in the photograph.

Gauze strips not only remove disturbing secretions and saliva, but are also handy for fixation of the tongue.

Air syringes or aspirators should also be mentioned; these allow an assistant to remove disturbing saliva bubbles, etc.

5.2   Visualization

A widely held misconception is that what we see corresponds to reality. We have the idea that the "world outside" is projected to somewhere in the back of our heads. Naturally, visual perception is a far more complex process which communicates many physiological and psychological influences; this process has by no means been completely researched.

Before pressing the shutter release, it is very important—not just in dental photography—to carefully consider a number of points. Visualization comprises the mental framing of the image before it is taken and the careful assessment of the image in the viewfinder. If an image is made without this visualization, the resulting photograph can be disappointing. Only after the image is made, for instance, does the operator discover that the occlusal plane runs diagonally through the image, or moustache hairs hang down into the picture, or even calculus was overlooked during focusing, simply due to having "eyes only for the subject". However, if visualization becomes a habit, photographs will rapidly improve.

Points which must be checked before pressing the shutter are:
- Composition and framing of image.
- Orientation of image.
- Cosmetic issues.
- Point of sharpest focus.

5.2.1   Composition and framing of image

In terms of composition of the image, the rule of thumb is: the most important aspects in the center, the least important on the edges or eliminated altogether, e.g., the nose, which is included in palatal photographs, can sometimes ruin the whole effect of the image. Such things are easy to eliminate if the viewfinder is deliberately checked.

5.2.2   Orientation of image

In general, the photographer should get used to taking the image in the correct axis. This means:

- The optical axis should run through the occlusal plane. Photographing from below or above distorts the perspective of the incisors.
- In lateral views, try to photograph perpendicular to lateral teeth (with the aid of a mirror).
- Occlusal views should be as nearly perpendicular to the camera as possible (also with the aid of a mirror).
- The occlusal plane should be parallel to horizontal frame of the photograph. See Figs 5.12 to 5.15.

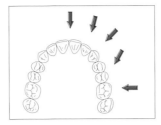

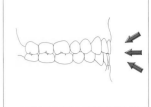

Fig. 5.12   The optical axis should be achieved in intraoral photography so that it is either directly from the front, lateral, or at an angle of 45 degrees to the dental arch (green arrows). Non-defined alignment of the optical axis leads to images which cannot be reproduced (red arrows).

Fig. 5.13   Viewed from the side, the optical axis should be a continuation of the occlusal plane (green arrow) and should not be aligned with the teeth from above or below (red arrows).

The correct orientation is an important factor in producing reproducible images. Subsequent images should not be identical to the initial image, but should be taken from the same angle and at the same reproduction ratio. This means that the viewer does not have to reorientate him- or herself when looking at a series of images.

Fig. 5.14   Leonardo da Vinci already knew about the effect of the viewing angle on perspective (a). If one photographs from "below" into the dental arch, there is shortening of the perspective (b) and conversely, the front teeth appear longer (c).

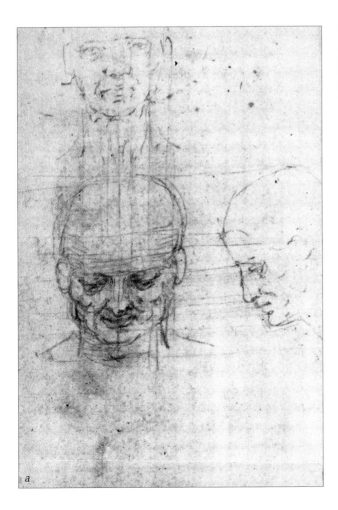

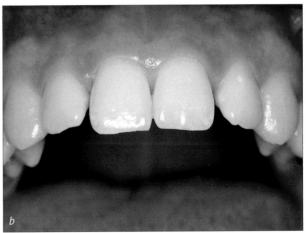

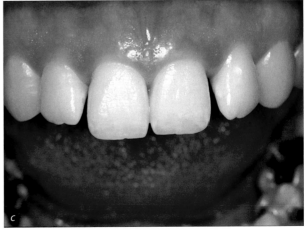

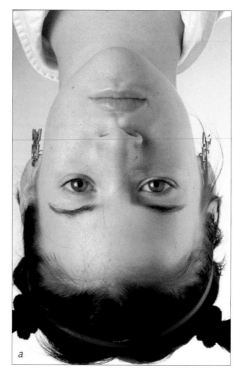 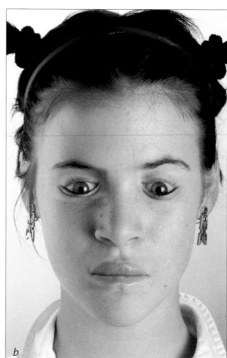

Fig. 5.15   Mouth and eyes were manipulated in this image. The distortions of this manipulation cannot be detected if the image is upside down (a). If the image is in the correct position, the manipulation can be seen (b).

Furthermore, the correct orientation of an image is important for physiological reasons in perception. Things which are horizontal—in keeping with the arrangement of our eyes—are easier for us to see than things which are diagonal or upside down.

5.2.3   Cosmetic issues

Calculus or disturbing plaque layers should be removed before the image is taken if they are not the subject of the photograph. Not only can plaque and calculus reduce the impact of an image, they can also reduce its brilliance, which arises in part from reflections from clean teeth.

5.2.4   Point of sharpest focus

The problems of depth of field have already been discussed under technical considerations. The entire dentition can only be photographed completely in sharp focus if the focal plane is positioned carefully. Therefore, do not focus on the front of the dentition. In a frontal view, the point of focus should be around the canines.

The person looking through the viewfinder is responsible for the end result of the image. He or she must take care that the above points are kept in mind, that no cheek holder creeps into the image, that the mirror shows no fogging and is correctly positioned.

5.3 Standard views

Reproducible conditions for photography are sensible because they not only save time, but also achieve consistent results. For these reasons it makes sense to take the basic intraoral views in a standardized approach. The basic intraoral views can differ for an orthodontist or periodontist. It is important to continue to follow the same standardized procedure once chosen.

General guidelines

Psychologically speaking, the oral cavity is a personal, private area. In a way, photographing this area makes it public. Even though most patients are relaxed about this, some patients may feel their privacy is being infringed upon. Therefore, it is not only important to ask the patient's permission to do this (generally granted), but also to communicate to him or her the reason for the photographs. This helps create a relaxed and quiet atmosphere, which is advantageous, since dental photography can be stressful and uncomfortable for a patient.

The patient should sit, leaning back slightly, in the chair. The height of the chair should be adjusted so that the patient's head is somewhat lower than the head of the photographer. Awkward positions over the patient can be avoided by asking the patient to turn or tilt his or her head.

Format, position and framing

All standard views are done in horizontal format.

A stable position for the photographer is important, since the camera is hand-held and not placed on a tripod. The upper arms are held against the upper part of the body, with the left hand supporting the front of the lens. The eye is not pressed directly against the eyecup, but slightly in back of it. The other eye should be open (Fig. 5.16). The photographer's leg should be supported by the outside edge of the patient's chair in order to find a secure, comfortable position.

Select the magnification ratio according to the desired frame and focus by moving the camera back and forth—not by turning the focusing ring! The magnification ratio frequently has to be adjusted slightly in order to fill the frame with the standard view. Fewer corrections are necessary with increasing experience.

A grid focusing screen is helpful in framing the image and orienting the camera. The middle of the image is placed on the central crosshair, then a check is made to see if the occlusal plane is horizontal. Finally, the edges of the viewfinder are checked to ensure that there are no disturbing details (nose, retractors, edges of mirror, etc) or whether the positions of the retractors and mirror have to be altered. If necessary, the focus plane

Fig. 5.16 *Relaxed and secure camera position.*

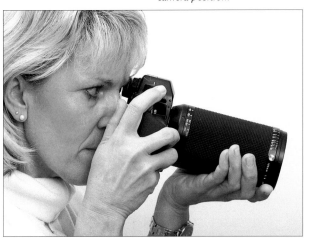

is moved from the front point of the object somewhat in the distal direction in order to make the most of the depth of field.

Several photographs should be made of the same subject, since in close-up photography, even small changes in position can negatively affect the image.

Lighting

Since focusing at close range in the dark oral cavity is very difficult, the operating light is used for illumination. However, it should only be directed at the edges of the mouth. Using a maximum amount of supplementary lighting of the oral cavity would result in overexposure when using cameras which do not have TTL flash. Cameras with TTL flash measure the light reflected from the subject. This would not create overexposure, but this would cause a slight reddish-yellow color shift, since the operating light generally has a halogen bulb which has a lower color temperature.

Fig. 5.17   Frontal view of the dental arch. Position of retractors (a), diagram of composition (b) and result (c).

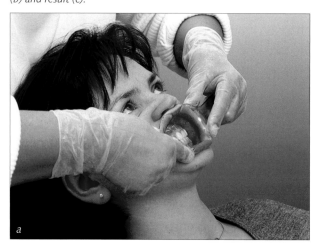

5.3.1   Frontal view (anterior-posterior)

Two variants are possible here, depending on the application of the image. These differ in their magnification ratios and framing. The procedure for taking these images is practically the same.

Variation 1: Overview of the entire dentition

The overview is preferred for general purposes and orthodontics (Fig. 5.17).

The center of the image is the contact point of the central maxillary incisors. The reproduction ratio is 1:1.8 or 1:2. The edges of the photograph are in the vestibulum oris.

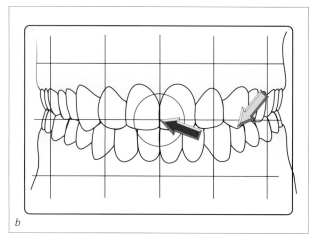

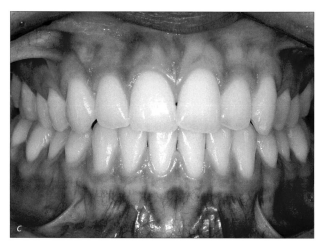

Variation 2: Frontal view of the anterior teeth

This segmental view is generally selected in periodontology, but also for prosthetic dentistry (Fig. 5.18).

The center of the image is placed on the contact point of the central maxillary incisors. The magnification ratio is about 1:1.2. The lateral edges of the photograph are on the distal edge of the canines. If a magnification ratio of 1:1 is chosen the lateral edges of the photograph go through the center of the canines.

The retractors are inserted symmetrically and applied outward as much as possible, with the handles pulled forward slightly. This opens the buccal corridor, that is, the cheeks no longer lie against the buccal surfaces of the molars. Finally, the lips are tautened by moving the retractors in parallel to the front. This prevents the middle of the lips "hanging" in the middle of the photograph. Pressure from the thumb or index finger is applied on the cheek retractors to prevent them from slipping when the lips are tautened.

In both variants, the center of the image is the contact point of the central maxillary incisors. To maximize the depth of field, focus on the canines (variant 1, overview) or on the mesial contour of the lateral incisors (variant 2, detail view).

Care should be taken that the occlusal plane is parallel to the horizontal borders of the frame (check focusing screen) and, when viewed from the side, the occlusal plane should be a continuation of the optical axis of the camera.

Lighting is provided by ringflash, bilateral flash system, or side flash located in the 12:00 o'clock position. In a normal bite, this produces a fine shadow contour below the maxillary incisors.

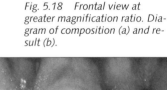

Fig. 5.18 Frontal view at greater magnification ratio. Diagram of composition (a) and result (b).

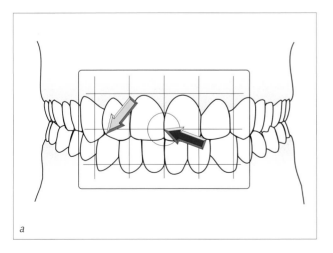

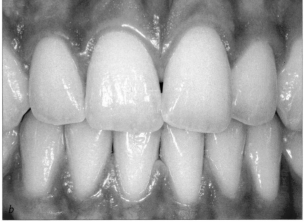

5.3.2 Oblique lateral view

This view is preferred over the purely lateral view for a quick overview, since it can be taken without using mirrors, making work much easier.

Two retractors are used. The side being photographed is uncovered toward the distal by maximum tension on one rectractor, while the second is used only to keep the lips apart (Fig. 5.19).

The reproduction ratio is about 1:1.5. The head is turned slightly away from the camera. The center of the image is around the canine. The edges of the image are the central or lateral incisor on the side away from the camera and—depending on how far back the lips can be moved—the mesial contour of the second molar. Focus is on the first premolar.

The camera is positioned so that the occlusal plane is parallel to the horizontal edge of the photograph and in the center of the image.

For illumination, a ringflash, a flash bracket system, or a point flash can be used, which is positioned so that light "comes from the front teeth" (9:00 and 3:00 o'clock positions).

Fig. 5.19   Oblique lateral view. Position of retractors (a), diagram of composition (b) and result (c).

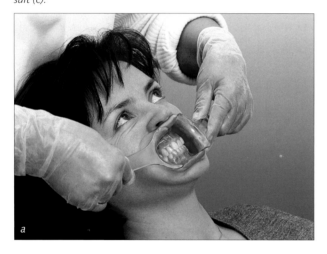

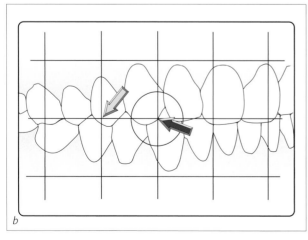

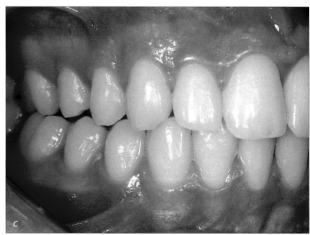

5.3.3   Lateral views

Purely lateral views are used especially for orthodontic, periodontal and prosthetic documentation. Mirrors are always required. A sufficiently wide lateral mirror is inserted on the side to be photographed until the posterior border lies distally of the last tooth in the vestibule. It is turned to the outside as far as the cheeks and lips will allow. Care should be taken that the edge of the mirror does not rest on the gingiva firmly since this can be very painful. To avoid this, the patient can be asked to hold the mirror, while the mirror position is gently manipulated by the photographer or assistant.

To prevent part of the final tooth near the end of the mirror being photographed directly along with the mirror image, the mirror should be moved outwardly and slightly parallel to itself. Mirrors with glued-on handles are particularly well suited to this. The mirror is turned so that the occlusal plane runs across the middle. A retractor is used loosely on the opposite side to hold the lips in position without stretching them.

If no sufficiently wide lateral mirror is available, then a narrow lateral mirror can be used in combination with a wire retractor. The camera and mirror are positioned so that the optical axis is as perpendicular as possible to the mirror image (Fig. 5.20). The occlusal plane runs horizontally in the middle. The center of the photograph and focus point are around the second premolars or the first molars, depending on the framing of the image. If a reproduction ratio of 1:1 is selected, the side edges of the photograph are mesial to the first premolar and distal to the second molar. If the canines are also to be photographed, a reproduction ratio of 1:1.2 should be selected (Fig. 5.20). As always when using mirrors, the mirror image should be in sharp focus. The edges of the mirror and adjacent structures are not photographed.

Fig. 5.20   Lateral views. Position of retractors and mirror (a), diagram of composition (b) and result (c).

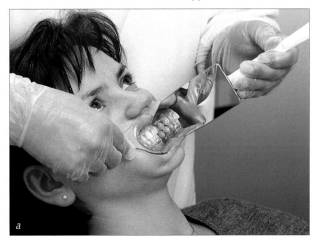

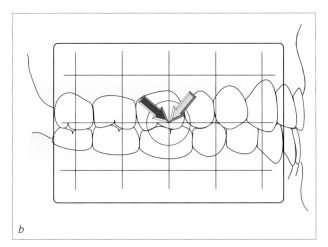

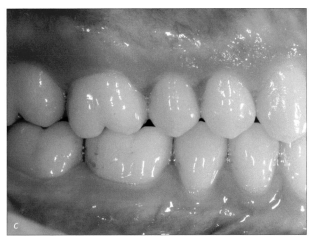

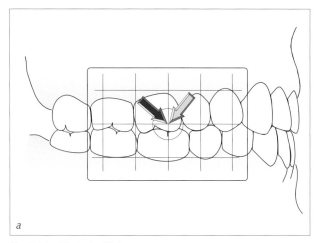

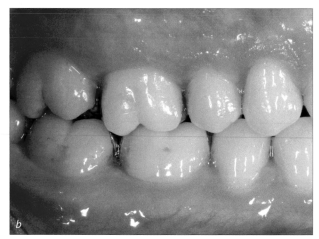

Fig. 5.21 Variant with larger reproduction ratio of 1:1. Diagram of composition (a) and result (b).

Fig. 5.22 Occlusal view of mandible. Position of retractors and mirror. Index finger holds the lower lip against the retractor (a). Diagram of composition (b) and result (c).

Lighting is provided by a ringflash or flash bracket system. If a single side flash is used, it is positioned on the side of the mirror (9:00 and 3:00 o'clock). This makes the posterior teeth appear particularly plastic.

5.3.4 Occlusal mandibular view

This is a photograph from an occlusal view of the entire dental arch of the mandible, taken with the aid of a mirror (Fig. 5.22). In order to have as much room as possible in the corners of the mouth for the mirror, the retractors—which have been shortened on one side—hold the lower lip away from the teeth so that it is not visible in the mirror.

The palatal mirror is inserted with the broader end toward distal in the case of adults. The patient is asked to raise the tongue to the palate and to breathe through

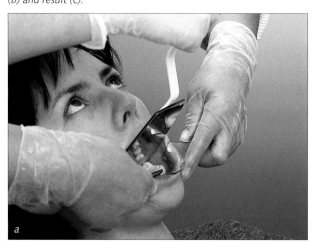

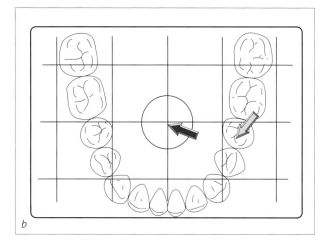

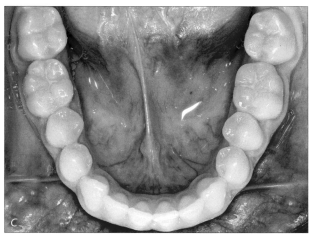

his or her nose. The mirror rests on the gingiva of the last molars. It is turned upwards with the mouth wide open until it touches the incisal edges of the upper incisors. To prevent the parts of the last molars being photographed directly in addition to the mirror image, the mirror has to be shifted in parallel to itself toward the maxilla.

The mirror and camera are positioned using the viewfinder so that the optical axis is exactly perpendicular to the mirror image of the occlusal plane of the dental arch. The center of the image is at the intersection of the sagittal plane with the line crossing the second premolars, which is positioned horizontally in the center of the image. Focus is on the fissures of the posterior teeth. For adults, a reproduction ratio of about 1:2 is preselected.

If only one sideflash is used, this is employed in the 12:00 o'clock position.

5.3.5 Occlusal maxillary view

The entire dental arch of the maxilla can be photographed with the aid of a palatal mirror. This photograph is less difficult to take than that of the mandible. The palatal mirror rests on the gingiva distally of the last molars and turned down as far as possible until it touches the lower incisors (Fig. 5.23). The upper lip is held as far out as possible using the retractors which have been shortened on one side, so that the lip is not longer visible on the mirror image. The patient is asked to breathe through the nose.

To avoid photographing parts of the last molars in direct view in addition to the mirror view, the mirror must be moved parallel to itself towards the mandible.

Using the viewfinder, the mirror and the camera are positioned so that the optical axis is exactly vertical to

Fig. 5.23 Occlusal view of the maxilla. Position of retractors and mirror (a). Thumbs hold the upper lip against retractor. Diagram of composition (b) and result (c).

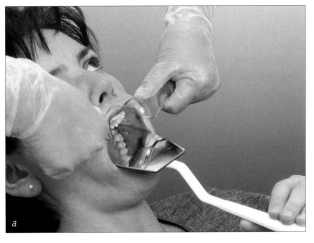

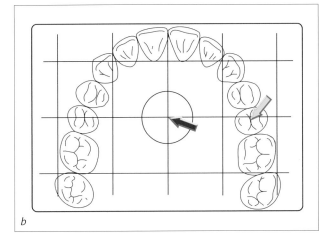

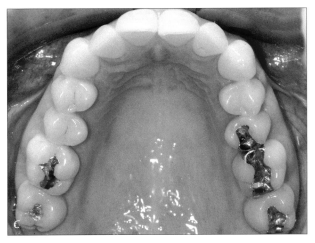

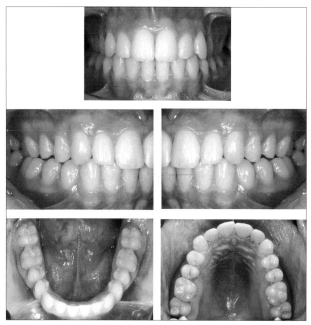

Fig. 5.24   Complete photo status with oblique lateral views of the posterior teeth. Recommended for quick overview.

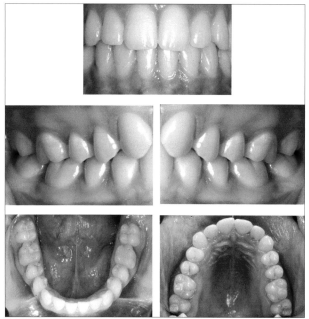

Fig. 5.25   Complete photo status with larger reproduction ratio. Recommended, for example, for routine documentation in periodontology and prosthetics.

the mirror image of the occlusal plane of the dental arch. The center of the photograph is at the cross-section of the sagittal plane with the connection line between the second premolars running horizontally in the middle of the image. Focus is on the fissures of the posterior teeth. For adults, a reproduction ratio of about 1:2 is preselected.

If only one sideflash is used this is turned to the 6:00 o'clock position.

Depending on the view selected, the above photographs produce different photostats consisting of five images each (Fig. 5.24 and 5.25).

5.4 Supplemental segmental views

In addition to the standard views of the two dental arches, segmental views are photographed to show details. Here too, the basics should be adhered to in order to achieve reproducible images:

- Images with correct axis: perpendicular to the occlusal plane or row of teeth.
- Occlusal plane always horizontal.

5.4.1 Frontal view of jaw

Frontal views of the upper and mandible are especially useful for prosthetic and periodontal purposes. The same procedure is used as with photographing a frontal view, differing only in that the patient has his or her mouth open. The center of the image is in the area of the interdental papillae of the maxillary or mandibular central incisors. The reproduction ratio should be about 1:1 or 1:1.2 (Fig. 5.26).

A black background is particularly useful for these photographs, as it isolates the front teeth.

Fig. 5.26   Frontal view of the anterior maxilla. Position of retractors. The thumbs prevent lips from slipping out of retractor (a). Result (b). Analogous procedure for mandible (c and d).

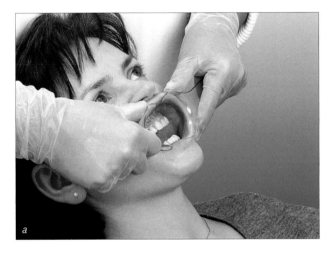
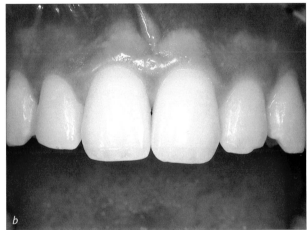
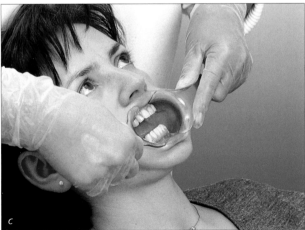
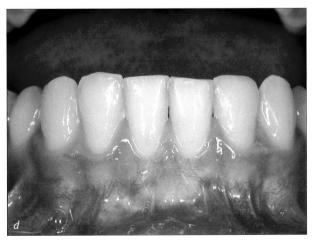

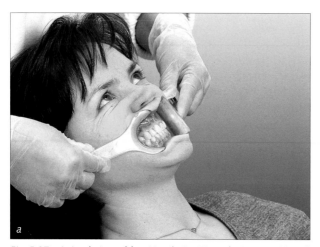
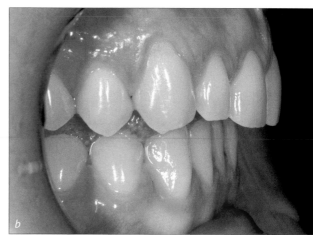

Fig. 5.27   Lateral view of front teeth. Position of retractors (a) and result (b).

*Fig. 5.28   Oral views of the front teeth groups. Position of mirror and retractors for maxillary photograph (a) and result (b).
Position of retractors and mirror for mandibular view (c) and result (d).*

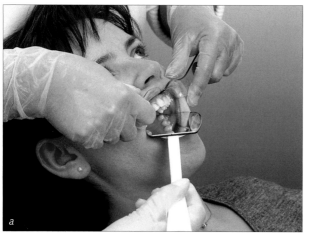
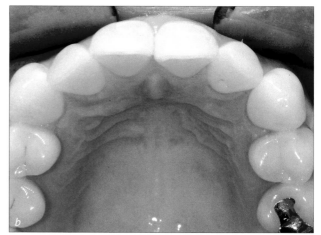

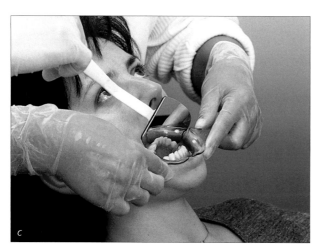
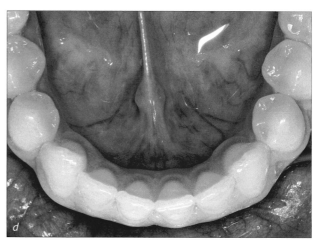

5.4.2   Lateral view of the front teeth

This view is taken in particular to document the amount of overbite of the front teeth (prosthetic dentistry, orthodontics). Both corners of the mouth are held back by lip retractors (Fig. 5.27). The recommended reproduction ratio is 1:1. This means that the lateral edges of the images are approximately between the first and second premolars on the one side, and in front of the incisors on the other side. The occlusal plane is horizontal. The same lighting is used as for a lateral view, that is, the main light is from the front teeth side.

5.4.3   Oral view of the front teeth

A photographic mirror is used to photograph the oral aspects of the front teeth. Use either a palatal mirror or the wider end of a lateral mirror. The patient should hold the tongue against the palate for photographs of the mandible. The mirror and camera should be positioned so that the optical axis is vertical to the mirror image of the occlusal plane (Fig. 5.28). The reproduction ratio is between 1:1 and 1:2.

In this type of photograph, it is especially important that the lips, cheeks, cheek holders, nose and other extraneous elements are not photographed as well.

5.4.4   Oral view of the posterior teeth

A buccal mirror is used to photograph the oral aspects of the premolars and molars. This mirror is placed distal to the final tooth to be photographed, inclined sideways, and rotated along its longitudinal axis until it is possible to take the photograph (Fig. 5.29). The repro-

Fig. 5.29   Oral views of posterior teeth are produced with the buccal mirror which is introduced at an angle of about 45 degrees toward the side teeth (a). Result for maxilla (b) and mandible (c).

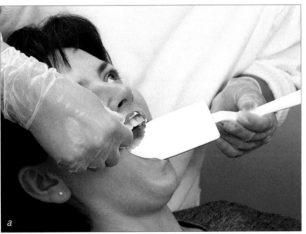

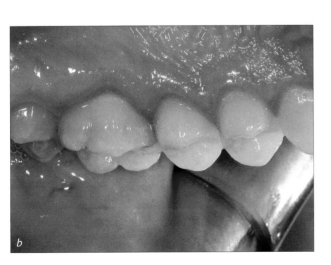

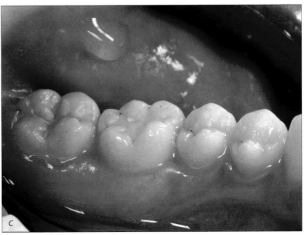

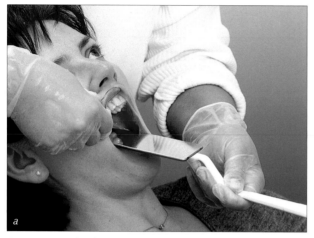
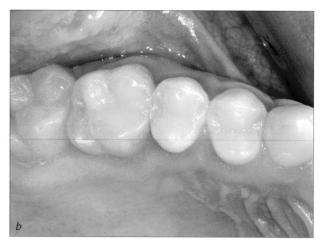

Fig. 5.30   Occlusal areas are also photographed with a buccal mirror. Position of mirror (a) and result (b).

duction ratio is 1:1 or 1:1.2. This brings the lateral edges of the image to mesial of the first premolar or the canine and distal of the second molar. The mirror and camera are positioned so that the optical axis is vertical to the mirror image of the teeth.

5.4.5   Occlusal view of the posterior teeth

The procedure in this case is the same as for occlusal views. The lateral mirror is used instead of the palatal mirror. The mirror end rests on the distal aspect of the last tooth to be photographed and then turned as far as possible in the direction of the other jaw (Fig. 5.30). The reproduction ratio is 1:1 to 1:1.2. The optical axis is perpendicular to the mirror image of the occlusal plane of the row of teeth.

5.5   Reproducible conditions – Making a series of photographs

If the aim is to show a course of treatment, all photographs should be taken under the same conditions. This includes the reproduction ratio, direction of the photograph, and the framing. This ensures that the person viewing the series does not have to reorient him- or herself with each new image (Fig. 5.31). If these photographs are made in one sitting, this is not a problem: determine the point on which the crosshair of the focusing screen rests and leave other settings of the camera the same.

It is frequently not clear from the outset that one image can become part of a series. There are a number of ways of ensuring that these images are reproducible. In general, the basic instructions on setting up the camera should always be adhered to. If the file of the first image can be opened and looked at on the screen it will be no problem to take the following shots in the same way. If certain standard views

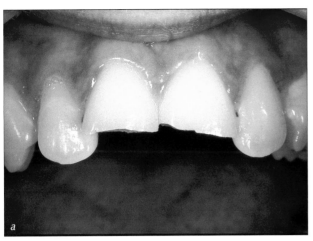
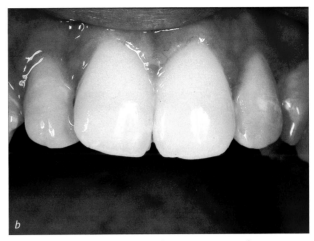

Fig. 5.31   *When taking a series of images, the basic position should not alter so that the viewer does not have to reorientate him-
or herself with each new image. Front teeth after sports injury (a) and after reattachment of tooth fragments (b).*

have been agreed upon in the dental practice, these can
also be noted in the records.

Another method is to note the key data used in photographing groups of teeth on the patient's card. This data should provide information about the framing of the
image, including:

- Position of the image center.
- Magnification ratio.
- Direction of camera.

Front view	+
Lateral view left and right	⊣ or ⊢
Maxilla occlusal view	∩
Mandible occlusal view	∪
Posterior teeth maxilla right	⌋
Posterior teeth maxilla left	L
Posterior teeth mandible right	⌐
Posterior teeth mandible left	Γ
Maxilla frontal view	⊥
Mandible frontal view	T

5.5.1   Position of the image center

The center of the image can be defined as the intersection of two lines, whose position can be reduced to only a few possibilities. The verticals either run through the
middle of a tooth or through the contact point of two
teeth (Fig. 5.32). This can be written down as either
tooth numbers or the numbers of the two teeth in question (e.g., 14 or 1121). The horizontals run either at the
level of the transition from the middle to the incisal third
(abbreviation "i") or the transition from the middle to
the cervical third (abbreviation "c"). A center of the image which lies on the contact point of the central maxillary incisors would thus be indicated as 1121i.

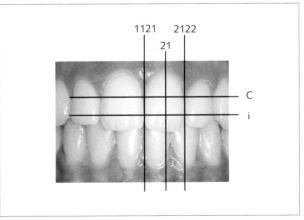

Fig. 5.32   *The center of the image can be imagined as the intersection of two straight lines. The vertical lines either run through
the middle of the tooth or through the neighboring contact points.
The horizontal lines either run through the top of the papillae or
the contact point in the incisal third.*

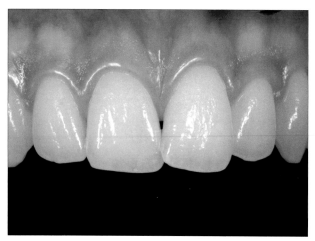

Fig. 5.33   *A photograph from the front could be abbreviated 1121c 1:1b.*

5.5.2   Magnification ratio

This is generally noted using the standard ratios, e.g., 1:2.

5.5.3   Direction of camera

In general, the images should be taken from buccal, lingual/palatal or occlusal (abbreviations b, l, p, o).

In summary, the abbrevation 1121c 1:1 b characterizes a front view of the anterior teeth in a reproduction ratio of 1:1 (Fig. 5.33).

This method appears complicated at first sight, but is easy to use and has been proven effective in our practice.

Always remember:
- Direction of the optical axis always perpendicular to the dental arch or to the tangent of the arch.
- Occlusal plane parallel to horizontal edge of the photograph.

5.6   Extraoral close-ups of the mouth

Especially for esthetic purposes, extraoral close-up views of lips and teeth give valuable information about the appearance of teeth and restorations framed by their natural surroundings. In principle, alignment of the camera is the same as for intraoral views. The patient is sitting in an upright position, the optical axis of the lens and the occlusal plane are on the same level.

The magnification ratio is between 1:2 and 1:3. The occlusal plane is horizontal. Lighting of the image is crucial. Ringflash gives poor results. Lateral lighting is better, especially when diffusors are used to increase the flash area.

5.6.1 Frontal view, lips relaxed

With a magnification ratio between 1:2 and 1:3, there is some space on both sides of the mouth, a part of the philtrum is visible, as well as an area of the skin below the lower lip. Nose and chin are not visible (Fig. 5.34).

The lips are in a relaxed position and slightly opened (so-called emma position). To add some specular highlights, the patient is asked to lick the lips. The use of lip

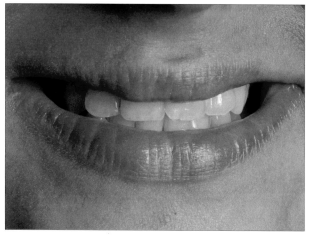

Fig. 5.34   *Frontal view, lips at rest.*

gloss or lipstick can give the image a dramatic appearance. But sometimes the appearance of the mouth is far from natural. Teeth are partly visible, the contact point of the central maxillary incisors is the center of the image and the focus point as well.

5.6.2 Frontal view, natural smile

With this view, the amount of gingiva of the maxilla can be evaluated, as well as the contour of the lips and its relationship to the contour of the incisal edges of the upper teeth (Fig. 5.35). Framing of the image, focusing, and camera alignment are as in the frontal view with relaxed lips. The patient is smiling, exposing the teeth of the maxilla. Front teeth and premolars are visible, sometimes the first molars.

With a full smile, parts of the lower teeth and the buccal corridor are visible.

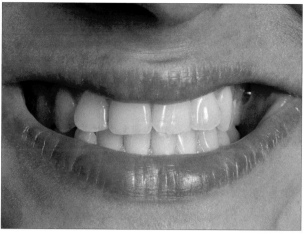

Fig. 5.35   Frontal view with a full, natural, and relaxed smile.

5.6.3 Oblique lateral smile view

This view gives some information about the relationship between lips and teeth and the angulation of the teeth. The image center and focus point is the lateral incisor (Fig. 5.36). Framing, patient position and camera alignment are as described above.

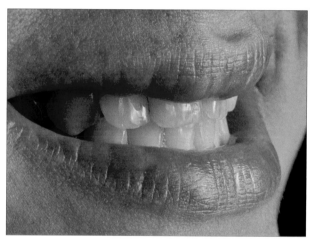

Fig. 5.36   Oblique lateral view, patient smiling.

5.7 Tips for photographing skin and oral mucosa

Often it is the dentist who first is confronted with changes in the skin or oral mucosa (Fig. 5.37). She or he is the person who starts therapy or who at least paves the way for further therapy or diagnostic measures.

A camera should be available in the practice as a matter of course for stomatological treatment of the patient just as the X-ray system is for general dental treatment. Photographs of changes in the oral mucosa are especially important in diagnosis and in monitoring the progress of treatment.

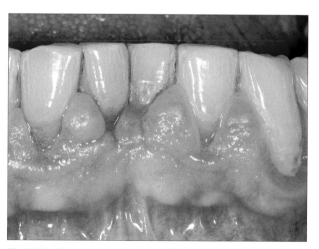

Fig. 5.37   Documenting changes of the oral mucosa is an important part of intraoral photography.

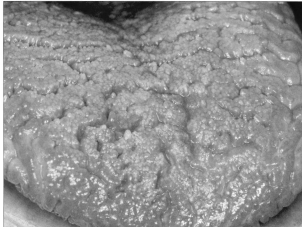

Fig. 5.38   Flat lighting emphasizes the texture of the tongue.

It is important that the lesion is accessible to the camera. For this purpose, retractors, photo mirrors, dental mirrors, spatulas and gauze strips are useful. The magnification ratio should be noted to allow comparison of size. It is recommended to keep the initial photograph in the patient's records. Surface characteristics can be more clearly shown through suitable lighting. Light from a flat angle shows form and structure of a change (Fig. 5.38). Axial light (ring flash) gives good color rendition, but does not emphasize the morphology.

5.8   Photography of surgical procedures

Photography of oral surgery involves a number of points which are briefly discussed here.

Equipment

The same equipment is required as for clinical photography. It is especially important that no trailing cables compromise the sterility of the operating area. For the same reason, a long subject-to-camera distance is required. If the operation area is in the mouth cavity, a ring flash is acceptable and less problematical to use. Otherwise, a side flash or a flash bracket system produces more plastic results.

Image composition

If the person performing the operation is not the photographer, the photographer should be briefed on the significance and procedure of the operation.

Fig. 5.39   In photographing during an operation, it is important to keep the area as free of blood as possible.

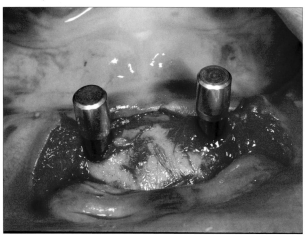

It is important that the operating area and its surroundings are cleaned by thorough rinsing and aspiration and by changing the visible operation cloths (Fig. 5.39). Superfluous instruments should be removed in order to focus on important aspects.

If highly polished instruments are used they can lead to reflections and thus to incorrect exposures. Images can be spoiled if TTL flash units are used, as the extremely bright reflections can affect the overall image brightness. This is not the case with manual exposure settings. If the surfaces of the instruments are made matte or the chrome surfaces turned, this problem can be alleviated. Manufacturers produce most modern instruments with matte surfaces.

The image should be framed to correspond to the point of the view of the person performing the operation, thereby facilitating later orientation. Scale can be indicated by placing objects of a known size in the photograph. Detail views, which are difficult for the uninformed observer to grasp, can be supplemented with an overview.

5.9 Applying photography in the dental practice

Experience has shown that photography is only performed systematically in the dental practice if its routine is not greatly disturbed. Most practices generally operate under considerable time pressure. Since photography is time consuming, even when well organized, it must be ensured that it takes as little time as possible.

It is important to ensure that the camera and aids (mirrors/retractors) are at hand. If the camera first has to be "assembled", the image is generally not taken. Extra batteries and storage media should also be available. As far as possible, photography should be delegated, which does present problems if special details must be recorded.

Image filing and archiving will be discussed later in detail. In many cases it is helpful to photograph the patient's record card with his or her name, thereby avoiding any confusion of images.

Portrait and profile photography

6

Dental portraits are predominantly used for documentation in orthodontics, surgery, and prosthetic dentistry. If these images are to be used for documentation, then the patient must be positioned in accordance with strict guidelines. If the images are to be used more to present an esthetic impression of dental treatment, there is more flexibility in positioning the patient.

6.1   Technical prerequisites

6.1.1   Camera

The same camera can be used for portraits as is employed in intraoral photography. It is especially important to use at least an 80-mm lens in order to avoid distortions

Fig. 6.1   Portraits with different perspectives using lenses with different focal lengths: 28mm (a), 55mm (b), 105mm (c) and 200mm (d). The most natural appearance results from using a 105-mm lens.

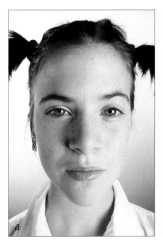
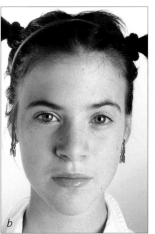
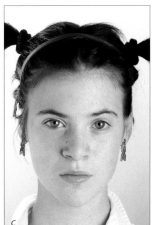
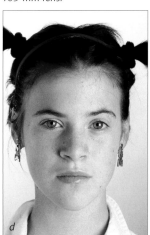

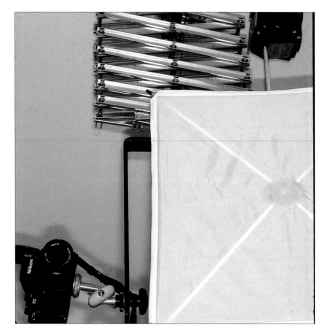

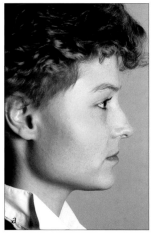

Fig. 6.2 *A scissors arm allows the camera and flash to be hung from the ceiling, thus saving space.*

Fig. 6.3 *Suitable background colors for portraits are gray (a), blue (b) and black (c).*

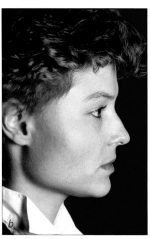

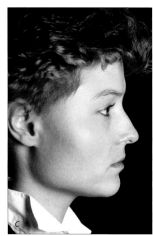

in the portrait (Fig. 6.1). When using a digital SLR camera with a crop factor of 1.5 or higher, a 60 mm lens would also be appropriate.

If portraits are taken frequently in the practice, then it is recommended that a specific area be set aside for this purpose. Patient and camera positions can be marked on the floor in order to ensure reproducible results. Rail systems with an adjustable arm fixed to the wall or ceiling can be useful for this purpose (Fig. 6.2).

Unlike in intraoral photography, the vertical format should be used to completely fill the frame.

6.1.2   Background

The background must allow a full assessment of the profile. It should be without structure and non-reflective. Gray or black decorative felt or cardboard have proven useful for this purpose (Fig. 6.3). It must always be ensured that no objects of the practice appear in the image.

If a white background is desired, this must be illuminated separately by its own light source. In this case, an exposure compensation (plus correction) may be necessary. When using black backgrounds there is the risk that dark-haired patients will not stand out sufficiently from the background.

The National Cleft Audit Photography Group (www.imi.org.uk) published national guidelines in 2004. The group recommended the use of black or white backgrounds.

6.1.3   Lighting

For the most part, macro flashes used in intraoral photography are too weak and are therefore only a compromise. Ring flashes should not be used at all, as they result in a completely flat reproduction of the face, and because of their low power and resulting large apertures, they achieve images with too shallow a depth of field (Fig. 6.4).

Regardless of whether constant light sources (studio lights) or flashguns are used, the light source should be bright enough to allow apertures of between f/11 and f/22. In order not to light the portrait too harshly, the light source should be made larger, either by using a diffuser (soft box) or indirect flash by using a styrofoam sheet or a reflector (Fig. 6.5). Some digital SLRs offer a wireless flash function. The main flash is triggered by an infrared device positioned on the camera or by the camera flash itself. An alternative option is to use a slave flash triggered by the camera flash.

It is also possible to bounce the flash off a white wall or the ceiling, although this frequently results in images without much contrast.

In general, it is sufficient to light the face with one light source. The side away from the light can be filled in using a reflector. If the main light source is a flash, it can be triggered via a cable. It is also possible to trigger the flash without a cable using a slave which is triggered by the camera's flash. If the flash is not TTL controlled, the correct aperture must be determined at the outset by a flash meter or by bracketing. Since the camera-to-patient distance and the flash-to-patient distance always remain constant, the setting determined can always be reused.

A second light source is required only if the background needs to be lit separately. This has the advantage of eliminating any shadow in the background and illuminating the background more brightly. A small secondary flash triggered by a slave cell is useful for this purpose.

Three-point lighting

A classical and more advanced technique of lighting is "three-point lighting". It is similar to the lighting technique described above. A main light (key light) comes from a point 15 to 45 degrees to the side of the camera and also 15 to 45 degrees higher than the camera angle. A second light – the fill light – softens and extends the illumination provided by the key light. It comes from the opposite side and should be lower than the key light and about half to one-third as bright. The fill-in light can be provided by a reflector as well. A third light, also called back light or rim light, creates a defining edge. It helps to visually separate the person from the background. For this, a spot light is used coming from above or the side, adding some reflections to the person's hair (see Fig. 7.45).

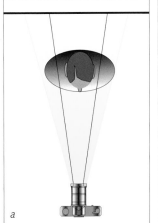
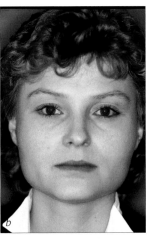

Fig. 6.4   Ringflash is not suitable for portrait photography. Diagram of lighting (a), result (b). The photo does not appear three-dimensional, has a shallow depth of field and exhibits "red eye".

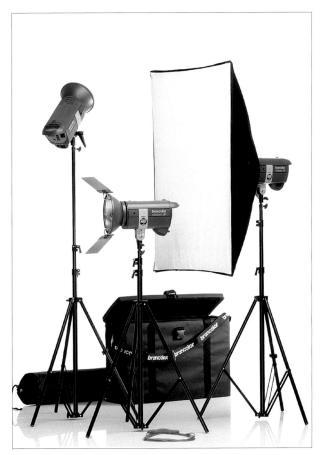

Fig. 6.5   Diffusors increase the size of the light from the flashgun, making the image softer and more pleasant (Photo: Bron color).

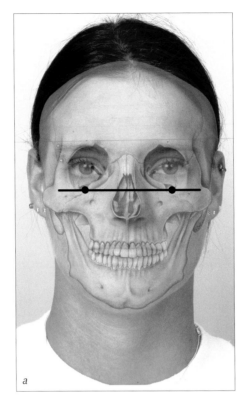
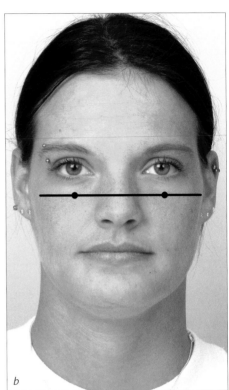

Fig. 6.6 The positioning of the head is done according to anthropological reference points (a). In a front view (b), positioning is done according to the horizontal connecting the orbital points or the bipupillar line.

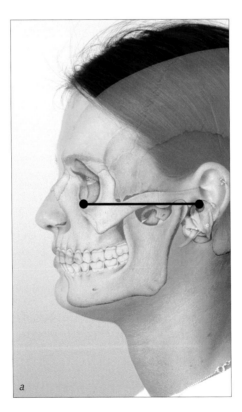
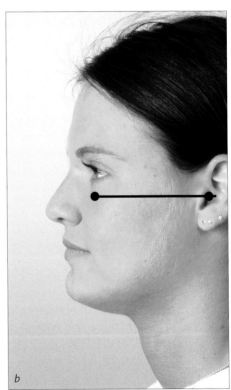

Fig. 6.7 In a lateral view, the Frankfurt horizontal (a) is positioned horizontally (b).

6.2   Standard views

Standard views are used to ensure reproducible images. The accurate positioning is achieved by using anthropological reference points (Fig. 6.6 and 6.7). The most important anthropological reference points are the tragion, orbitals, glabellars and nasion. These have corresponding points on the skin. The upper part of the tragus corresponds to the tragion and the orbital points are the width of the eyelid below an eye which is relaxed and looking straight ahead. The main reference points are the "Frankfurt horizontal" (tragion-orbital) and the orbital plane.

It is sensible to brief the patient shortly about the purpose of the photographs. Eyeglasses should be removed to avoid reflections. If the hair covers the ear it should be pulled back. Ears should be visible so that the tragus may be aligned with the camera.

Magnification ratios

It is recommended to always use the same magnification ratios for certain views. Then the development of patients (especially children) can be judged more precisely.

The following magnification ratios are recommended:
- Full facial views   1:8
- Close up lip/nose views   1:4
- Intraoral views (cleft patients)   1:2

6.2.1   Frontal view (Norma frontalis)

The magnification ratio is 1:8. The frontal view permits assessment of the proportions, form and symmetry of the face (Fig. 6.8).

The head should be positioned so that the orbital plane and/or the bipupillar line is horizontal in relation to the horizontal plane of the photograph. A focusing screen with a grid is very useful for this. The mid-vertical grid line should pass through the mid-sagittal plane (median plane) of the face. The mid-horizontal passes through the Frankfurt horizontal plane.

The patient should look directly at the camera in a relaxed manner. The camera should be about at the height of the middle of the face and in portrait format. Space should be left on all sides between the face and the sides of the photograph. The upper edge of the photograph should be just above the top of the head and the lower frame line around the larynx.

Focus on the patient's eyes. Light should come diagonally from the front, leaving the patient's shadow out of view of the camera. The side away from the light is filled in by a styrofoam sheet or a reflector. It is, of course, possible to use more than one light source and to illuminate the face symmetrically.

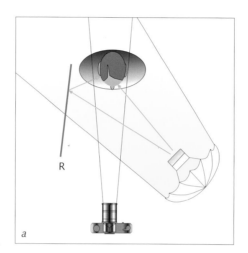

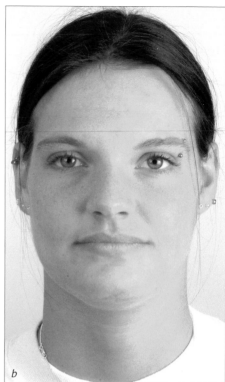

Fig. 6.8   Frontal view. Diagram of the set-up (a) and the result (b).

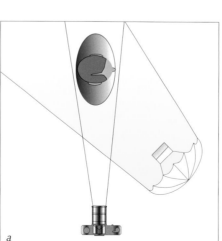

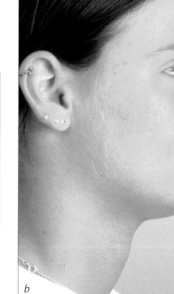

Fig. 6.9   Lateral view. Diagram of the set-up (a) and the result (b).

6.2.2   Lateral view (norma lateralis)

The magnification ratio is 1:8. Profile photographs allow assessment of the profile and the classification according to certain basic types of face (Fig. 6.9).

The patient's head should be positioned so that the Frankfurt plane is horizontal and parallel to the horizontal frame of the photograph. The patient should look straight ahead in a relaxed manner, keeping his or her jaw closed in a typical manner and the lips also relaxed. A mark on the wall or a mirror hung there can aid in this positioning. When photographing children, a third person can be helpful by asking the child to look at him.

For reproduction reasons, it is recommended that the head be turned slightly (3 to 5 degrees) toward the camera (Fig. 6.10). The image should be framed so that the upper edge of the photograph is just above the part in the hair and the lower around the throat. Showing the back of the head is not necessary. The remaining free space should be in front of the profile. Focus on the patient's eye.

Lighting for lateral views should always fall on the patient's profile (light always from the point of the nose). This has the advantage of clearly showing the mandibular margin and keeping the patient's shadow out of the picture (Fig. 6.11). If the portrait is lit from the back of the head, the angle of the jaw is not shown clearly and the nasal labial line will be unflatteringly lit (pouchy cheeks).

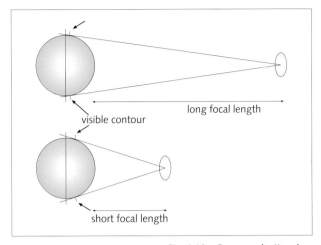

Fig. 6.10   For reproductional reasons, the subject's head should be turned slightly in the direction of the camera to correctly show the contour of the face.

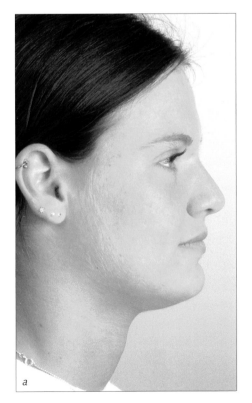

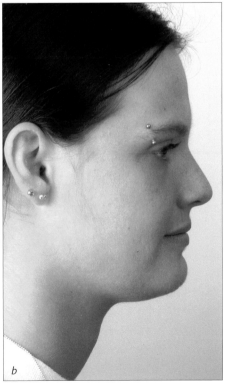

Fig. 6.11   With lateral photographs, it is important to always allow the light to fall on the profile from the "nose side". Thus, the angle of the jaw is shown nicely (a). If the light comes from back of the head, the profile is shown unfavorably (b).

6.3   Additional photographs

6.3.1   AP view with spatula/AP view mouth open

Magnification ratio 1:8
For documentation of an uneven bite, facial views can be taken with the same settings as described earlier. A wooden spatula held by the teeth can demonstrate an uneven bite. Optionally, the same facial view is taken with the mouth wide open. Irregularities of the temporomandibular joints can be shown.

6.3.2   Oblique facial views

Magnification ratio 1:8.
Especially in surgery on the jaw and in prosthetics, portraits are taken from a three-quarters position in which the sagittal plane of the patient and the optical axis of the camera are positioned approximately 45 degrees to each other (Fig. 6.12).

The other aspects are similar to the above.

Difficulties can arise in reproducing the head position of the patient for this shot. It is recommended that the patient turn his or her head away from the camera until the contour of the eye farthest away from the camera appears to touch the lateral visible contour of the orbita (Fig. 6.13). Another recommendation is to turn the head away until the tip of the nose is aligned to the cheek.

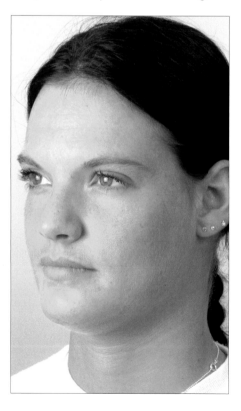

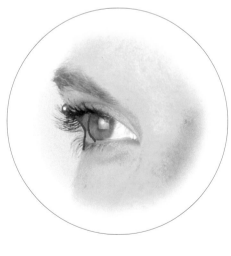

Fig. 6.12   Three quarters profile. The oblique lateral view is oriented as the frontal is: bipupillary line horizontally.

Fig. 6.13   To find a reproducible head position, the head is turned away so far that the outer contour of the eye does not overlap the skin contour.

If there is a certain place where these photographs are always taken, a 45-degree angle can be measured on floor of the studio and marked.

6.3.3   AP views taken at magnification ratio of 1:4

Especially for cleft patients, some closer views are recommended to show more details of the lips. They are taken in portrait format and are aligned according the general rules explained before. Magnification ratio of 1:4.

AP view at 1:4
The vertical grid is aligned through the midline of the face, the horizontal grid passes along the base of the nose. Lips are relaxed and closed (Fig. 6.14).

AP view at 1:4, lips blowing
Same image composition as before. The patient is asked to purse their lips or whistle.

Head tilted back ("Lips, worm's-eye view")
The head is tilted back about 45 degrees. To obtain a reproducible inclination of the head the base of the nasal alar should be aligned at 90 degrees to the camera lens axis (Fig. 6.15).

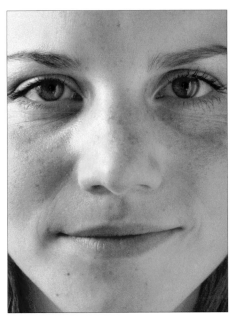
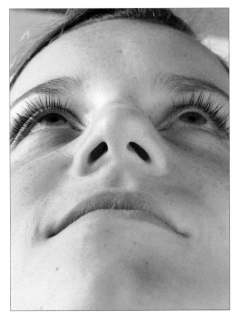

Fig. 6.14   Closer frontal view at magnification ratio 1:4.

Fig. 6.15   Frontal view with head tilted back (45 degrees).

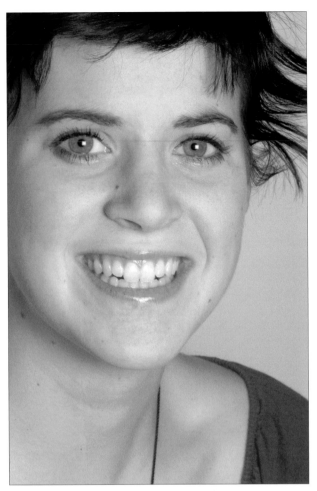

Fig. 6.16   Photographs to illustrate esthetic characteristics give subject and photographer more latitude.

Fig. 6.17   An angled mirror allows frontal and both lateral views to be photographed simultaneously.

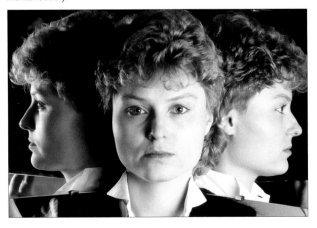

6.3.4 Photographing the target bite

In orthodontics, it is often a therapeutic goal to change the position of the mandible. In order to assess the extent of the changes in the soft tissue profile in advance, the patient assumes the mandibular position which is desired. Such images also contribute in remotivating patients and their parents when their compliance decreases, by once again visualizing the improvement in the profile.

6.3.5 Esthetic purposes

Documenting the esthetic effect of reconstructions is an important task in dental photography. A three-quarter view is often used for this purpose and the patient encouraged to smile. The photographer may need to encourage the patient to do this ("Smile!" "Say cheese!" "Please look up slightly!") since very few patients are relaxed and spontaneous in front of the camera (Fig. 6.16).

Computer simulation programs have largely replaced earlier methods of using photo montages and models to picture the effect of surgery on soft tissue morphology and the profile.

6.4 Additional accessories

The appliances used to anchor the subject's head in the early days of photography due to the long exposures required have largely been dispensed with.

A self-made angled mirror (two folding mirrors with wooden frames) are recommended for documentation of the frontal and the two lateral views on one shot (Fig. 6.17). However, it usually takes longer to set up the mirror than it does to make three separate exposures.

If it is necessary to document dimensions exactly, a millimeter scale can be included in the photograph; this is held up to the middle of the face in profile photographs.

The photo background by Hinz is designed to document the patient's name, number, and date of photograph; the photograph is taken in horizontal format (Fig. 6.18).

Checklist for portrait photography

- Camera is in vertical format.
- Magnification ratio is set to 1:8 (full face views).
- Aperture f/11, f/16 or f/22.
- Focal length 100 mm.
- Camera level with the middle of the face.
- Patient's head aligned (bipupillar plane or Frankfurt horizontal).
- Hair is pulled back.
- Lights for profile photographs positioned on the nose side (lateral and oblique views).
- Focus on eyes.
- Background is checked.

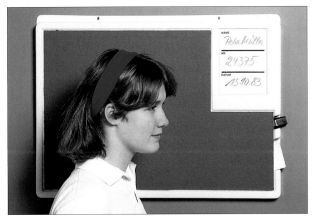

Fig. 6.18   The Hinz photo background (Photo: ZFV-Verlag).

Photographing small objects for dentistry and dental laboratory

7

Many objects which are commonplace in our everyday dental practice are worth photographing. These include dental instruments, models, teeth, gross specimens, and other things. Many of these objects are very small, highly reflective, and often have a very bright surface. These present problems in photography.

The purpose of photographing these is for documentation, patient information, and the production of illustrations for lectures and publications. As in the case with photography for other purposes, the goal is to present the maximum amount of information, fill the frame, and create images with optimum perceptibility. For these reasons, the following points covered below are of particular importance:

- Special equipment.
- Placement of the object.
- Selection and arrangement of a suitable background.
- Proper lighting of the object.

Advantages of digital photography for small object photography

Using a digital camera for object photography is a totally new approach to this field. Anyone who has experienced a learning process using a conventional camera will see that the learning curve is much steeper with a digital camera. This is only true if the photographic basics are understood.

- You can see the results on the LCD monitor at once and therefore the whole process is much more interactive.
- Using the histogram function, exposure can be controlled effectively.
- As there are no film costs, you can experiment until you get the result you want, exploring the possibilities of your equipment.
- White balance setting of your camera allows you to work under almost any light. Unlike in conventional photography, you do not need daylight-balanced lighting in order to match colors. Nor do you need expensive studio flashes to control the lighting effects and color reproduction. You can use simple and inexpensive tungsten light in combination with reflectors.

7.1 Camera equipment

If a digital SLR camera is available, this is also the best choice for object photography. Because a crop factor must be taken into account for most DSLRs, a focal length of 50 mm (macro lens) is the best for most situations, as the effective focal length will be between 75 mm and 100 mm. A focal length of 100 mm could result in a very long working distance, causing problems especially when copy stands are used.

The camera should be equipped with a grid line viewfinder screen facilitating camera alignment. A polarizing filter (circular type) is necessary to eliminate reflections on glass plates. To prevent stray light entering the lens and decreasing image contrast, a lens hood should be used. A cable release helps to prevent camera shake. Alternatively, the self-timer function of the camera can be used.

Advanced viewfinder cameras are the second choice, and work quite well for object photography. They should offer the following features:

- Macro function should be available.
- Manual focus to allow use of the full range of depth of field.
- A flash hot-shoe allows connection to more powerful flashes.
- Aperture and manual exposure mode help to control exposure.
- Exposure compensation helps to find the right exposure.
- An AC adapter prevents your camera going into sleep mode.
- A good monitor plus an enlarging function allow basic control of your images. The final control has to be done on the computer monitor.
- A self-timer allows triggering of the shutter without using a cable release.

7.2 Placement of the object

In contrast to clinical photography, object photography can be undertaken with a stabilized camera, that is, by using a tripod or copy stand. This has the advantage of allowing the image to be assessed at leisure in the viewfinder; a constant light source can be used in this instance also (see below).

Fig. 7.1   This vertical shot does not provide the viewer with sufficient information (a). An angled view (b) is better and aids in recognition of the object.

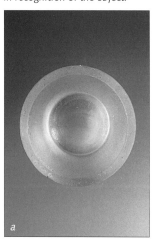
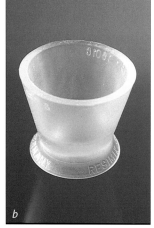

The objects should be placed so that even an uninformed observer can see and easily recognize them. This means, for instance, that they have a clear contour and are presented so that they are perceived in three dimensions (Fig 7.1). In most cases, this is an oblique view from above. The objects should also be placed to make the best use of the depth of field. If possible, the object should be placed perpendicular to the optical axis. In order to increase perceptibility of the image, the objects should be placed so that the axis of the object is parallel to the upper and lower edge of the photograph.

Various means are available to help position the camera and objects to ensure the above considerations are met.

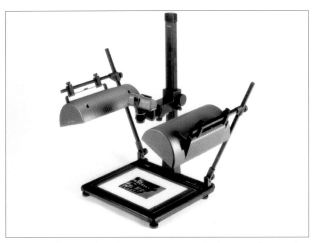

Fig. 7.2   The Copylizer from Kaiser Fototechnik is a professional copy stand system with an integrated light box in the base board (Photo: Kaiser).

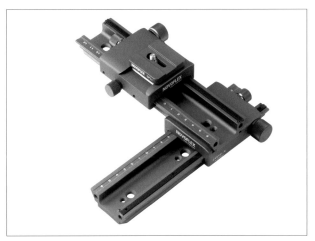

Fig. 7.3   A cross-focusing rack is a valuable tool for adjusting the camera position precisely (Photo: Novoflex).

7.2.1 Camera stabilization

Copy stand

Purchase of a copy stand (e.g., Copylizer, Kaiser Fototechnik) is recommended if object photography is undertaken frequently (Fig. 7.2). Such systems are modular and can be expanded if required. A few points should be kept in mind when buying such a system:

- Sufficient stability.
- Large enough baseboard.
- Long enough vertical column.
- Area lights/soft lights.

A baseboard with an integrated lightbox is very useful. The camera arm should allow the camera to be positioned in several axes. A useful feature is an object holder, a glass plate which can be moved vertically and inclined in two axes (see Fig. 7.14).

Cross-focusing racks can be helpful for macro work, when shooting with high magnification ratios (Fig. 7.3).

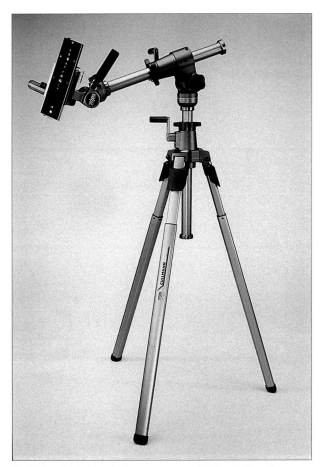

Fig. 7.4   Stable tripod with a macro arm (Photo: Cullman).

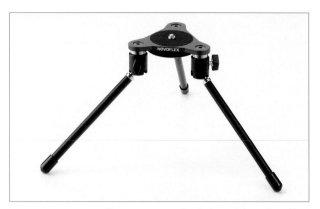

Fig. 7.5   It is especially important to check the stability of small tripods (Photo: Novoflex).

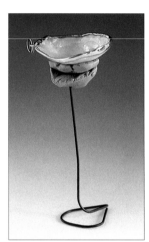

Fig. 7.6   Simple means—here wire and kneaded rubber—can be used to hold small objects in position.

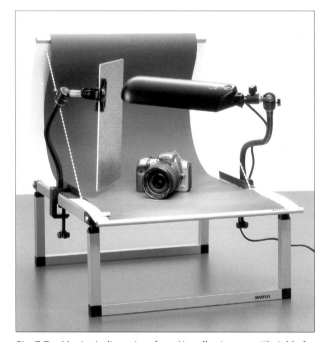

Fig. 7.7   Magic studio system from Novoflex is a versatile table for small object photography (Photo: Novoflex).

Tripods

A tripod allows more flexibility in camera positions than a copy stand (Fig. 7.4). Tripods which stand on the floor should have a macro arm, that is, a horizontal arm which allows the camera to be moved by millimeters. Tripods today are made out of metal or are stable systems of carbon fiber. Tripods, especially ones suitable for the worktop, should be checked for stability (Fig. 7.5).

7.2.2   Holding the object

Adhesives are available from photography stores which aid in fixing an object in a particular position (haftplast, Hama). Silicon impression material or soft wax as used in dentistry are also suitable (Fig. 7.6). Alligator clips as used in electronics are also inexpensive means of anchoring small objects. Rod sets, for example, from Novoflex, are also available from photographic suppliers. Matte black paint reduces reflections and the visibility of the means of fixing the object in the picture if a black background is used.

When photographing from the vertical, a wire run through a cardboard can allow an object to be fixed so that it "floats" in front of the background. Spherical tables are used to allow objects to be rotated in all directions. Flash brackets or a model table of a parallelometer from a dental laboratory can also be used.

Professional equipment suppliers offer shooting tables of various sizes, e.g., the Novoflex Macrocopy stand or the Magic Studio (Fig. 7.7). The Top-Table system from Kaiser is a "classic" among these tables; it can be used for many purposes and allows objects to be photographed in isolation (Fig. 7.15).

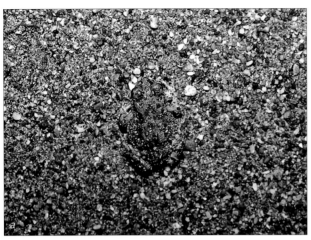
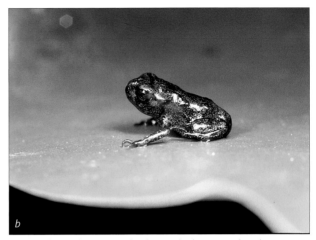

Fig. 7.8   Objects can be perceived only if they contrast with their background. If not, they cannot be detected. This principle—known as mimicry in biology—is demonstrated here with a sand frog (a). The survival of animals which stand out from their backgrounds depends only on large numbers.

7.3   Selecting and arranging suitable backgrounds

The most important criterion for perception of an object is that it stands out from the background (Fig. 7.8). A suitable background isolates the subject and emphasizes its contours. In general, the most suitable ones are those which have a single color, are matte, and lack structure. The arrangement of the background depends on the camera direction (Fig. 7.9). When photographing vertically, the base is also the background. When photographing horizontally, the base flows into the background. This

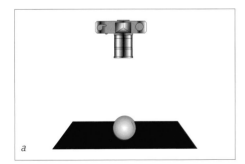
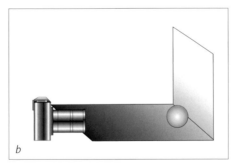
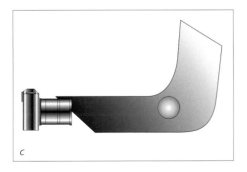
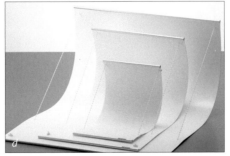

Fig. 7.9   With a vertical photograph (a), the base is also the background. In photographing horizontally, a sharp division between background and base should be avoided (b), since this creates an irritating line in the photo. A curved surface is much better (c). Curved backgrounds are available in different sizes (d) (Photo: Novoflex).

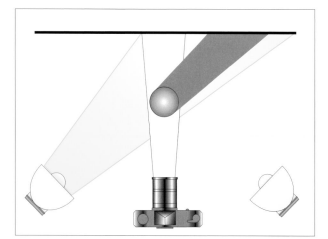

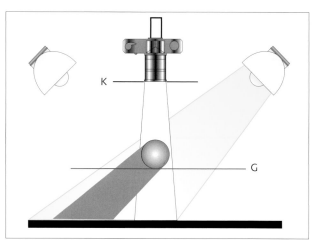

Fig. 7.10   Diagram showing how to isolate an object when photographing horizontally. The distance between the object and the background and position of the light source is set so that the object's shadow is outside the camera's view.

Fig. 7.11   When photographing vertically, a glass support is used to isolate the object. Here too the position of the light source and the distance from the base are set so that the object's shadow lies outside the camera's view.

should be set up to curve to avoid a disturbing horizontal line in the picture. This type of arrangement is used in the design of special tables for photography. It is also possible to produce individual arrangements using cardboard, plexiglas, or velvet.

7.3.1   Isolating an object

It is generally advantageous to isolate an object optically. It gives the impression that the object is floating without a visible shadow and focuses the observer's attention completely on the object. In psychological terms, this is the so-called figure-ground-segregation. We perceive the content of the picture as the "figure" and the remainder as the "base". The better ground and figure are separated, the greater the impact the picture has and the easier the perception. This isolation is achieved by an appropriate combination of background arrangement, placement of the object, and lighting.

When photographing horizontally, the object-to-background distance should be large enough and the main light positioned so that the object's shadow is outside the viewing field of the camera (Fig. 7.10). The object is placed directly on the base.

With vertical shots, the objects are isolated using a glass plate about 15 to 20 cm above the base (Fig. 7.11). If the lights are arranged properly, the object's shadow is out of the camera's viewing field. The main advantage of this type of isolation is that the base color does not affect the object's color, which is especially important in dental photography. This can be achieved using simple

Fig. 7.12   Isolation of a small object using a simple glass plate.

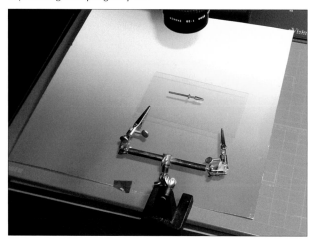

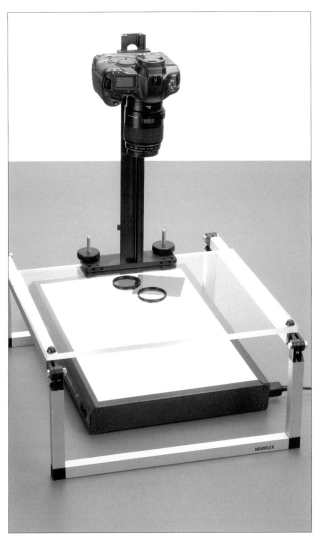

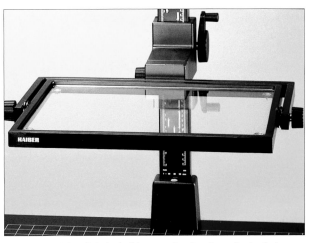

Fig. 7.14   Kaiser Fototechnik's copy stand system also includes a holder for objects. Attached to the column, it can be vertically adjusted and rotated in two axes (Photo: Kaiser).

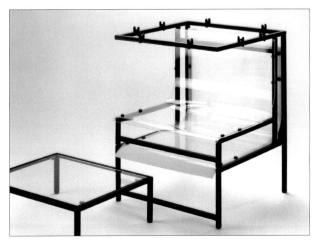

Fig. 7.13   The Novoflex Magic Studio system allows the isolation of objects in front of the background (Photo: Novoflex).

Fig. 7.15   The Kaiser TopTable system is a good aid if object photography is frequently done (Photo: Kaiser)

glass plates, a Jobo Variocopy table, the Kaiser copy stand object holder, or the Top-Table system, depending on the size of the object (Figs 7.12 to 7.15).

The TopTable system consists of a curved opaque Perspex sheet on which objects are placed directly or on colored cardboard backgrounds. An additional table, with a clear Perspex sheet, can be mounted on top of the basic table. The objects placed on this combination seem to float above the surface of the table or the background attached to it. There is also a table with a flat crystal glass plate to go on top of the basic table. It is used, for example, for photographing objects which present hygienic problems such as pathological specimen. A strong holding frame helps hold colored or diffusion foils and lighting equipment.

Using glass plates to isolate objects presents problems with reflections. If the camera is vertical in relation to the glass plate, it can be reflected in this (Fig. 7.16). This problem can be solved by fitting a piece of black cardboard under the camera with

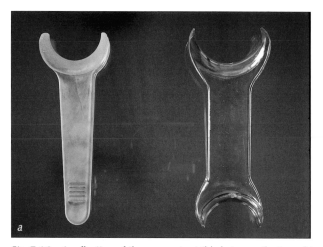

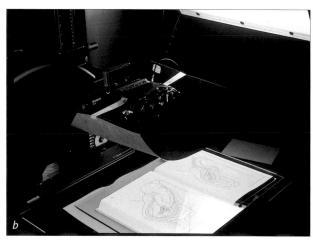

Fig. 7.16   A reflection of the camera is visible between the two objects (a). This reflection can be easily eliminated by placing a piece of black cardboard in front of the camera with an opening cut out for the lens (b).

Fig. 7.17   Reflections from an object frequently ruin a photo (a). This problem can be solved by using a polarizing filter. Unpolarized light vibrates transversely in all planes around the beam axis. Using a polarizing filter restricts the vibrations to one plane: the light is polarized (b). A second polarizing filter with a "grid direction" perpendicular to this blocks this polarized light. Reflections from glass and the surface of water mostly consist of polarized light (c). These reflections can be eliminated by using a polarizing filter (d).

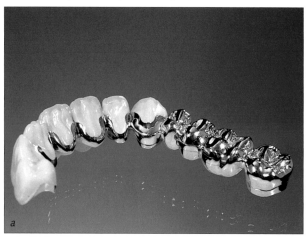

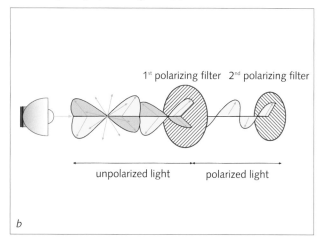

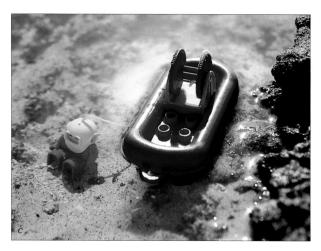

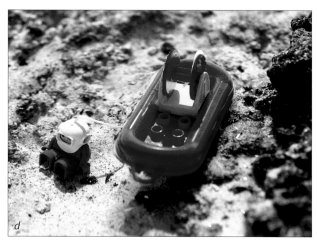

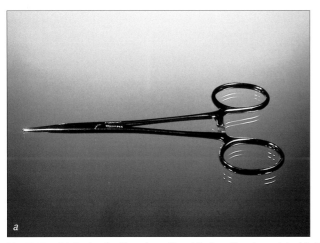
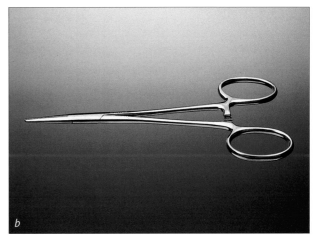

Fig. 7.18   Distinct reflections from the object on the glass plate (a). The same object, photographed using a polarizing filter and a light tent: the reflection has disappeared (b).

a hole cut out for the lens. Reflections from objects on the glass surface present a more serious problem (Fig. 7.17 and 7.18). Such reflections consist of polarized light unless caused by metal. Reflections from objects onto glass plates are eliminated by using a polarizing filter. This is fitted in front of the camera lens; the photographer looks through the viewfinder while turning the filter until the reflections are eliminated. Sometimes it is necessary to change the angle of the optical axis to the glass plate to completely eliminate reflections.

BACKGROUND

Polarizing filter

Neutrally colored filter which only lets light through which oscillates parallel to the polarizing plane of the filter. This increases contrast and achieves images with greater color saturation and separation. Its significance in dental object photography lies in the fact that polarizing filters can eliminate reflections from shiny, non-metallic surfaces which consist of polarized light. The reduction of reflections depends on the angle of the polarizing filter to the reflecting surface. An angle of about 35 degrees is the optimum, depending on the type of material. It is possible to completely eliminate reflections, even from metallic surfaces, by also polarizing the light used to make the image. Cross-polarizing filters are available for opthalmology, but these create unnatural and strange looking images in dental photography.

Digital cameras which have polarizing elements in the camera meter's light path (semi-permeable mirrors, beam splitters, etc) need circular polarizing filters. In contrast to the normal linear polarizing filter, a circular polarizing filter splits the light into two phase-shifted components which oscillate at 90 degrees to each other, permitting exposure measurement independent of the polarization direction.

Aside from eliminating reflections, special applications for polarizing filters include photoelastic study of stresses and the representation of double refractive phenomena.

7.3.2   Background color

There is no universal background which is suitable for all purposes. Selection of a particular background depends on many factors, such as the color of the object and the purpose for which the photo is being made (print, projection, etc.). In general, it is better to restrict the number of backgrounds, making it easier to put together series of photographs without subjecting the observer to too many colors. Uniform backgrounds allow selection of the object with one mouse click during image editing processes performed later.

White background

Especially objects which are dark can be photographed particularly well against a white background. White backgrounds are often used as they reproduce well in printing. However, white backgrounds can create problems in presentations because they tend to blind the observer. Especially when alternating with dark images, white backgrounds can lead to visual fatigue.

A white background is created either by placing the light source under the object (for example, a light box) or simply by using white paper or styrofoam under the glass plate which is used to isolate the object (Fig. 7.19). This must be lighted separately to avoid creating a gray background. The brightness of the white background should be about two stops higher than the brightness of the object. The object should not be placed directly on the white background to avoid "washing out" the object colors and structures.

Fig. 7.19   Set-up for achieving a white background (a) and the resulting image with "plus correction" for exposure (b).

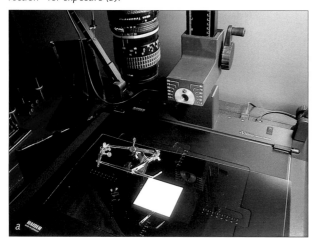
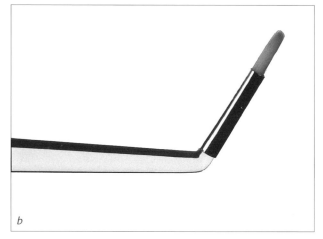

It is important to mask off the area around the object which is out of the viewing field of the camera in order not to lose contrast in the photo through flare light entering the lens. Photographic suppliers offer special masks for this purpose, but black cardboard can also be used.

Especially when using white background, it is important to have a clean lens in order not to obtain low contrast results.

Other problems with using white backgrounds are covered below.

Black background

A black background not only creates a pseudo three-dimensional reproduction of the object which appears to float on the background, but it also dramatically increases the luminous power of the object's colors. Fine nuances of color are rendered well, since the object's color is not affected by that of the background (Fig. 7.20). Another advantage of a black background is that it almost intrinsically eliminates shadows.

A black background is produced by using black cardboard or black velvet; the objects are placed on these or they are laid on the glass support which is used to isolate the object (see below).

Placing small objects on a mirror creates a black background behind the object automatically, if flash is used. In this case, the object is shown twice.

Black backgrounds can be problematic if the object's color does not contrast sufficiently with them. Showing a long series of images with low brightness can tire the viewer during presentations.

Black backgrounds can also cause difficulties in exposure measurement. Since the camera does not "know" what it is photographing, the exposure is set so that it always creates average image brightness. A small bright object on a black background thus leads to overexposure of the object, since the overall brightness which is required to produce an average exposure has to come from this small object (Fig. 7.21). In this case, it is helpful to use spot metering on the object or a "minus correction" by using the exposure compensation of the camera. The amount of correction depends on the size of the surface of the bright object in relation to the

Fig. 7.20   A simple piece of black cardboard through which a wire is passed attached to the object to create a black background (a). The final image does not give any indication of the simplicity of the arrangement. Placing the object on a mirror is another simple technique for black backgrounds (c).

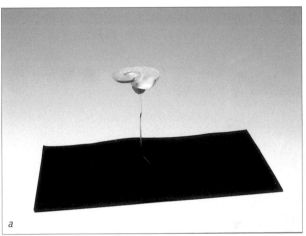

a

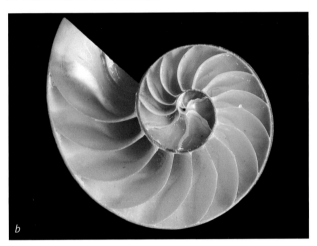

b

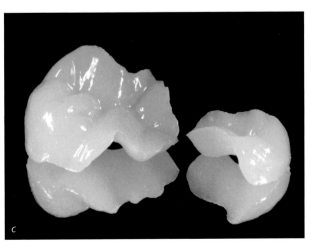

c

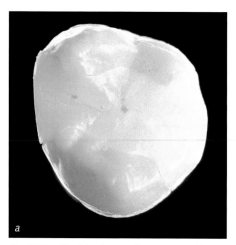
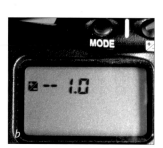
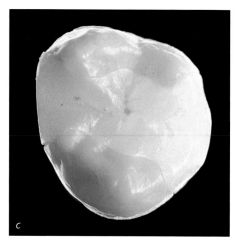

Fig. 7.21   Black backgrounds can cause objects to be overexposed (a). A minus correction (b) achieves correct exposure (c).

overall image area. In case of doubt, exposure bracketing in 1/3 stops leads to the correct exposure.

Vice versa, a white background or a white object with a large surface can lead to exposure problems. A white plaster model or teeth which fill the frame require a "plus correction" to achieve correct exposure.

Gray background

If there is a universal background, then it is gray, since it does not cause problems in determining exposure. Gray also does not affect the color nuances of the object (Fig. 7.22).

A gray background is created using gray cardboard, upon which the object is placed. White paper placed at a suitable distance under an object can also result in a gray background due to the reduction in brightness. Illumination with polarized light also can be used to create a gray background (see below). It has to be kept in

Fig. 7.22   A gray background can be created in the same way as a white one (a). The drop in brightness between the object and the background creates the bright gray color (b).

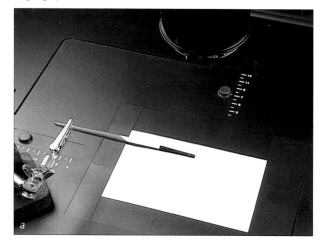
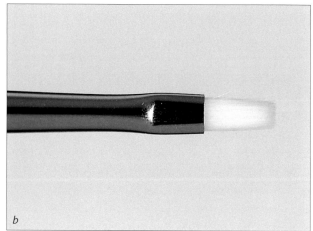

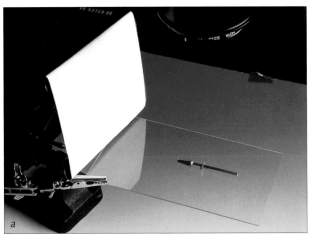
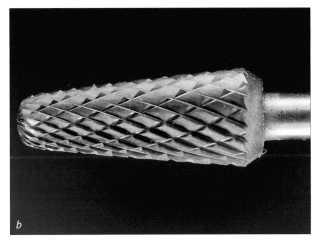

Fig. 7.23   Arrangement for a color background (a). The small field of view and the short exposure makes the background appear very dark and without gradation, although a graduated background was used (b).

mind that colored objects, when photographed against a gray background, may not appear sufficiently isolated if printed in black and white.

A further advantage of gray backgrounds can be that color correction is very easy using an image editing program afterwards.

Colored backgrounds

Colored backgrounds take advantage of the visual attraction of color, and focus the observer's attention on the image (Fig. 7.23). Special color boards are available from photographic suppliers; these are placed under the glass support which is used to isolate the object. It is advantageous to restrict the number of colors used, in order to facilitate creating image series for presentations.

A number of factors are important in selecting colors:

The background should isolate the object. Placing a yellowish gold object on a yellow background for instance makes little sense. This is especially important if the image is later to be reproduced in black and white (Fig. 7.24). In this case, lightness of object and background should be different.

Background and object colors should be harmonious. For example, a red object looks better on a blue background than on a green one (Fig. 7.25).

The background color should not dominate the image, and should remain in the background visually as well. Therefore, red should be avoided as a background

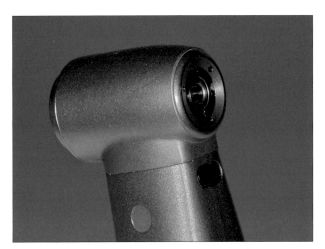

Fig. 7.24   Insufficient isolation of an object in front of a background with a similar color.

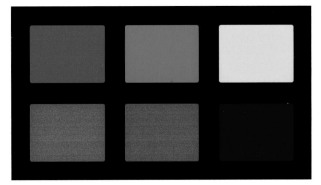

Fig. 7.25   Many color combinations appear harmonic, others are not harmonic and should be avoided. Generally the combination of blue and yellow is tolerable, but the complementary pairs of cyan-red and green-magenta are mostly felt not to be harmonic.

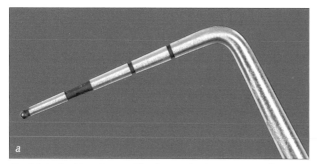
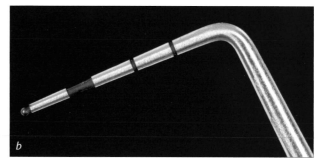

Fig. 7.26   Red is not a good background color, since visually it springs into the foreground (a). Blue is a good background color as our eyes are not very sensitive for blue (b).

color. Physiological factors of perception play a role in this. Just as in the case with camera lenses, the human eye focuses different colors on different planes. Red, for instance, is not a background color, as it is optically perceived to be in front of the object (Fig. 7.26 a,b). Renaissance painters already knew and observed this. In paintings of the Virgin Mary, she was always clothed in a blue gown; the more "earthly" saints or their companions who were closer to us were always clothed in red. For the same reason, it is best to avoid too many colors in an image in order not to overtax the observer visually. This is especially obvious in title slides with many colors, which quickly tire the viewer by making him or her focus on the various colors at various planes.

The background color should not affect that of the object (Fig. 7.27). This is avoided by isolating the object and using a glass support which is about 15 cm above the colored background.

Other sensory physiological and psychological factors should also be considered. The phenomenon of simultaneous contrast makes an object on a brighter background appear darker than on a darker one (Fig. 7.28). In a series with varying background colors, the successive contrast can lead to false color perception.

Fig. 7.27   If an object whose color is important is placed directly on a colored background, its own color will be significantly changed (a,b).

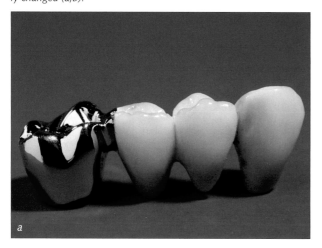
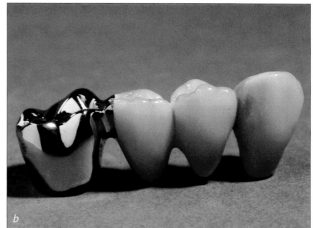

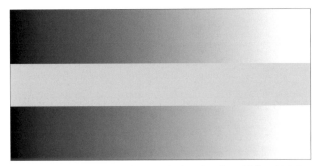

Fig. 7.28   Simultaneous contrast is a sensory physiological phenomenon which demonstrates that the color perception of an object is also influenced by the background color.

Fig. 7.29   Contrast in brightness: the band in the middle which is uniform gray not only appears to vary in brightness, but also in width.

Another physiological sensory phenomenon makes brighter objects appear larger than darker ones. A woman's "little black dress" makes her appear thinner than her other dresses (Fig. 7.29). If lighter and darker parts of an image are to have the same value optically, the brighter portion of the picture should take up one third of the image and the darker two thirds.

It is difficult to assess the emotional impact of an image since individual conditioning also plays a role. However, red generally has a strong impact and attracts attention (used for signals), blue is soothing, understated, and sober.

Gradient backgrounds

Gradient backgrounds from one color to white or—not as good—from one color to another avoid making objects appear as if in a catalog. They give the image a certain depth. As a rule, the brighter part of the background is at the top and the darker at the bottom (Fig. 7.30).

Gradient backgrounds can be created through lighting, but it is easier to buy special "fading effect" backgrounds from a photographic supplier. It is important to match the size of the card to that of the object. Photographing an individual crown against a 2-m long background does not make sense, since the blending occurs over the entire length of the card. In a small section of the image, the blending is not evident. All background effects and colors can also be created by image editing programs.

Fig. 7.30   "Fading effect" backgrounds are pleasant to look at because they correspond to our everyday perceptions, for example, in the appearance of the sky.

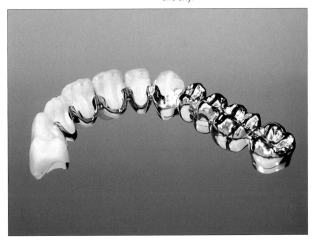

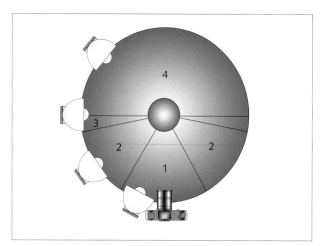

Fig. 7.31   Lighting is divided into axial front lighting (1), incident lighting (2), texture lighting (3) and backlighting (4).

7.4 Adequate lighting for objects

One of the most difficult tasks in dental photography is correctly lighting an object. The main function of lighting is to give an object presented on a two-dimensional image the appearance of a three-dimensional object, in other words, to reveal the shape. The second main consideration is texture, the visibility of which is dependent on the strength and direction of the lighting. The third consideration is tone and color.

The type of the light source and its direction must be carefully considered from various aspects. Light sources are divided into daylight and artificial light, and the latter into flash and constant light sources.

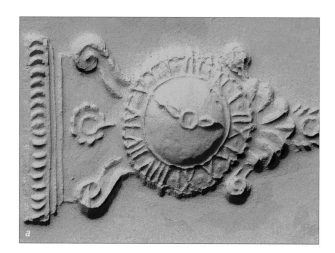

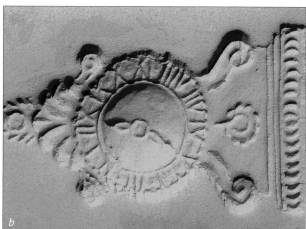

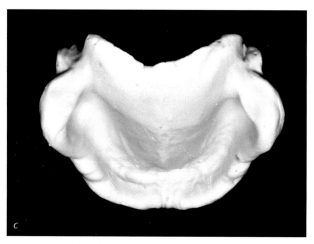

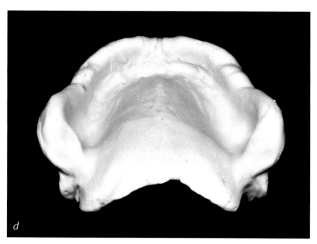

Fig. 7.32   The distribution of light and shadow edges influences our perception of depth. If the edge of the shadow is below and the light above, the object appears raised (a), otherwise as recessed (b). For this reason, in photographs of impressions, the recessed areas frequently appear raised (c and d). Thus, in object photography, the light should always come from above to create an image with correct rendering of the third dimension.

Light can be either incident or back lighting. Incident lighting is either axial (e.g., by using a ringflash), oblique, or texture lighting, which clearly emphasizes the surface details of the object (Fig. 7.31). In general, lighting should be as simple as possible. As a rule, a single light source is sufficient in most cases. It should also be noted that the main light should come from above. Since in the course of our evolution we are accustomed to having light from above from the sun, the pattern of light and shadows give us an idea of the three-dimensional quality of the object (Fig. 7.32). A rim of light on the upper part of the object and shadow underneath are perceived as a raised surface and the opposite as a depressed one. If this principle is ignored it can lead to irritating optical effects. An image of an impression, if lit improperly, can appear to be a dental cast and vice versa.

7.4.1   Types of lighting

Daylight – "Northlight"

Using daylight to light an object seems at first completely old-fashioned and insufficient. However, using daylight from a northern direction can achieve completely professional results without having to invest practically any money (Fig. 7.33).

In the early days of photography many photographers had studios which had north-facing windows and a window in the roof which faced north. The northerly direction avoided the sun shining in directly. For us, light from the north also has the most constant color temperature throughout the day and time of year, and largely avoids color casts.

Fig. 7.33   Photography using north light. In the early history of photography, photographers worked in north-facing studios (a). This prevented the sun shining in directly. A north-facing window is just as suitable for today's object photography (b). This ensures that the light has the most consistent color. With some experience, the photographer can achieve fine results which do not reveal their simple set-up (c).

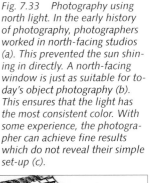

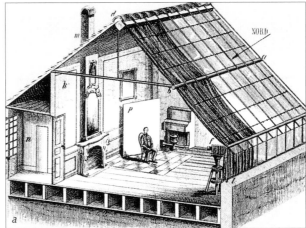

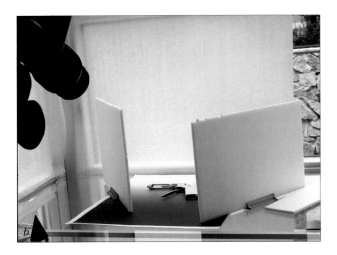

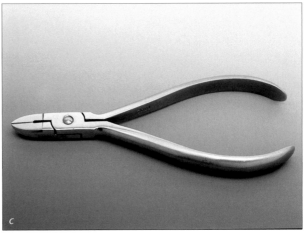

Photographing with light from the north is very simple. A work table is set up near a north-facing window. The light can be diffused by fixing drawing paper or a special diffusion foil to the window. The object is positioned, possibly isolated on a glass plate. The camera is placed on a tripod. The image is framed through the viewfinder and the aperture selected for the required depth of field (checked by using the depth of field preview button). Still checking through the viewfinder, the photographer illuminates the side of the object away from the light source using small reflectors (styrofoam from a hardware or home hobby store or reflectors from photographic suppliers). The shutter is triggered using a cable release to avoid camera vibrations or via the self-timer. To begin with, an exposure bracketing series is useful, though later this is necessary only with objects which are difficult for exposure metering. Exposure should be checked using the camera's histogram function. With some practice this type of inexpensive lighting can achieve very good results.

This type of work can be improved by a custom white-balance setting and/or a gray card.

A disadvantage of north lighting is dependency on daylight. In order to solve this problem, artificial light must be used.

Artificial light

If object photography must be performed frequently, artificial light is more commonly used. This type of lighting is divided into flash lighting and constant light sources. Both can be used and have their advantages and disadvantages. Digital photography takes away most of the stress caused by color rendition under different lighting conditions.

Electronic flash

Electronic flash is frequently used, as flashguns suitable for dental photography are available anyway (Fig. 7.34). Other advantages are the daylight character of the light (its color temperature is balanced for the flash white-balance setting of the camera) and the short duration of the flash, which eliminates the problem of camera shake. Electronic flashguns are compact, do not take up much room, and are available in a wide range of types.

A disadvantage of flashguns is that the effect of the light cannot be assessed because of its short duration. The photographer must be quite experienced to achieve the best possible distribution of light and shadow, or take a lot of exposures to achieve a good image.

Fig. 7.34   If electronic flash is used for technical photography, the beam of light should be spread by using a diffuser.

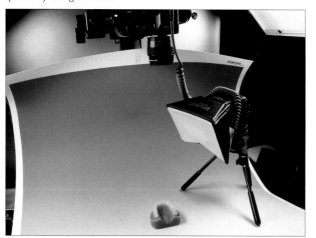

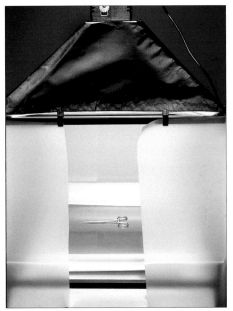

Fig. 7.35 *Studio flash lights have a built-in constant light source which can be used as modelling lamp. This allows control of the distribution of light and shadow.*

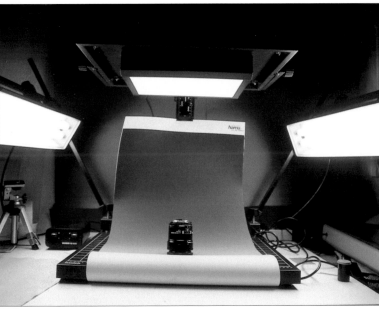

Fig. 7.36 *Constant light sources such as the light banks and the light box mounted above allow the illumination to be checked in the viewfinder.*

Studio flash

Professional flash units overcome this disadvantage of electronic flash by adding a constant light source to the flash tubes (Fig. 7.35). While looking into the viewfinder, the photographer can adjust the flash position until the desired light-shadow combination is created. The object is then photographed using flash. The flash output is ascertained in advance using a flash meter. Such studio flash units are available in a very great variety, with many accessories which concentrate or diffuse the light. The purchase of such lighting units for dental photography is worthwhile only if they are frequently used.

Continuous light

Continuous light allows the photographer to assess the effect of the lighting and the distribution of light and shadow in the viewfinder before the exposure is made (Fig. 7.36).

When using conventional silver halide photography one of the major problems was color rendition depending on the type of light source. Each source of light has a different color temperature.

In digital photography this problem can be solved easily by white-balancing the camera.

7.4.2   White balancing

There are different ways to capture images with natural looking colors.

If the color temperature of the light source is known, the white balance system of the camera can be preset according to this value.

Some examples:

- Incandescent light   3000 °Kelvin
- Fluorescent light   4200 °Kelvin
- Flash light   5400 °Kelvin

In many cases, this procedure will give satisfactory results, but it is not the most precise way.

Custom white-balance setting

Especially when working under mixed lighting conditions, it is recommended to meter the color temperature using the digital camera. Afterwards, the system adjusts the image so that its colors appear as if shot in daylight.

The procedure in detail depends on the individual camera (look into the camera's manual), but in principal it is always the same. The camera is aimed at a white piece of paper or a neutral gray card in the same light which is used to take the subsequent pictures (Fig. 7.37). A "white balance shot" is done, telling the system how to neutralize the following shots.

Getting perfect results is easy when every light source has the same color temperature. Problems arise if there is a mix of ambient light (e.g., daylight) and tungsten light. Even a carefully set custom white balance cannot avoid areas—especially those in shadows or at a larger distance from the light source—which are contaminated by the ambient light and are thus not properly color balanced.

Fig. 7.37   White balancing can be done by using a gray card, which fills the frame of the camera (a). After removing the gray card, the object can be photographed.

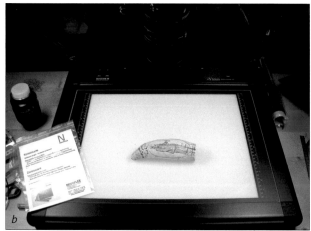

There are different ways to avoid these problems:

- Block out daylight as far as possible.
- Use artificial light with a color temperature of daylight (e.g., 5000°Kelvin fluorescent bulbs).
- Take the first photograph with a gray card included. This gray card can be used by the image editing program to neutralize the colors. Changes can be stored and used afterwards for the other images of this session.

7.4.3 Checking exposure – using a gray card

With a digital camera, not only can you optimize color rendition, but also image exposure.

A gray card is a piece of paper, cardboard, or plastic with a defined reflectivity (nearly 18%). This corresponds with a middle gray. If you take a shot of the gray card under the same lighting conditions as your object shots are performed, you can adjust exposure by manual setting and you can check it afterwards using the histogram (Fig. 7.38).

Advanced cameras offer the possibility to show a histogram of the images. If your camera does not offer a histogram function, you should check it using an image editing program as long as you are able to repeat the shot. A histogram is a bar graph; here, it shows the distribution of brightness levels in the image. In more detail, it shows how many pixels have which of the possible 256 brightness levels. The horizontal axis shows the brightness levels beginning with 0 (shadows) and ending with 255 (highlights). The vertical axis shows the number of pixels that have each of the 256 levels. The higher the peaks of the curve, the more pixels have that corresponding brightness level.

The distribution of the pixels is important for checking an image. If there is an even distribution of the pixels in the middle three-quarters of all possible brightness

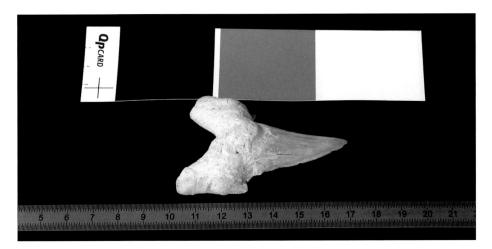

Fig. 7.38   The first shot of an object can be done with a gray card and a millimeter scale in the viewing field of the camera. This helps to find the correct exposure and a neutral color, and also gives information about the size of the object.

levels, the image has a broad dynamic range (also called tonal range) and sufficient contrast. If the pixels clump together in the middle of the scale, the image has low contrast and a narrow tonal range. The distribution of the pixels depends on the exposure of your image and on the image's content.

A high-key image (very light image content) or an overexposed image shows the peaks of the histogram curve shifted to the right. Digital imaging chips are like color transparency film in this regard. Once the highlights are blown out, image information is lost. A low-key (dark content) or underexposed image has the majority of its pixels on the left side. Digital imaging has a remarkable ability to extract detail from the shadows. It is best to expose digitally as much toward the right side of the histogram as possible without blowing out the highlights. In other words, overexposure is preferable to underexposure in terms of maximizing dynamic range and minimizing digital noise.

If your shot of the gray card is exposed correctly, the histogram only shows a spike just in the middle of the horizontal axis. There is no even distribution of gray values, as the gray card only has middle gray values. If the peak is more to the left, the image is underexposed; if more to the right, the image is overexposed.

Then you can compensate exposure take the gray card away and take your object shots under the same lighting conditions.

In addition, you can use a gray scale (e.g., Kodak Gray Scale) to check if your camera captures the whole range of tone values. Such a gray scale shows twenty increments between white and black. An overexposed image shows white tones which cannot be separated sufficiently; an underexposed one does not separate the dark tones.

BACKGROUND

Maximizing image information

Many modern DSLRs record a 12-bit image. (To increase confusion, this is often referred to as 16-bit image, but in reality the camera records 12 bits in a 16-bit space.) That means that such a camera is capable to record 4,096 discrete tonal values (2^{12}). If a digital image has a dynamic range of five or six stops, these 4096 tonal values are not distributed evenly over these five stops. The first stop (the brightest) contains half of the available amount (2048 tonal values). Each subsequent stop records half again of the remainder. Because each f/stop records half the light of the previous amount, only one-half of the remaining data space is available.

From this table, the following information can be derived: Half of the data of a 12-bit image reside in the brightest stop. If you do not use this range, because you underexpose your image, you waste half of the available encoding levels of your camera. On the other hand,

12-bit raw file	
First f/stop, brightest tones	2048 levels available
Second f/stop, bright tones	1024 levels available
Third f/stop, mid-tones	512 levels available
Fourth f/stop, mid-tones	256 levels available
Fifth f/stop, dark tones	128 levels available
Sixth f/stop, darkest tones	64 levels available

if you overexpose the image, you blow out the highlights (past the right edge of the histogram). Blown-out highlights contain no image information, which was exactly the case in slide photography.

When shooting digitally, exposure should be adjusted in a way that the usable range of the scene is as far to the right of the middle of the histogram as possible without blowing out the highlights. When working in RAW mode, exposure can be adjusted during RAW conversion to a more pleasing image. In this manner, a maximum of the data space available has been used.

Trying to bring back details after underexposing results in wasted bits and the risk of substantially increased noise in the mid- and dark tones.

7.4.4   Direction of light

The direction of light is also as important as the type of light source. Typical examples are given below which can be achieved with either continuous light sources or electronic flash. The direction of the light is the main factor in the character of the image and the rendering of the object's shape, texture and color.

Incident light/oblique lighting

The most common practice is to light the object from above using incident light (Fig. 7.39). Generally, this requires only one light source. Light falling from one side is supplemented by reflectors which illuminate the side of the object away from the light. Such reflectors can be obtained from photographic suppliers (e.g., Lumiquest Table Top Reflector System). Small styrofoam sheets are just as good for this purpose and less expensive; these can be positioned next to the object. If the sheets are moved closer to the object the light is intensified; if moved further away the image has more lighting contrast (Fig. 7.40). Instead of styrofoam sheets, shaving mirrors and wrinkled aluminium foil can be used.

Fig. 7.39   Object photographs generally require only one light source. The unlighted side of the subject is illuminated by a reflector (R) (a). This principle is also used in professional photography (b).

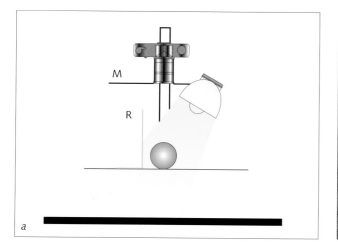

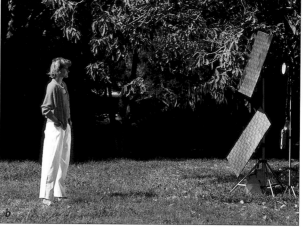

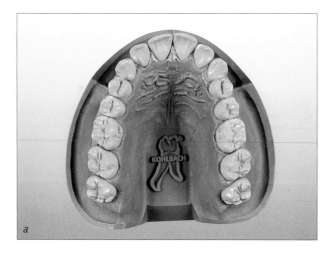

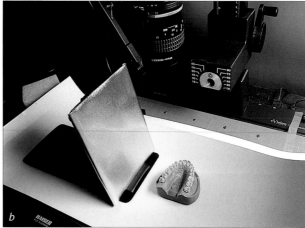

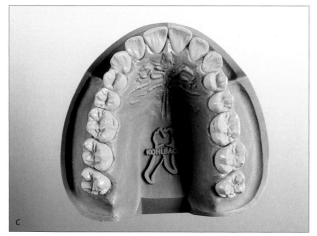

Fig. 7.40   Symmetrical lighting frequently results in images which are not sufficiently plastic (a). If a single light source and a reflector (b) are used, the images appear more three dimensional (c).

Lighting an object symmetrically from the right and the left side leads to a flat appearance, since the object is largely without shadows, giving very little information about the three-dimensional nature of the object (Fig. 7.41). Using the built-in flash normally does not yield the best results, as the light is very hard and cannot be modified either in its direction or its surface. Ring flash gives very flat results. It can only be recommended if objects are very small. To increase directionality of light, single flash reflectors can be switched off or their light output can be reduced. Another possibility is to take the ring flash off the camera and hold it to one side of the object manually.

Twin flashes (e.g., Canon, Olympus, Nikon) can be used in a symmetrical arrangement or to produce unsymmetrical lighting, which often gives better results.

Modern digital camera systems allow the use of dedicated flash. Here, the direction of the flash is more variable and indirect lighting via reflectors is possible.

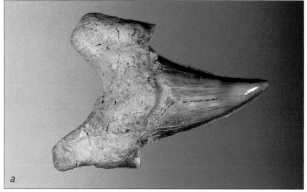

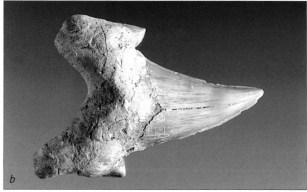

Fig. 7.41   Symmetrical lighting of a fossil using a copy stand (a). A better result is achieved using direct lighting with a reflector illuminating the shadow details (b).

Diffuser-reflector lighting

This is essentially the same type of lighting as oblique lighting, only with diffused light. Using a point flash with a small reflector rarely achieves satisfactory results. To achieve pleasant lighting, the size of the light-emitting surface and the object should be in a good relation to each other (Fig. 7.42). A very small light source leads to harsh lighting with a lot of contrast and marked divisions between light and shadow. A typical example of this is illumination by the sun on a cloudless day which results in unflattering portraits. It is better when the emitting surface of the light source is increased, as is the case on an overcast day.

The emitting surface of the light can be increased by placing a diffuser, that is, a transparent medium which scatters light, in front of the light source (Fig. 7.43). The hard light hits the diffuser and a part of it goes through, making the diffuser the light source. Very good dif-

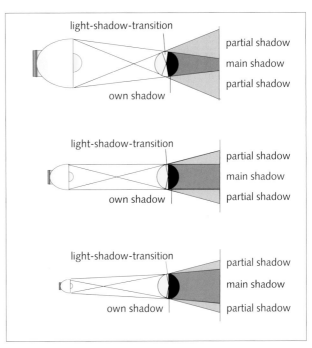

Fig. 7.42   *The illuminating surface of a light source should be significantly greater than the object. Only in this way can soft transitions between light and shadow and pleasant lighting effects be created.*

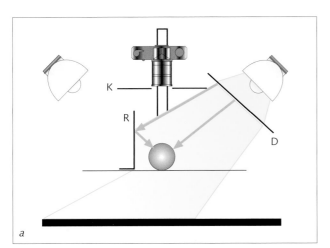

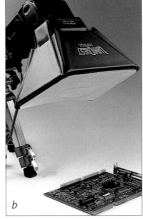

Fig. 7.43   *Diagram of lighting using a diffuser and reflector, which achieves the best results in technical photography (a). The light-emitting surface of a flashgun can be increased using a soft box (b). This produces less harsh lighting (d), in contrast to the image made without using a soft box (c).*

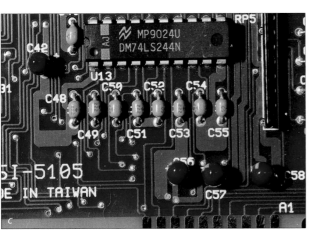

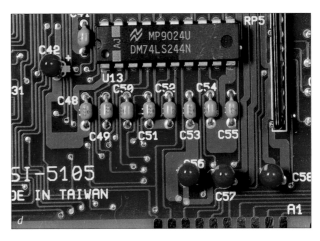

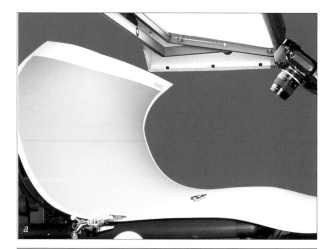

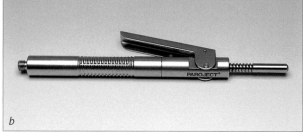

fusers can be made using stretchers (art supply stores) and vellum attached to them by tape. Special diffuser gels and accessories for flash units (e.g., soft boxes) are designed for this.

Another way to increase the reflective surface of a flash and to soften its light is to use a flash reflector or to bounce the flash light off styrofoam sheets or specially designed umbrellas.

The same principles of enlarging the light surface can be applied to continuous light sources, giving us the chance to control the lighting effect (distribution of light and shadows) before taking the picture just by looking into the viewfinder.

Light banks and light boxes, formerly used for checking slides, have very large illuminating surfaces; these generally have a "diffuser" in the form of an opal screen (Fig. 7.44). If the size of the illuminating surface is increased and one or more reflectors are moved closer to the object, it is possible to bathe the object in light and achieve the effect of a light tent.

Fig. 7.44   A light box is ideal for incident lighting since it puts out a broad, soft light. Check to make sure it is daylight balanced (a). Images taken using this simple arrangement do not betray this simplicity (b).

Three-point lighting

A more sophisticated lighting arrangement for objects is the three-point lighting.

The main light, also called key light, comes from one side and a little bit above the object. A second light, the fill light, comes from the other side and illuminates the shadow areas created by the main light. It is 2 or 3 stops less intense and gives the

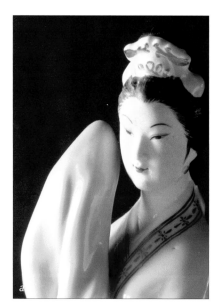
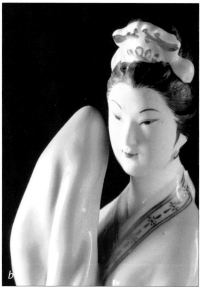
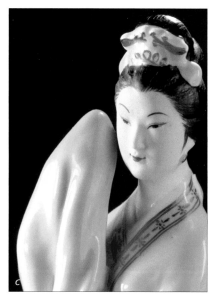

Fig. 7.45   Three-point illumination. One main light (key light) illuminates the object (a). A second one (or a reflector) serves as a fill light (b). A third one coming from behind and above illuminates the contour of the object (c).

shadows more detail. The function of the fill light can also be fulfilled by a reflector. The third light comes from behind the object and creates a bright contour. Its function is to let the object stand out in front of the dark background (Fig. 7.45 a-c).

Sometimes a background light can be necessary in order to control the lightness of the background, or to eliminate shadows cast on the background.

Light tents

Objects made of highly polished metal and chrome instruments not only reflect the light source(s) but also their dark surroundings, as these are far removed. This creates very light highlights and practically black surfaces, making it difficult to assess the object's surface and its natural color. It is therefore advisable to photograph such highly reflective objects using a light tent (Fig. 7.46). The combination of reflective and diffusing surfaces creates large reflections on the metal surface, leading to a better rendering of the object's surface.

Such light tents are sold by photographic suppliers in many types and sizes (Fig. 7.47). With a little skill and talent for improvisation, however, the photographer can build her or his own light tent from materials available from hardware stores. All light tents are principally cylindrical, conical, cubic, or semi-round forms which can be made of transparent paper or other transparent materials. Plastic drinking cups with the bottom removed or white silk which is intended for silk painting can be used. The photographer is limited only by his or her imagination. Conical and cylindrical paper shapes have proven themselves; these can be made in different sizes for different reproduction ratios. Since light tents create not only large reflective areas but also diffuse lighting which is practically without shadows, the objects can often be placed directly on a photo cardboard without creating irritating shadows.

If the object needs sharper contours, a black piece of cardboard can be glued in the transparent cylinder; its reflection falls on the surface of the object as a shadow adding some modelling on that side. Another way to increase plasticity is positioning a light source in the light tent (Fig. 7.48). Examples of light tent photographs are shown in Figs 7.49 to 7.52.

Using a dulling spray is another means of improving the appearance of highly polished metal surfaces.

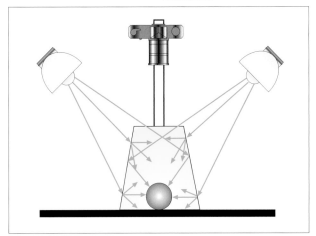

Fig. 7.46   A light tent surrounds the object from all sides and thus creates large, enclosed reflections.

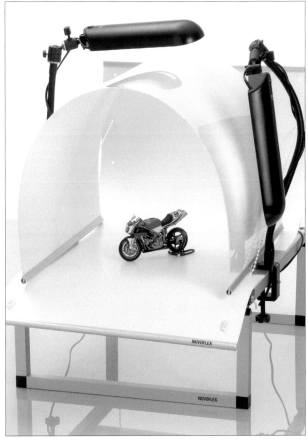

Fig. 7.47   A light dome generates even reflections on the subject (Photo: Novoflex).

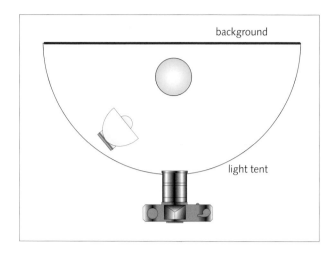

background

light tent

Fig. 7.48
A light source within the light tent provides more directional light.

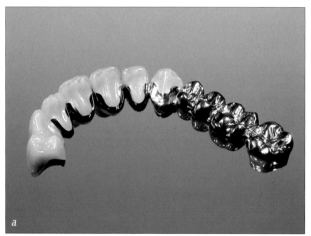

a   b

Fig. 7.49   *A highly reflective object photographed without (a) and with (b) light tent.*

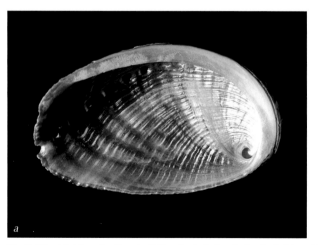

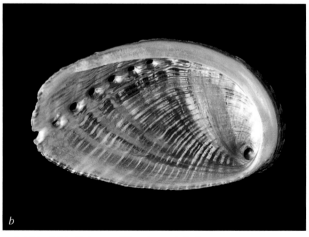

a   b

Fig. 7.50   *Highly reflective shell illuminated directly by flash (a) and in a light tent (b). Color rendition is much better.*

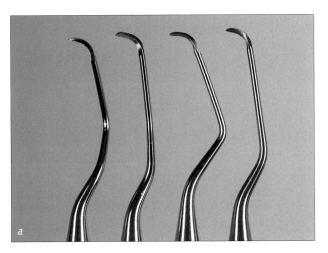

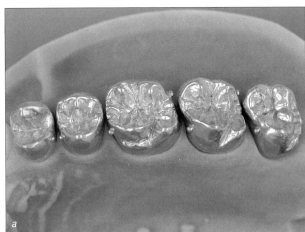

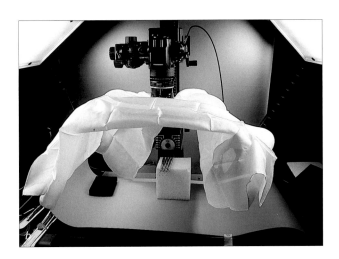

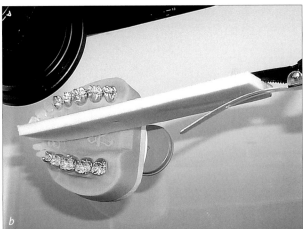

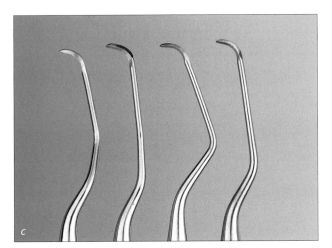

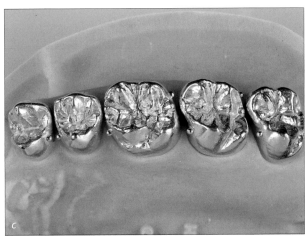

Fig. 7.51   Curettes lit by two light banks (a), set-up of a simple light tent (b) and the result of photographing using the light tent (c).

Fig. 7.52   Sometimes the illumination using a light tent is too "soft" (a). In these instances, a simple reflector (b) can be used to improve results (c).

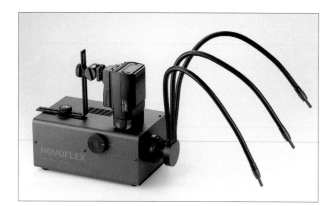

Fig. 7.53   *Novoflex Cold Light Source Macrolight Plus (Photo: Novoflex).*

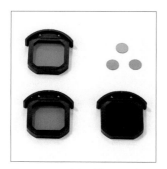

Fig. 7.54   *A blue filter can be placed in front of the light source to provide daylight balanced light. Light output can be reduced if necessary by using a gray filter (Photo: Novoflex).*

Especially for lighting coins, it is recommended that a thin glass plate should be placed 45 degrees to the optical axis and photographed through. The glass plate is lit from the side and part of the light is directed vertically off its surface onto the coin.

Rendering surfaces of small objects

A photographer trying to recreate the morphology of a tooth's surface in a light tent soon discovers that this is possible only to a limited extent, since there is not much contrast on the predominantly white occlusal surface. To do this, a flat, directed light (texture lighting) is required in order to show the surface morphology by creating shadows. Various manufacturers produce fiber-optic light sources for this purpose (Figs 7.53 and 7.54). The most important qualities to look for in this type of equipment is the rigidity of the light conducting arms, the variety of accessories, and the ability to change the color temperature of the integrated halogen light source permanently by using a blue filter in front of it. One recommended system is the fiber optic light source from Novoflex; its light arms are positioned on the top and thus their position is easily retained. This system not only has color and polarizing filters which are placed in front of the light emitting arms, but also a slot in which a conversion filter can be left long-term. An electronic flash system can be used in place of the halogen light source; its flash can be directed into the light pipes through a mirror system. This arrangement allows moving objects to be photographed. Very creative solutions for lighting, especially of very small objects, can be achieved in this manner (Figs 7.55 to 7.57).

Moving light / painting with light

Very interesting results can be obtained using a long exposure with the illumination provided by a moving light. This type of lighting can only be used in a darkened room. It needs some experience, but as we can check the results immediately when using a digital camera, it is worth trying. Results are not as reproducible as with a standard technique but look very interesting.

Transmitted lighting

When the light source is positioned behind an object, we call this transmitted lighting; this is naturally useful for (semi-)transparent objects.

As in microscopy we use the term bright field illumination when the object's surroundings appear bright. If they are dark or black, they are termed dark field illumination.

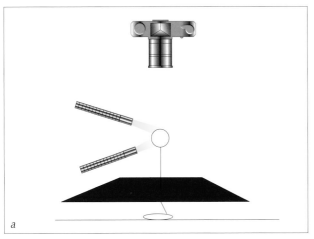

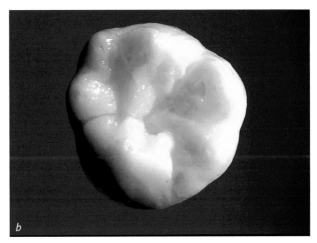

Fig. 7.55   *Fiber optic light sources permit individual and creative lighting effects using only one piece of equipment. Arrangement of fiber optic light sources (a) and the result (b).*

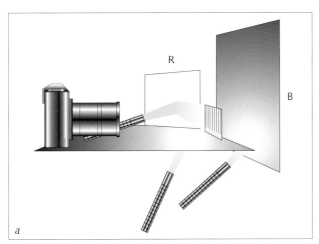

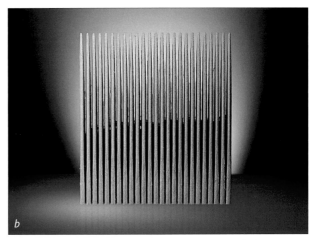

Fig. 7.56   *This image too does not reveal the secret of its simple set-up. Diagram of the fiber optic light sources (a) and result (b).*

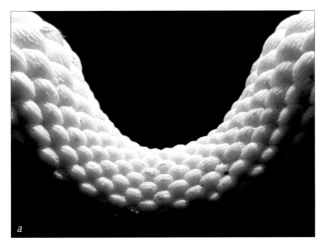

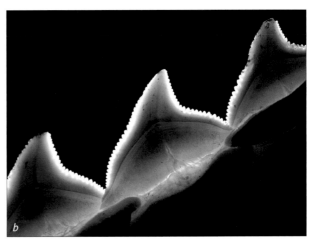

Fig. 7.57   *The texture of these ray teeth is emphasized by fibre optic illumination (a). The semi-transparent shark teeth are transilluminated with a fiber-optic light source (b).*

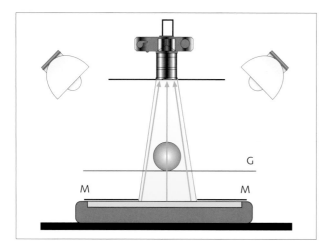

Fig. 7.58   Diagram of a transmitted light arrangement (bright-field illumination). The object is placed on a glass support (G) and is illuminated from beneath. The light box outside of the camera's view is masked off with black cardboard (M) to prevent stray light from entering the lens.

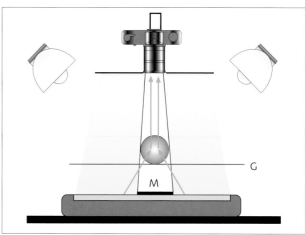

Fig. 7.60   Set-up of a dark-field illumination. The background of the object is covered using an opaque mask (M). The object is lit by the light surrounding the mask.

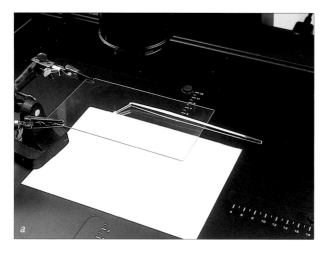

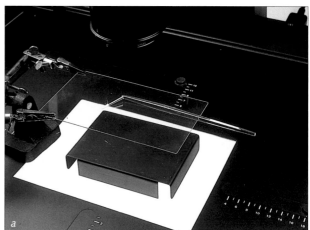

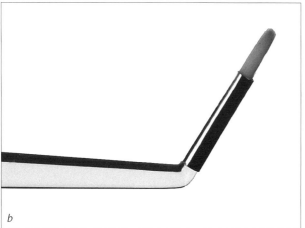

Fig. 7.59   A simple arrangement for a bright field illumination photo (a) and the result (b).

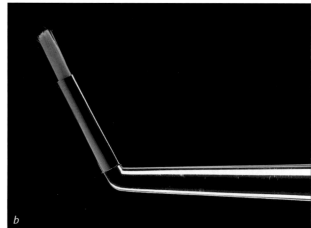

Fig. 7.61   Set-up for a dark-field photo (a) and the result (b).

Bright-field illumination

In this instance, the light source is in back of or below the object within the camera's field of view. This light, coming from behind or below, passes through the object and the light which passes the object to the side creates the brightness around the object (Fig. 7.58). This allows transparent or partially transparent objects to be photographed.

To avoid flare and unnecessary loss of brilliance due to the dispersed light falling on the lens, the area surrounding the camera's field of view should be covered with black cardboard (masking).

A plus exposure correction should be used when photographing an object with a white background in order to achieve correct exposure (Fig. 7.59).

Dark-field illumination

In this case, the light source (for example, a light box) is behind or under the object; however, its surface, about the size of the camera's field of view, is covered with black cardboard so that it is opaque (Fig. 7.60). The object itself is about 10 cm in front of or above the light source. This allows the light rays from the light source to strike and illuminate the object (Fig. 7.61). This type of illumination achieves striking effects. Filigree and objects with partially transparent surfaces are particularly suitable for this and show up very clearly against a black background. Minus corrections of exposure must be made to avoid overexposure, depending on the size of the object's surface in relation to the frame.

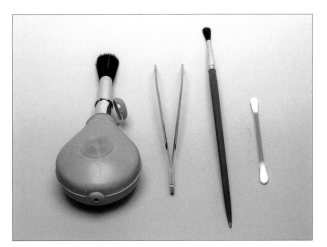

Fig. 7.62   Small tools helpful in cleaning off dust particles for dark-field illumination photos.

Glass supports must be free of dust and dirt when used to photograph objects in isolation, since dust particles also light up in the dark field and make the image unusable (Fig. 7.62). Dust can be removed by using canned air, soft brushes or Q-tips.

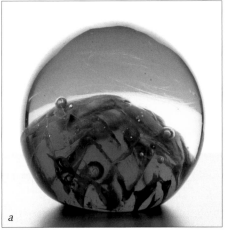
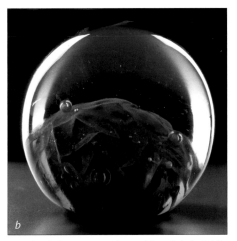

Fig. 7.63   Transparent objects appear differently in bright-field illumination photos (a) and dark-field illumination photos (b).

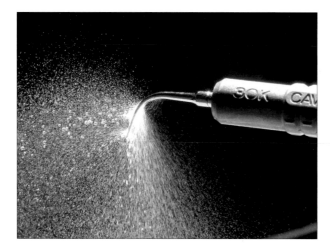

Fig. 7.64   Very fine structures such as the spray droplets are illuminated in dark-field illumination photographs. The spray would merely be visible in a bright field illumination photograph.

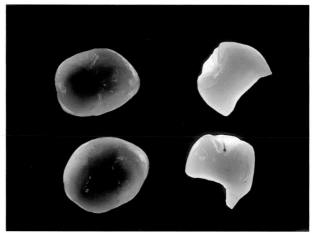

Fig. 7.65   Dark-field illumination photo to illustrate the varying transparency of metal ceramic crowns (left) and Procera crowns (right in photo).

The room should be darkened to improve the visability of the dust particles. Once the photographer's eyes have become adjusted to the dark, he or she can use the depth of field preview button to check for dust and remove it with a small brush or cotton tip. A minus correction is required for dark field illumination to achieve a truly black background (Figs 7.63 to 7.65).

Photographing with polarized transmitted lighting

This type of lighting, which is very easy to achieve, results not only in very impressive images, but also allows the background brightness to be infinitely varied. A polarizing filter sheet is placed in front of the light source and the second polarizing filter on the camera lens (Figs 7.66 and 7.67). The light falling in the direction of the camera is polarized by the polarizing filter. The photographer rotates the second polarizing filter on the camera lens while checking in the viewfinder. If the polarizing axes of the two filters are perpendicular to each other, all the light is cut off. However, the direction of the oscillations of the light passing through the object are altered and are thus not blocked completely by the polarizing filter on the camera lens. The result is that the object appears in its natural colors in front of a background which appears to be bright, gray, blue or black, depending how the filter is rotated (Fig. 7.68).

Materials which are double-refractive appear in all colors of the rainbow in polarized transmitted light. Sections of teeth, for instance, can be photographed very impressively in this manner (Fig. 7.69).

Inner stresses of plastic objects can also be shown when they are photographed using two crossed polar-

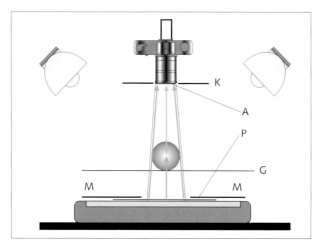

Fig. 7.66   Polarized transmitted light creates interesting effects. A polarizing filter (called a polarisator = P) is placed on the light box; the second one, the analyzer, is fitted on the lens (A).

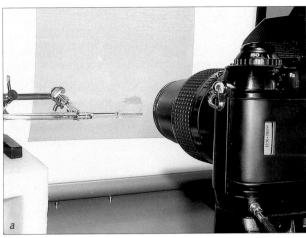

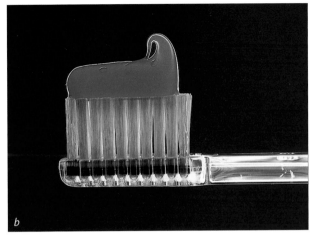

Fig. 7.67   *Photographing horizontally using polarized transmitted light (a). A polarizing sheet has been fixed to a light box stood vertically. A second polarizing filter is fitted to the lens. If both polarizing filters are adjusted so that they are nearly perpendicular, the background appears dark blue (b).*

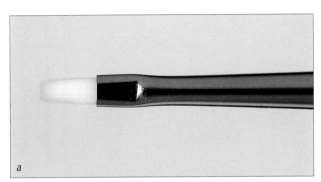

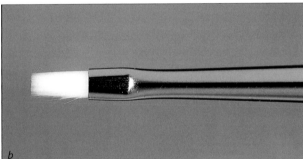

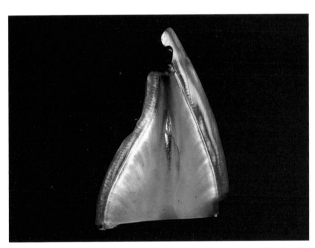

Fig. 7.69   *Many materials are double refractive, such as this tooth, which is shown as a section in all the colors of the rainbow.*

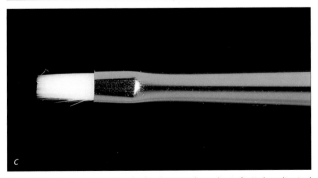

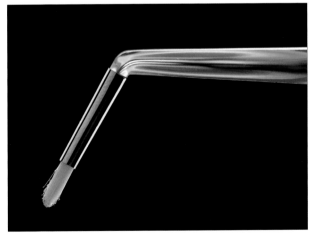

Fig. 7.68   *The brightness of a background can be infinitely adjusted by using polarized transmitted lighting. The brightness varies in accordance with the adjustment of the polarizing filter on the camera (a-c). The surface of the object was additionally lit from the top.*

Fig. 7.70   *Polarized transmitted lighting is also used for showing mechanical stresses. Internal mechanical stresses are rendered as color bands. The image shows this type of mechanical stress in the handle of a small brush.*

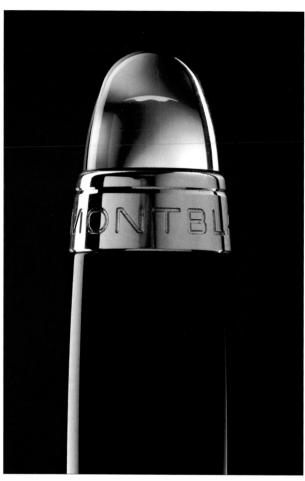

Fig. 7.71   Normal objects of daily life (like this cap of a pen) appear much more interesting in polarized transmitted light.

izing filters, which are known in photoelastic strain analysis as the polarizer and analyzer. The molecular formations occurring under mechanical stress cause varying degrees of shifts in the main oscillation direction of the polarized light and the analyzer thus blocks the light to varying degrees. The result is a rainbow of colors within the object; their arrangement gives some information about the stress peaks (Fig. 7.70). In this way, for example, implant forms were studied in order to investigate the load to bone.

Polarized transmitted lighting is a very simple lighting method that yields esthetic results (Fig. 7.71).

Photography of dental casts

8

The assessment of casts is one of the important bases of diagnosis and treatment planning not only in orthodontics, but also in prosthetic dentistry. For the purposes of organization and improvement of documentation, it makes sense in many instances to take photographs of the models. Due to its intrinsic problems, photography of casts is dealt with in a chapter of its own.

Special problems in photographing casts

Models not only provide information about the three-dimensional arrangement of the teeth in relation to each other, but also about their size and the size of the dental arch. Thus it is recommended that a millimeter scale placed about the level of the occlusal plane be photographed along with the model. This permits prints to be made subsequently at the correct scale. Alternatively, a fixed magnification ratio of 1:2 can be used permanently.

Casts are generally of uniform color and often white, with a very low level of contrast. Pretreatment of the models with soap, talcum powder, or special polish, which is normal practice to protect them from dirt, gives these models a shiny surface; this in turn improves the three-dimensional nature of the image due to the resulting highlights. Close attention should be paid to lighting in order to increase the three dimensional appearance of the model.

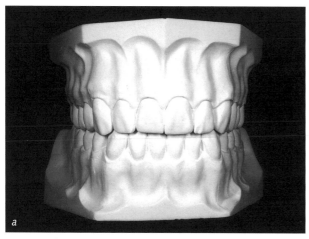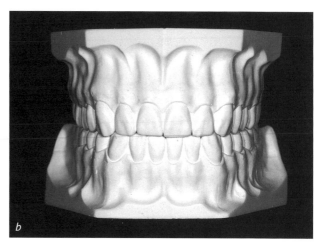

a   b

Fig. 8.1   If the focal leagth of the lens is too short—here a 50-mm lens—it distorts the perspective of the cast (a). A 105-mm lens repro-duces the cast as it would normally appear to us when viewed from a normal distance (b).

8.1   Technical considerations

8.1.1   Camera

There are no specific requirements for the camera other than those for clinical photography. It is important to use a lens with a focal length of about 100 mm in order to avoid distorted perspective (Fig. 8.1). A 60-mm macro lens can be used with a digital SLR camera with a cropfactor of 1.5. A focusing screen with a grid aids in achieving properly aligned photographs.

Fig. 8.2   Model on a copy stand. In this case too, only one light source is needed. The side away from the light is illuminated by using a reflector.

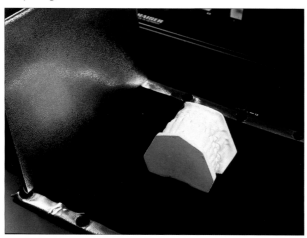

8.1.2   Stabilization of camera and model

The goal should be to produce images which are taken under defined and therefore reproducible conditions.

If models are photographed frequently, a copy stand should be purchased (Fig. 8.2). A prerequisite for speedy work is a correct trimming of the casts, which should always remain in the correct position without having to be supported. A copy stand can be fairly easily modified for photographing models. Two screw clamps can be used to attach a plate perpendicular to the groundplate. By rotating the entire copy stand almost 90 degrees, which brings the vertical column almost into a horizontal position, the models can be placed onto the plate so that they do not fall off

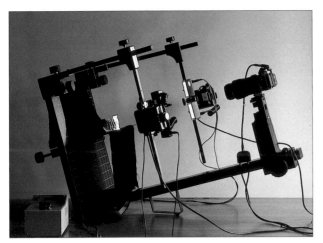

Fig. 8.3   *A copy stand modified with a perpendicular plate fixed to the ground board.*

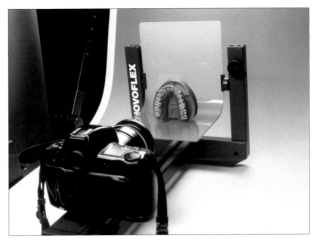

Fig. 8.4   *Macro/Reprostand from Novoflex.*

(Fig. 8.3). The Novoflex Macro/Reprostand is also suitable; this allows the camera to be attached in a similar manner to that of an optical bench (Fig. 8.4). However, the camera guide rail length must be increased.

8.1.3   Background

The most common background is black velvet or card-board, or a black plastic sheet (Fig. 8.5). The usually light-colored casts show up well against these back-grounds and the shadows they produce are not visible, as they are "swallowed".

If color backgrounds are desired, these can be select-ed and arranged in accordance with the principles cov-ered in the chapter on object photography.

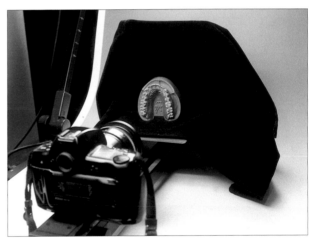

Fig. 8.5   *A black velvet cloth is used to isolate the model in front of a black background.*

8.1.4   Lighting

A single light source, whether electronic flash or a constant light source, is sufficient. A rotatable side flash attached to the camera or a side flash connected by cable are suitable. If a copy stand is used, its lights can of course be used. Figures 8.6 to 8.12 show typical lighting arrangements and their results.

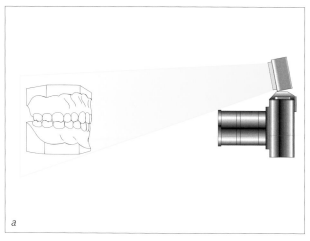
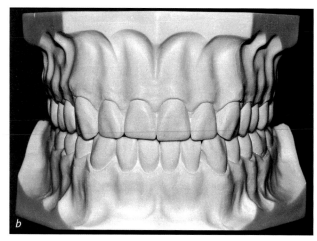

Fig. 8.6   *Frontal view of the model with flash in 12:00 position. Diagram (a) and result (b).*

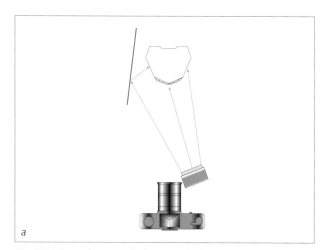
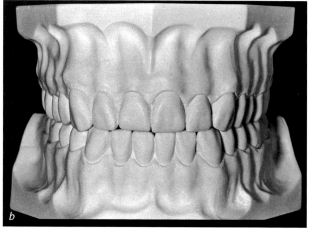

Fig. 8.7   *Frontal view with directional side lighting. The side away from the light is illuminated with a reflector. Diagram (a) and result (b).*

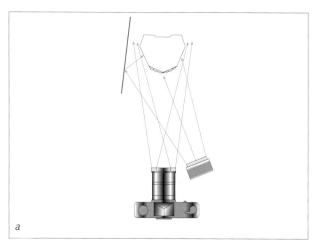
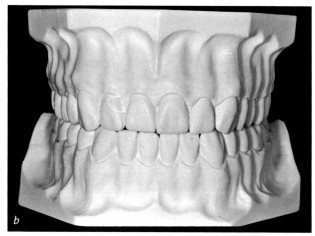

Fig. 8.8   *Frontal view with ring flash/point flash combination. Diagram (a) and result (b).*

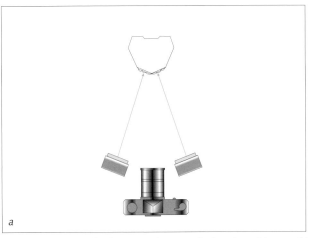
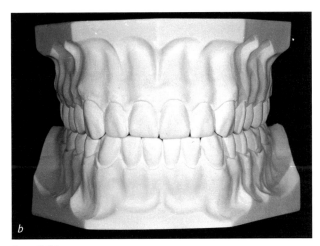

Fig. 8.9   *Photograph of a cast with a twin flash system. Diagram (a) and result (b).*

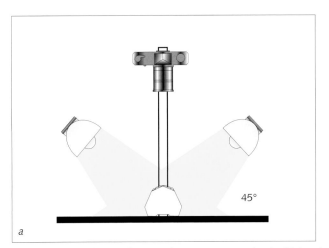
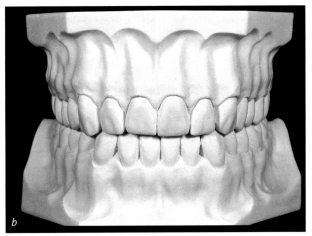

Fig. 8.10   *Frontal view of a cast taken using a copy stand with four lamps. Diagram (a) and result (b). If the top lamps only are switched, the light forms a shadow line below the maxillary incisors which clearly separate the maxilla and mandible.*

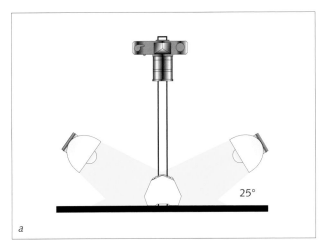
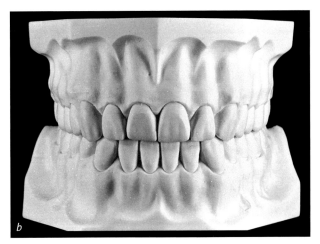

Fig. 8.11   *Light angled on a copy stand at a shallow angle increases the plasticity of the front teeth. Diagram (a) and result (b).*

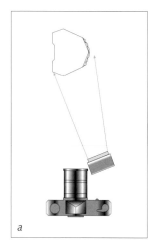

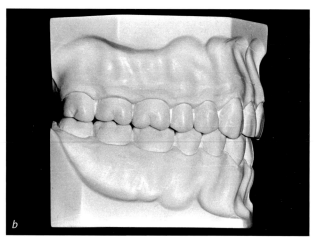

Fig. 8.12 When photographing a lateral view of a cast, the side flash should always be positioned on the side with the front teeth. Diagram (a) and result (b).

8.2   Standard images – Model status

The standard views correspond in general to those of intraoral photography: frontal view, two lateral views, two occlusal views. Thus, there are five standard views.

All images are made in horizontal format. If white models are photographed, an exposure compensation of about 1 to 1 ⅓ (Plus) stops is required so that the surface is reproduced brightly enough.

8.2.1   Frontal view

The center of the photograph is at the contact point of the upper incisors. Focus on the canines (Fig. 8.13). The occlusion plane is horizontal. The model is illuminated with a flash fitted to the camera at the 12:00 o'clock position or a light source from the side plus illumination of the opposite side using a reflector. If the photographer has a copy stand with two lights on the right and the left, the lights on the mandibular side should be switched off. This achieves a fine shadow contour below the maxillary incisors.

Fig. 8.13 The composition in photographing the frontal view of a model should correspond to the conventions of intraoral photography. Diagram (a) and result (b).

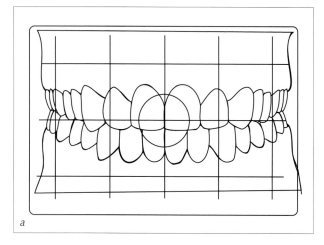

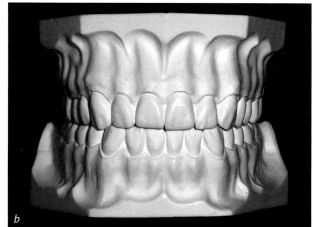

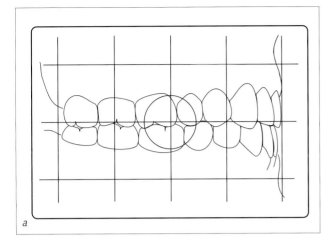

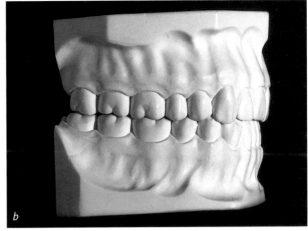

Fig. 8.14   Lateral view of a cast. Diagram (a) and result (b).

8.2.2   Lateral views

The center of the photo and the focus point are both around the second premolars or first molars (Fig. 8.14). Lighting should be from the side of the anterior teeth. The lighting should be angled so that the posterior teeth are separated by fine interdental shadow lines. This angle also makes the jugae alveolariae and the inserted ligaments visible.

8.2.3   Occlusal views

In this view, the center of the picture is at the intersection of the line joining the premolars and the sagittal plane (Figs 8.15-8.17). Focus on the fissures. Illumination is either with camera flash at the 12:00 o'clock position used with a reflector or with a side light plus reflector. If symmetrical lighting is provided by lights on a copy stand, it should be flat enough to clearly show the contours of the fissures.

Fig. 8.15
Mandible – occlusal view. Composition (a) and result (b).

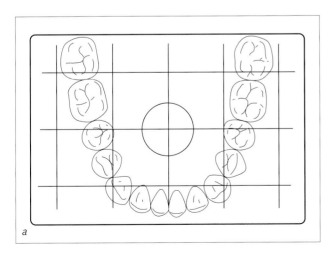

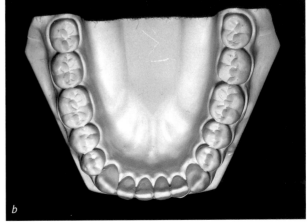

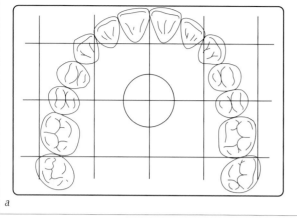

Fig. 8.16
Maxilla – occlusal view. Compositon (a) and result (b).

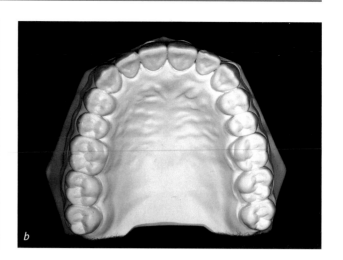

8.3   Special equipment for photographing casts

Only a few systems recommended in the literature and by commercial firms have proven of practical use. One of these is the Keil 3D model photo stand; this is an angled mirror which allows simultaneous photography of frontal and lateral views. Another system is the model photostat by Voss and the photo stand by Hinz which permit photography of the entire photostat in one image by the use of multiple exposures (Fig. 8.18). The problem is: not every digital SLR camera allows multiple exposures. Therefore taking single shots and arranging them on one page using an image editing software will be the normal procedure if a print for the patient's file is requested at all.

Checklist for photography of models
- Camera with 60/100-mm macro lens.
- Magnification ratio of 1:2.
- Exposure compensation +1 or 1 1/3 stops for white models.
- Positioning of the model using grid focusing screen.

Fig. 8.17
Both occlusal views can be photographed in a single image.

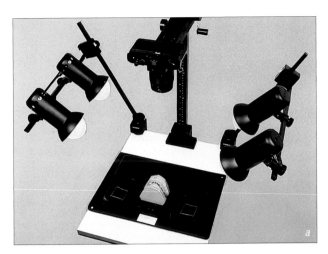

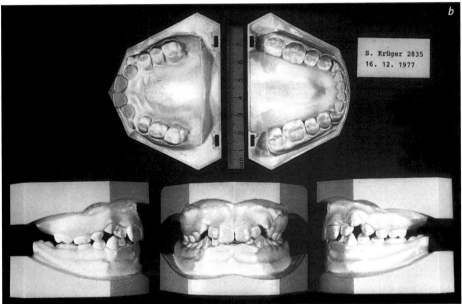

Fig. 8.18   *Hinz photo stand (a)*
and the resulting image with the
standard arrangement in one
photograph (b)
(Photos: ZFV-Verlag).
The same effect can be achieved
by putting together single shots
using an image editing software.

Copy work   9

The term "copy work" means the reproduction of images, text or objects for which the third dimension is not important (e.g., coins). In dental photography copies are used for instance for:

- Reproducing originals (text or images) for lectures or publications.
- Reproducing patient records relating to treatment in order to save space.
- Reproducing patients' photos for the dental technician.

The copying of radiographs is treated in a separate chapter due to its specific requirements.

9.1   Technical considerations

9.1.1   Camera

A camera suitable for clinical photography can also be easily used for copying. The focal length of the macro lens depends on the size of the original to be copied. Since there are no major perspective problems to be expected with flat documents, a 50 or 60 mm macro lens can also be used. Due to the crop factor of the camera, in most cases, the 50/60-mm lens is the better choice if the vertical column of the copy stand is not extremely long.

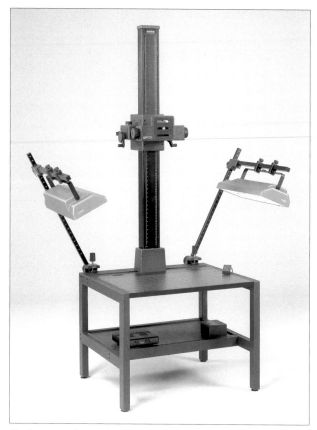

Fig. 9.1   For those who photograph frequently, a copy stand is
a sensible acquisition – and not
only for copying (Photo: Kaiser).

9.1.2   Camera stabilization – copy stands

In principle, it is possible to stabilize the camera using a tripod, but if a lot of copy work is required, it is better to purchase a copy stand, which—as has already been demonstrated—can also be used for other photographic purposes (Fig. 9.1).

The following criteria should be considered in the purchase of a copy stand:

- Good overall stability.
- Modular design.
- Large enough baseboard.
- Tall enough vertical column.
- Even illumination.

Many types of copy stands are available from photographic suppliers for the dedicated amateur or professional photographer.

One of the major advantages of digital photography is that the camera can be white balanced to a large extent independent of the color temperature of the light sources (Fig. 9.2). Opal lamps have a color temperature of about 2400°K to 2800°K. Nitraphot lamps have a color temperature of 3200°K. Daylight lamps have a color temperature of 5000°K.

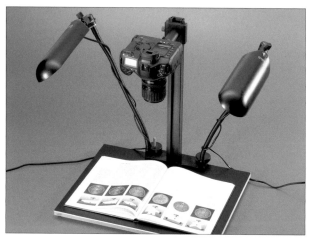

Fig. 9.2   Using a digital camera, every type of artificial light source
can be used as the camera can be white balanced (Photo:
Novoflex).

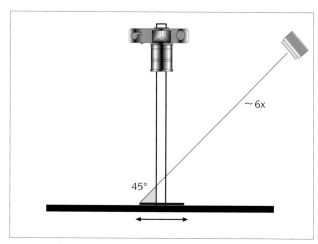

Fig. 9.3   If only one flashgun is available, it should be positioned
at a distance six times the width of the original. Only in this way
can an evenly lit copy be made.

Constant light sources can be used, or electronic flash. If only one flash is available, this should be placed as far away from the document as possible to achieve uniform lighting. As a rule of thumb, the distance between the flash and the document should be about six times the width of the document (Fig. 9.3).

9.2 Practical considerations

9.2.1 Lighting and framing

The original is placed on the baseboard and the camera fixed on the copy stand. Its exact vertical placement can be checked with a spirit level, but it is even simpler to use a mirror placed on the base board. By looking through the viewfinder, the camera position can be altered until the lens opening is directly in the mirror.

The lamps should be positioned symmetrically. The axis of the light should be about 40 degrees to the base plate to prevent reflections from the document's surface entering the lens (Fig. 9.4). The symmetry of the illumination can be checked by noting the shadow of a pencil placed in the middle of the original (Fig. 9.5).

The copy is framed by moving the camera vertically on the column and then adjusting the focus. The shutter is released using a cable release or the camera's self-timer with the setting for aperture priority ("A" marking) and the aperture set at f/8 or f/11. If the original shows black print on white background, an exposure compensation (plus correction of 1 to 2 stops) is necessary to avoid results which are too dark. Some digital cameras offer a special "copy program", which can be preselected.

A more precise method is to use a gray card for exposure metering, especially if the originals are particularly light or dark.

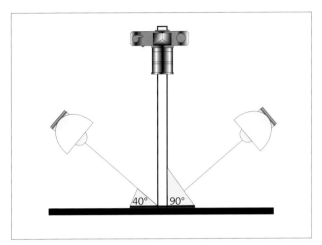

Fig. 9.4   The lighting should be set up so that reflections do not strike the camera. A lighting angle of 40 degrees to the base board can achieve this.

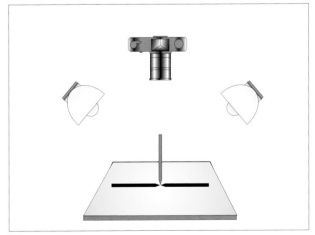

Fig. 9.5   If the shadows of a pencil placed in the middle of the original are symmetrical, it can be assumed that the lighting is also symmetrical.

9.2.2   Measuring exposure with a gray card – substitute readings

Light meters, either hand-held or those built in to the camera, are calibrated to give settings that will produce an average image brightness, i.e., this is for an object which reflects just under 18% of the light falling on it. The exposure is set so that the object is rendered as a mid-gray. If the object is brighter than average, the resulting image is too dark. Using a gray card is helpful in such cases; this is a sheet of cardboard or plastic which reflects light at approximately 18%. Instead of the object, the exposure is measured with the gray card (substitute reading).

To do this, the camera and the original are placed in position and the image framed (Fig. 9.6). The gray card is then placed on the original. The camera is set for manual exposure ("M" symbol) and the aperture set to the "copying apertures" of f/8 or f/11. Using the viewfinder, the shutter speed is adjusted to achieve the proper exposure. The gray card is then removed from the original and the photograph is taken.

The result is that the original is reproduced at its correct brightness and the camera light meter is not fooled into trying to achieve an "average" exposure for the image. The shutter speed can be used for copying originals of a similar size as long as the other parameters (aperture and placement of the lamps) remain the same. Setting exposure with a gray card is to be preferred to using the camera's automatic exposure function as it achieves better results.

If a digital SLR camera is used, the histogram function helps to check exposure as described in chapter 7.4.3.

 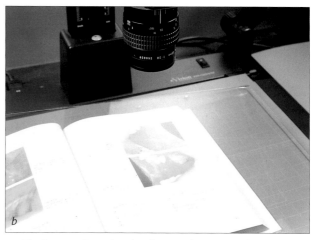

Fig. 9.6   A gray card is helpful in copy work in achieving correct exposure. The image is framed and with manual exposure, the aperture set at the "copying apertures" of f/8 or f/11 and the shutter speed adjusted to create the correct exposure (a). The gray card is then removed and the image is made (b).

9.2.3 Improving color reproduction

Color reproduction depends on the color temperature of the copy stand lamps and on the white balance setting of the camera. There are different ways of neutralizing the colors. White balancing the camera is an easy and fast way to obtain neutral colors. The specific procedure depends on the individual camera model. The general procedure is always the same. The camera on the copy stand is aimed at a white sheet of paper or a gray card, which is illuminated by the copy stand lamps. Then the "white balance shot" is triggered. By this, you "tell" your camera that this white or gray piece of paper is neutral. The camera meters the color temperature and adjusts the settings for the following pictures according to this metering.

Another method is also possible. A gray card is placed beside the original in the first image. Original and gray card are photographed. Then the other pictures are taken without gray card. The first image (original with gray card) is opened in Photoshop (or other image editing program). The LEVELS menu is opened, showing three eyedropper tools. The middle one is the gray one. It is selected and moved over the gray card in the image. Clicking adjusts the color of the whole image. This adjustment has to be saved, and afterwards it can be used for all other pictures taken under the same conditions.

Fig. 9.7   Uneven originals can be flattened using a glass plate. The black cardboard in front of the camera prevents reflections on the surface of the glass.

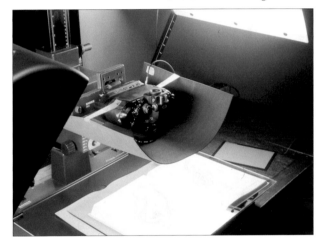

9.3   Tips for problematical originals

- Uneven originals should be flattened under a glass plate (Fig. 9.7). However, care should be taken to avoid unwanted reflections. Reflections of the camera itself can be avoided by using a black cardboard shield with an opening for the lens, placed in front of the camera.
- If there is print from the reverse of thin originals shining through, this can be remedied by using a sheet of black cardboard underneath.
- Transparent paper originals can be copied by laying a white sheet of paper underneath to improve the contrast of the print.
- Damaged originals can be copied by using a sheet of paper with the same color as that of the original.
- A book holder is useful if books are frequently copied; this also flattens thick books (Fig. 9.8).

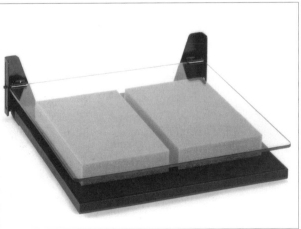

Fig. 9.8   If copies are frequently made from books, a book holder is a good investment (Photo: Kaiser).

Copying radiographs   10

Radiographs belong to the most important sources of information in dental diagnostics. It may be necessary to copy them to illustrate publications and lectures, but also to copy important treatment documents for colleagues or the dentist's own records.

Within the last few years, digital radiography has become increasingly popular. It can be useful to digitize conventional radiographs just by copying them with a digital camera. This avoids the use of two different techniques simultaneously. Special films and processes are available to produce contact copies. This section deals with photographic techniques of copying using digital cameras.

In principle, copying radiographs is the same as copying originals with transmitted light. Thus, a light source which shines through the radiograph is needed in addition to the equipment for copying.

10.1   Camera stabilization

Radiographs are by nature unsharp (two layer films, fluorescent dispersed illumination, patient movement). To avoid intensifying this blur, hand-held copying should be the exception for "emergency cases" due to its relatively long shutter speeds. The camera must be stabilized. A copy stand is of course the most suitable for this, optimally one with a light box integrated in the base board (Fig. 10.1). Alternatively, a tripod which allows the camera to be mounted for a vertical shot can also be used.

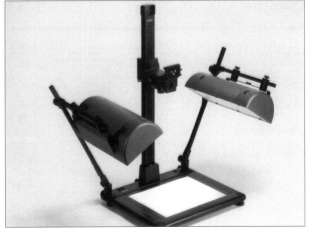

Fig. 10.1   The Copylizer is a modern copy stand with an integrated light box in the base board (Photo: Kaiser).

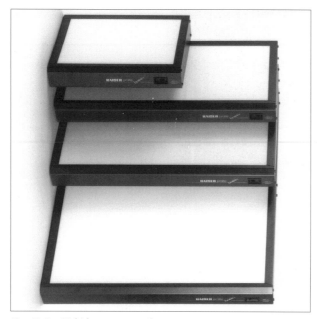

Fig. 10.2 Light boxes are available in various sizes. (Photo: Kaiser).

10.2 Accessories for transmitted light

Any light box which provides even lighting is suitable for copying radiographs. This includes those used for viewing radiographs, which are normally found in the practice anyway, and slide viewers (Fig. 10.2). Slide viewers generally have daylight balanced light sources. Radiograph viewers for the most part have fluorescent tubes; using them with daylight balanced cameras results in a greenish-blue color cast. The better white balance setting is "fluorescent light". Another choice is to white balance the camera individually (for details, see the instruction manual of your camera) or to use the camera with its black and white mode.

It is important that the area around the radiograph be masked off with black cardboard (Fig. 10.3). This prevents stray light from entering the lens and reducing the brilliance of the image. Masks with various size openings are also available for this purpose from photographic suppliers (Fig. 10.4)

An electronic flash can also be used if necessary. The radiograph is placed on a glass plate about 15 cm above a styrofoam sheet which is illuminated by two flashguns.

Dental x-ray films can also be copied with a slide copier, since they are about the same format as 35-mm slides.

If copies need to be made only occasionally, x-ray film can be copied by using a window (optimally north-facing). The x-ray film is fixed to the window with transparent tape and the camera is attached to a tripod.

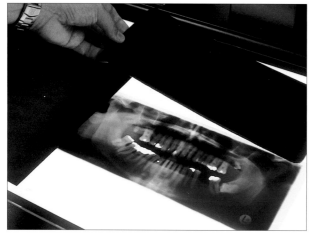

Fig. 10.3 To prevent stray light from entering the lens, which reduces the brilliance of the image, the area surrounding the radiograph is masked off with black cardboard.

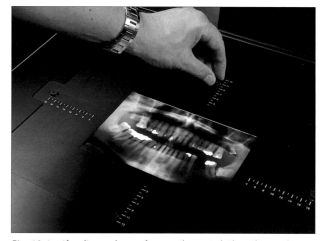

Fig. 10.4 If radiographs are frequently copied, then the mask frame from Kaiser is worth considering (Photo: Kaiser).

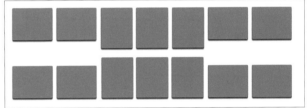

Fig.10.5 Radiograph holders with opaque frames between the individual images are very well suited for copying as they help avoid incorrect exposures.

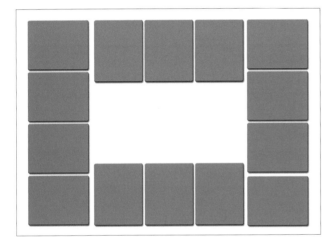

Fig. 10.6 There are various ways of arranging x-ray films, which results in different sizes of these individual images.

10.3 Arrangement for copying

The aim of the copy is to fill the frame as much as possible. For a dental radiograph, a reproduction ratio of 1:1 is necessary.

Series of radiographs are best copied by attaching the individual images one by one to a transparent sheet. Overlapping areas of the images can be cut away and the edges covered with black tape. Using the conventional radiograph holders allows a lot of light between the individual images and leads to exposure problems. In order to avoid, this radiograph archive holders with opaque individual frames are available (Trollhätteplast, Sweden) (Fig. 10.5).

When copying a series of dental x-ray films with 14 individual frames, an approximately 45% increase over the individual films can be achieved by arranging the individual frames in a sequence other than the normal one (Fig. 10.6).

When making a panorama copy, consideration should be given as to whether it is necessary to reproduce the entire image, or whether, by leaving out the side portions, a better side ratio and thus a more format-filling copy can be obtained. If the original needs to be flattened, a glass plate can be used (Fig. 10.7).

Fig. 10.7 Diagram of an arrangement for copying radiographs. Flatness of the film (F) is achieved by laying a glass plate (G) on it. Areas of the light box around the film are masked off with black cardboard (M).

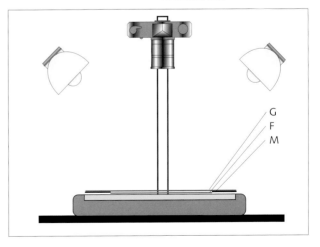

10.4   Step-by-step procedure

- Place the radiograph to be copied on the light source (light box) and cover the surrounding area with black cardboard.
- Set the white balance setting of the camera to "Auto".
- Determine the framing of the copy by changing the reproduction ratio.
- Set the camera to aperture priority ("A" symbol) and aperture to f/8 or f/11.
- Turn off ambient lights.
- Trigger the shutter with a cable release or the camera's self-timer.
- Use bracketing with apertures in increments of 1/3 for originals which pose difficulties (very dark or bright, high contrast). In general, however, this is not necessary.

From slides to digital images

11

We live in a period of different photographic techniques. Even if most professional photographers have switched over to the digital technique, there are of course people who use film at least from time to time or who have thousands of conventional slides with precious contents. Beside this, there may be reasons to hesitate starting digital photography right now. Many dentists have a conventional camera which works perfectly. Others do not have the time to start with a new technology, which digital photography is. Many want to wait until digital cameras are available at a lower price, although prices have fallen dramatically within the last months.

As always in such a transitional period, the old technique has to be transferred into the new one. There are different ways to do this:
- Picture CD.
- Photographing slides.
- Scanning slides.

11.1   Kodak Picture CD

The Kodak Photo CD built a bridge between conventional photography and the digital world. It was a professional digitizing and storage medium. Unfortunately, the Kodak Photo CD is not longer available. For amateur demands, the Kodak Picture CD may be appropriate. It can be used for dental photography to a limited extent.

The differences between Picture CD and Photo CD are displayed in the comparison chart below.

Feature	Picture CD	Photo CD
Intended for	The average picture-taker who wants to view pictures on a computer	Professional and commercial environments
Resolution	1 resolution at 1024 x 1536 pixels	5 resolutions ranging from 128 x 192 pixels up to 2048 x 3072 pixels. A 6th resolution is available with Kodak Pro Photo CD Discs (4096 x 6144 pixels)
File format	JPG	Image Pac (.pcd)
Input quantity	Single roll of color negative film (C41 Process)	Multiple rolls of film
Film type and size	Advanced Photo System (15, 25, and 40 exposure) 35 mm color negative film (24 and 36 exposure)	Black and white, color negative, or color reversal film (existing slides or negatives) *Kodak Digital Science Photo CD Master Disc* 35 mm or Advanced Photo System film *Kodak Pro Photo CD Disc* 35 mm through 4 x 5 in. film
Software availability	Software is included on the CD. Features include: easy access to pictures on your computer ■ convenient organization and storage of memories ■ picture enhancement features: zoom, crop, and red-eye reduction ■ e-mail capability ■ viewing pictures on-screen, creating slideshows, wallpaper, and more ■ ability to make reprints and picture	Software is needed to read and use the images
Ability to add images	No The CD is created at the time of film processing (one roll of film per CD).	Yes Up to approximately 100 images can be added to a Photo CD Disc at any time.

11.2   Photographing slides and negatives

Instead of using a film scanner, 35-mm film can be digitized by photographing the slides or negatives (see also Chapter 9).

Many advanced viewfinder cameras offer slide duplicating equipment as an accessory. For digital SLR cameras, slide duplicating equipment can also be used, as far as the camera sensor conversion factor allows (Fig. 11.1).

Novoflex offers a slide duplicator, which allows fast and easy digitalization of original slides from 35 mm up to 6 x 7 cm medium format. The digital slide duplicator reliably positions framed 35-mm or medium-format slides or film strips (Fig. 11.2).

This duplicating method is especially recommended if larger quantities of negatives or slides need to be digitized quickly with a digital camera. The high quality of today's digital cameras ensures good results in double quick time and many users prefer this method to scanning with a slide scanner.

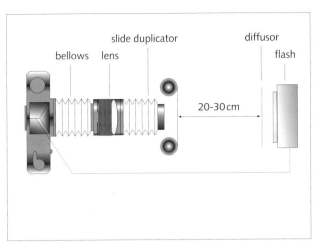

Fig. 11.1   *Diagram of slide copying set-up.*

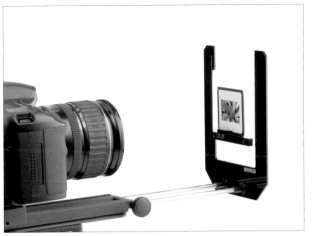

Fig. 11.2   *Slide duplicator for 35-mm format and medium format (Photo: Novoflex).*

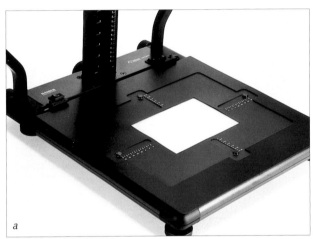

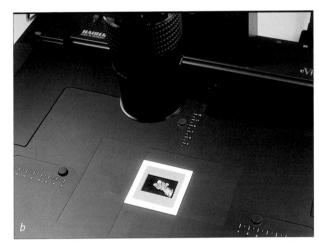

Fig. 11.3   *A mask frame on a light box is also very good for copying slides (a). If the area around the slide is left free to some extent, this also reduces contrast (b).*

Another simple method is to use a slide viewing box. It is recommended to check the white balance first, as color temperature of these boxes often generates a color cast. The camera is mounted on the copy stand with a light box integrated into the base plate. When taking a photograph of the slide on the lightbox, it is important that the field around the slide is masked by black cardboard or a professional mask in order to prevent light getting into the lens and causing flare (Fig. 11.3).

A third option is to use the color head of an enlarger. Some enlarger heads can be removed and used as a box to hold the slide (Fig. 11.4).

The quality of the results depends above all on the quality of the camera used. For most purposes, quality can be sufficient. High-end results can only be obtained by using a good slide scanner.

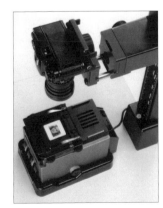

Fig. 11.4   *The color head of a color enlarger is well suited to slide copying since the color of its light can be changed as desired (Photo: Kaiser).*

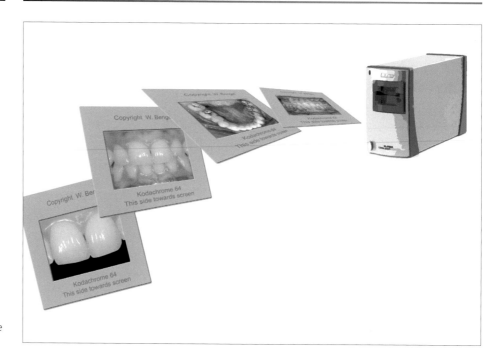

Fig. 11.5   A slide scanner is the best way to digitize slides.

11.3   Slide scanners

Good slide scanners are availabe today at reasonable prices (Nikon, Minolta, Polaroid, Mustek, Canon, Microtek etc). Selection criteria depend on qualities like price, scanning speed, resolution, and quality of the scan. As these properties change from time to time, it is advisable to gather information by reading test results in photographic journals (Fig.11.5).

Good scanners are connected to the desktop computer by USB 2.0 or FireWire IEEE 1394 cable. After connecting the scanner and installing the scanner software, the procedure is essentially as follows.

1. Slide scanner should be turned on before starting the computer. After turning on the scanner, it starts its self-calibration procedure, which takes a couple of seconds.
2. Adobe Photoshop (or other image editing program) is opened.
3. Select FILE > import > scanner, which is installed.
4. Insert slide into the scanner. Slide should be clean and not glass framed, it has to be inserted longitudinally with the emulsion surface face down (shiny surface up).
5. Scan software is opened, the basics settings are performed (film type as slides or negatives, colorspace).
6. Click on "Preview" to see a sample image.
7. Adjust settings of the scanning program (see instructions of the scanner).
8. Select the area to be scanned (crop area).
9. Click "Scan".

10. Scanned image will appear in the Adobe Photoshop window, where you can edit it, if necessary.
11. Close the scanner interface window and save the file or scan more slides.
12. Do not forget to remove the slide after scanning.

Beside scanning single slides, there are devices on the market that allow the scanning of negative strips or batch scanning of a number of slides in one session.

Scanning resolution

Scanning resolution depends on the later use of the image. Good scanners offer a sufficiently high resolution for all tasks (2700 dpi and more, top models have a resolution of 4000 dpi). Resolution must be extremely high as the dimensions of a slide are rather small and must be enlarged very much.

8-bit mode/16-bit mode

Good scanners offer the option to use a 16-bit mode. For average slides, the difference of the results will not be very impressive. But there will be a visible difference after having performed color and tone curve adjustments. The following procedure is recommended:

- Scan the slide in 16-bit mode as a TIFF file.
- Perform color and tonal adjustments.
- Change the mode to 8 bit.
- Store the final image as JPEG file.

Example for offset printing

If we want to make a 8 x 10 inch print from a 35-mm frame, and we need to print at 300 ppi for best results, we know we will need digital image pixel dimensions of at least 2400 x 3000. Knowing that the physical size of the 35-mm frame is slightly less than 1 x 1.5 inches, we can determine we would need to scan the film at 2400 ppi or higher capture resolution.

Example for computer monitors

If we want to use our images on computer monitors, we must know the monitor resolution or assume a common resolution we want to target for best results. If we assume most users will be utilizing screen resolutions of 1024 x 768, we would want to make our image resolution (pixel dimensions) 1024 x 768 for desktop wallpaper or full screen displays. For e-mail use, we would want to make them smaller, maybe 512 x 384.

The following table shows the resulting image pixel dimensions, megapixel resolution, file size, and print size at 300 dpi for scans of mounted 35-mm slides at the various scan resolutions. All numbers are for average crops from square opening 35-mm slide mounts. Negative scans will be slightly larger.

according to LTL imagery	Scan resolution			
	1000 ppi	2000 ppi	3000 ppi	4000 ppi
Pixel dimensions	1360 x 900	2710 x 1800	4050 x 2650	5420 x 3600
Megapixel resolution	1.2	4.9	10.7	19.5
File size	3.6 MB	14 MB	31.5 MB	57 MB
Print size at 300 dpi (in inches)	3 x 4.5	6 x 9	8.8 x 13.5	12 x 18

Enhancing the images

Good scanners/scanning programs offer techniques to improve image quality. Dust and scratch removal (e.g., digital ICE = Image Correction Enhancement) is performed by using infrared light in the film scanning process to identify and remove dust and physical defects in the film, such as scratches and pitting of the emulsion. As the emulsions of Kodachrome and black-and-white films are either entirely or largely opaque to infrared light, this technique does not work with these film types.

Another technology, called digital ROC (= recovery of color), is specifically designed to restore the color and tone of old, faded, and color-shifted films by extracting the original color information.

Another technique is the grain abatement technology (e.g., GEM = Grain Equalization and Management) which characterizes the film grain structure and then selectively eliminates or reduces its appearance without affecting image sharpness.

The advantage of a slide scanner compared with other methods of digitizing slidesis that you are completely independent. If you need a single slide scan, you can do it whenever you want.

11.4   Flatbed scanners/drum scanners

There are a number of flatbed scanners on the market with a transparency unit which permits slides to be scanned. In principle, such an adapter is a special scanner cover that diffuses light evenly through the slide or negative. Generally, the resolution is lower than the resolution of slide scanners. However, there are scanners on the market with a resolution which is comparable. Tests have shown clearly that the quality of the results in some cases is inferior when compared to the quality of slide scanners. The reason is that the resolution of the results sometimes does not reach the physical resolution mentioned in the data sheet of the flatbed scanner.

At the moment, the conclusion can be summarized as follows: flatbed scanners have the advantage of being cheaper, permitting scanning of printed pictures as well, and offering a quality which is sufficient for most purposes (Fig. 11.6). Better results can be obtained by high-resolution slide scanners.

Optimum results can be reached by drum scanners with a photomultiplier tube instead of a CCD. These tubes provide the highest quality scans with very good highlight and shadow detail. Their dynamic range is so high they can capture detail in both deep shadows and bright highlights; they also capture subtle differences in shading. Resolutions range up to more than 12,000 dpi. Not surprisingly, drum scanners are very expensive. They are used in specialized offices and lithographic companies.

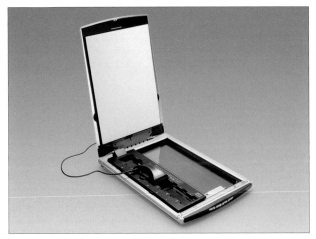

Fig. 11.6   Flatbed scanners with a transparency unit are the second choice for digitizing slides (Photo: Canon).

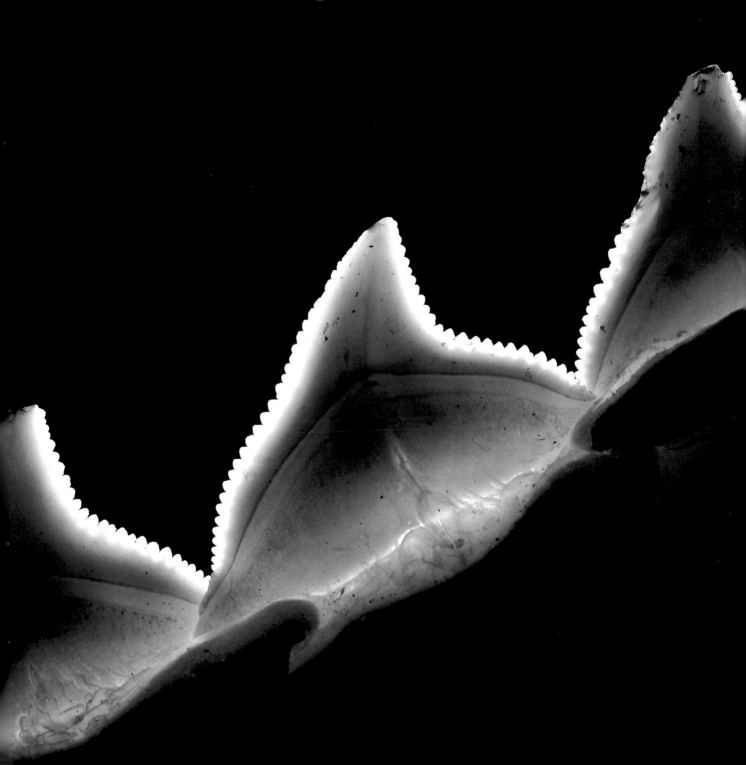

The digital workflow *Section C*

Workflow I: Image transfer 12

Workflow

Discussing the "workflow" without dealing with monitor calibration and color management does not make very much sense. As long as images remain in the dental office and are not used for publications or high-end printing, these two topics are of minor interest for the daily routine work. Therefore, they are discussed more in detail later.

Using a digital camera in the dental practice does not differ from employing a conventional SLR system. Although it is possible to connect the camera directly to the PC, image storage in the internal storage media has proven convenient. The camera is easier to manage and there are no annoying cables.

Before using the camera, some settings have to be checked:
- Number of remaining images?
- Battery status of camera and flash?
- Image resolution correct?
- Type of image data (TIFF, RAW, JPEG) correct?
- White balance set to flash photography?
- Aperture setting?
- Camera is set so that the rear LCD review shows an overlying histogram.

It is always good to have a spare battery and a second storage card at the ready. As in conventional photography, it is always recommendable to take several images of the patient or the object. In close-up photography, depth of field is very shallow and focusing is therefore always a problem.

After each single shot, the picture should be checked on the LCD screen on the camera back. Using the magnifying function, sharpness can be checked. Using the histogram function, exposure can be controlled. The last picture should be one of the patient's file, in order to know later which image belongs to which patient.

There are many options for a workflow of digital images. In principle, the procedure should be (Fig. 12.1):

- Transferring the images into a special file "NEW IMAGES".
- Making a copy of the image files "as they come out of the camera" on a CD.
- Deleting the "bad" images.
- Renaming the images.
- Editing the images.
- Adding keywords and captions.
- Transferring the image files to their final destination file in the image archive.
- Back-up of the image files on a second (external) storage medium.

After image data are stored in the computer and backed up, the data on the memory card can be deleted. The card is then removed from the reader and inserted into the camera again.

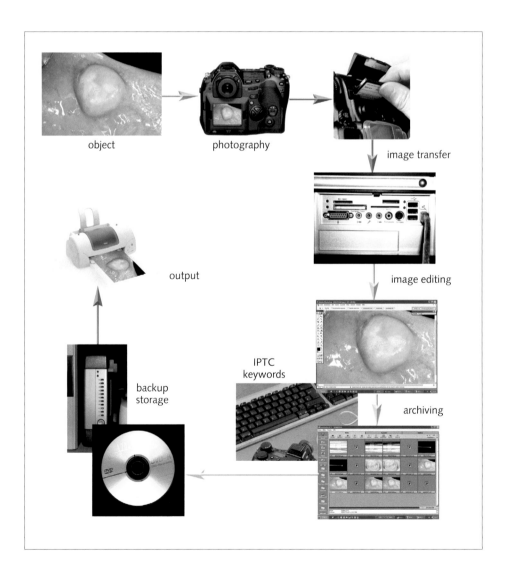

Fig. 12.1   Digital workflow from shooting the object to image output.

For this procedure different software tools are needed:
- Transfer software (optional).
- Image editing software (simple tasks can be done with most transfer programs).
- Archiving program/digital asset management.

Very often these software tools are purchased as a "bundle" with the camera. The beginner may start using only one software tool for all three tasks. The advanced user normally uses two or three different programs.

12.1 Transferring the images

Image transfer can be done by using a cable or the storage medium itself. Most cameras are sold with special transfer software, which can be used both for archiving and simple editing tasks. Examples are: Nikon View, Olympus Camedia Master, Canon Zoom Browser Ex, Fuji FinePix Viewer. The use of this software is not mandatory, as files can also be transferred using the Windows Explorer.

The target directory can be named "New Images" (or similar).

12.1.1 Transfer via cable

Some professional cameras offer a FireWire IEEE 1394 interface for very fast transfer, others use the USB interface. The USB version 2.0 is nearly as fast as FireWire. Only a few professional cameras offer both USB 2.0 and FireWire (e.g., Olympus E-1, Fujifilm FinePix S3 Prof.). The transfer process can be automated so far that it starts after a mouseclick in the moment the camera is connected to the PC.

12.1.2 Transfer via storage medium

To transfer the images to a PC, the storage medium is removed from the camera and either placed
- directly into the PC card slot or
- into an adapter (notebooks) or
- into a card reader with USB 2.0 interface.

The computer accesses this reader or the adapter as it would a normal drive.

There is normally no special transfer software needed to get the image data to the PC. After completing image transfer a copy of all image data "as they come out of the camera" is recommended, using a CD or DVD as storage medium.

These data are filed chronologically (one directory per day).

This copy has nothing to do with backups made after editing and adding key words. Irrespective of the file format (RAW, JPEG, TIFF) these files are in some respect "digital negatives" and should be protected of being accidentally erased.

12.2 RAW-file transfer and conversion

Nearly all DSLRs have the option of shooting images in RAW-file mode. These files can be converted into "normal" files by using the manufacturer's RAW converter or using a purchased third-party converter (Fig. 12.2, 12.3).

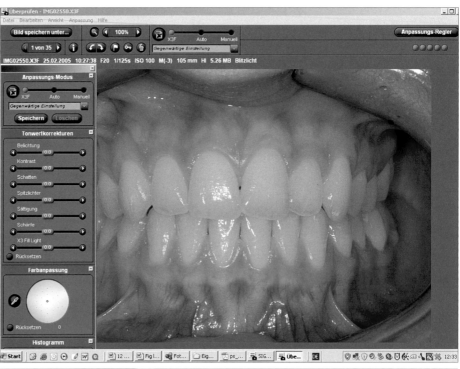

Fig. 12.2   The Sigma conversion program is simple to use. Sliders allow individual changing of all important parameters. Situation before improving the image.

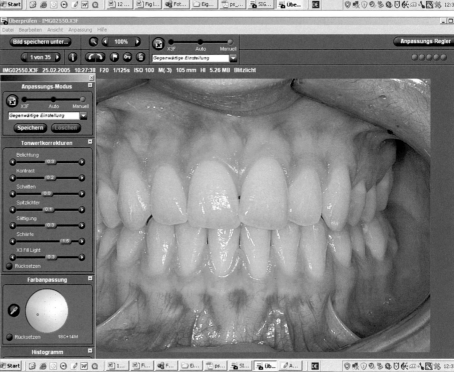

Fig. 12.3   Result after changing the image parameters, such as exposure, sharpness, contrast etc.

In addition, modern image editing programs (Photoshop CS, Photoshop Elements®) are able to convert these files. Otherwise, the specific program of the individual camera must be used (e.g., Canon Digital Photo Professional, Olympus Master etc.). To take advantage of the latest developments downloading the latest converters (e. g., Adobe Camera Raw) is necessery from time to time.

At the moment, nearly all DSLR cameras use a 12-bit mode. This mode is sometimes referred to as "16-bit mode". 12 bits allow a wider tonal range (instead of 256 brightness levels, 4096 levels are used). Therefore, the RAW converter has to be set to "16-bit mode", in order to get optimum results. Images should be kept in a 16-bit mode unless all image editing procedures have been performed. Afterwards, the image can be transferred into the 8-bit mode for storing, in order to save disk space.

Some basic adjustments have to be done during conversion: white balance, exposure compensation, color balance (setting the gray point), contrast (white and black points). Sharpening should be done later using the image editing program.

White balance

The most important first correction for any raw conversion is setting the white balance. By this, you can adjust the white balance of nearly any image, regardless of the color temperature under which it was shot. The Photoshop® Camera Raw Module has a slider-based adjustment. Other programs offer predefined color temperatures as "daylight", "tungsten light", "flash" etc. The Canon program offers a white balance setting by clicking with a pipette on a neutral (white or gray) area of the picture. In addition, finetuning is possible by moving within a color circle (Fig. 12.4).

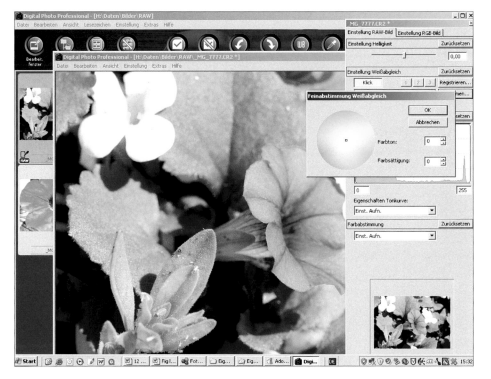

Fig. 12.4   The Digital Photo Professional program (Canon) is a RAW converter allowing the transformation of the Canon RAW files into JPEG or TIF files.

Exposure

Another very important adjustment is exposure. At this point, wide-ranging exposure adjustments are possible. These are far more extensive than the adjustments in Photoshop®.

Shadows, brightness, contrast, saturation

The settings of shadows, brightness, contrast, and saturation can be done in Photoshop® as well, with similar or even larger functionality.

Detail options

Clicking the Detail option at the top of the interface opens advanced settings: sharpness, luminance smoothing, and color noise reduction. The same options are offered when using Photoshop Elements® (Fig. 12.5). The main drawback of sharpening an image during conversion is that this is a global function. It is preferable to perform sharpening after conversion. Color noise artefacts caused by shooting at higher ISO speeds can be eliminated by applying luminance smoothing and color noise reduction, which works globally. To see the effects, the image must be at a zoom range of a minimum of 100%.

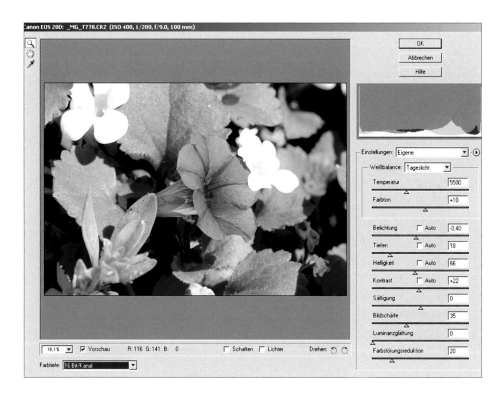

Fig. 12.5   Part of Photoshop Elements is a very good RAW converter.

Lens adjustments

Advanced programs (Photoshop®) offer the possibility of lens adjustments. By this, you can compensate for chromatic aberration and vignetting.

Calibration

Some cameras show a color bias, which can be neutralized by using the Calibrate tab. This enables fine-tuning of hue and saturation as well as possible shadow tints, which can sometimes be found in deep shadow areas. All settings can be stored in a custom setting, which can save a lot of time.

The raw files of the more important images should be filed along with the JPEGs or TIFFs, as these raw files are the digital negatives, which may be used later.

12.3 Which file format?

It is not necessary to use the raw file format for routine tasks. The question is, which is the best file format for dental photography? The answer depends on the individual situation. For daily routine in the dental practice, the JPEG format with the highest quality is recommended. This saves a lot of disk space. Images can be kept in a JPEG format during basic editing procedures and for the archive.

If storage space does not play an important role and if the camera offers the TIFF option, images are recorded using the TIFF format. This format can be kept during all editing procedures and also for archiving.

For special purposes and if the user knows how to fine-tune his or her RAW files, the RAW file format should be used. Shooting the pictures as RAW files, the user has all options to use all the information the image file contains. The image can be converted into a TIFF format, if long image editing procedures are planned. After that, the final result can be transferred into a JPEG for archiving, if disk space is an issue. If not, it can be archived as a TIFF. The RAW files have to be kept as well, as these files are the "digital negatives".

12.4 Deleting files

The most important tool for image archiving is the waste paper basket. This was true for conventional photographs and is also true for data files. When pictures can be displayed on the monitor using an image browser, the first task is to reduce the number of shots. For checking the pictures, the preview mode of the image browser is used to enlarge the image. One has to remember that some image viewing programs do not use the Windows waste paper basket, meaning that if an image is deleted, it cannot be reopened afterwards without the use of special programs and special skill.

Usually, a number of pictures are taken from every patient or object. Pictures which are technically unsatisfactory should be deleted. Only the best pictures should be kept. In slide photography, nearly perfect slides were also kept, just in case a copy was needed. This is not necessary in digital photography, as a copy can be made at anytime using the "original". Therefore: delete liberally and think of all the processing time and disk space you will save!

The next step is to edit the images using an image editing software program.

Workflow II:
Image editing – basic adjustments

13

There are hundreds of books dealing with image editing on the market (and nearly as many software programs). Only a general overview will be given here on the first steps necessary within the described workflow. In Chapter 17, you will find more information in detail. When talking about an image editing program, I normally refer to Adobe Photoshop®. Of course, other programs can also be used.

The following procedure has proven useful:
- Import image into Photoshop® (or other editing program).
- Align and crop image.
- Adjust brightness and contrast.
- Perform color correction.
- Remove dust spots.
- Sharpen the image.

The degree of image editing measures necessary at this stage depends – among other things – on the number of images to be archived. If hundreds of images are taken every day, it makes sense to organize the workflow in such a way that only an image selection is edited and stored in a special archive, while all images are stored in chronological order on a special PC hard drive.

For a normal dental office where the numbers of images are modest, all pictures should be treated in the same way.

13.1   Importing images into Photoshop®

The first step is to import the images from the directory NEW IMAGES into Photoshop®. RAW files are already in Photoshop®, if the program was used for conversion. Color space is Adobe RGB (1998), as this space is larger than sRGB. The files are left at their native resolution. If the camera allows, the images are imported in 12-bit mode ("16-bit mode"). This gives us more flexibility and better image quality.

Images can be opened in the editing program using the FILE > open command (CTRL.+O) or by using the Photoshop® BRIDGE program: FILE > Browser (SHIFT+CTRL:+O) and double clicking the selected image.

If a separate browser is used, images can be opened in Photoshop® by using the Drag and Drop function: an image is selected in the browser, then, with the left mouse tab pressed down, dragged into the Photoshop® working space.

13.2   Aligning and cropping images

Images which are not correctly framed can be aligned, and superfluous pixels can be eliminated by carefully cropping the image. This reduces the amount of data and is done with the crop tool; rotation can be done with the "rotate" command: IMAGE > Rotate Canvas > Arbitrary. Then the appropriate angle has to be entered (Fig. 13.1 a-c).

A very useful tool for aligning an image is the "Measure tool" to be found in the tool bar under the eyedropper (click and hold on the eyedropper).

If the occlusal plane is somewhat oblique (or the horizon of a landscape), you select the measure tool, click on the occlusal plane, and draw a line (mouse button pressed down) to a second spot on the occlusal plane (or horizon). The line is not printable. Then you go to IMAGE > Rotate canvas > Arbitrary and click. The Rotate Canvas Window opens, shows the angle by which the image has to be rotated in order to make the occlusal plane (or horizon) horizontal, then just click OK.

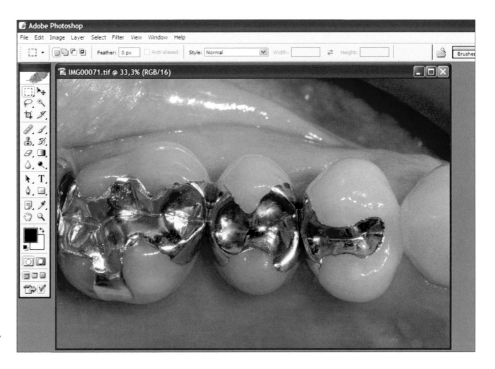

Fig. 13.1 a   This image is slightly oblique. It has to be aligned.

After this, the rotated image must be cropped (Fig. 13.2 a-d). The crop tool is simple to use. Width and height or a ratio aspect can be preselected. This is useful if an image is used later for a PowerPoint presentation. At this stage, only superfluous or disturbing image areas are cut off.

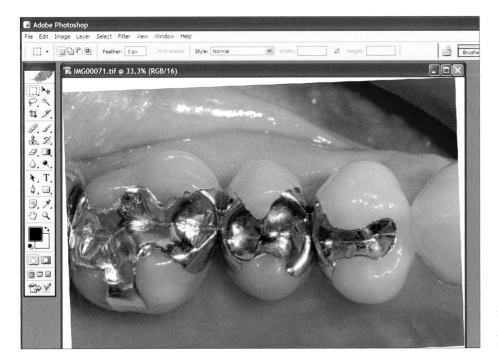

Fig. 13.1 b   Image is aligned. The white triangles have to be removed by cropping the image with the Cropping Tool.

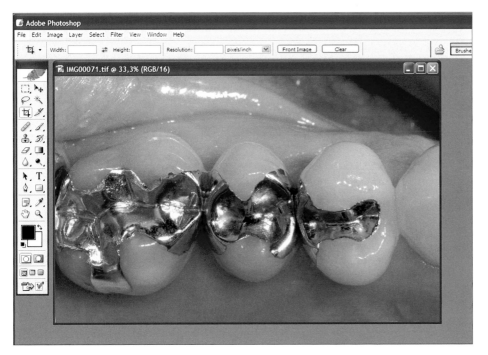

*Fig. 13.1 c
Image is aligned and cropped.*

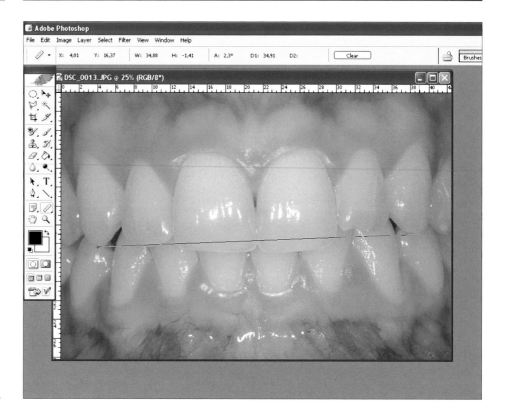

Fig. 13.2 a   The Measure Tool is to be found under the Eyedropper (click and hold). It can be used to find out the proper angle to align an oblique image.

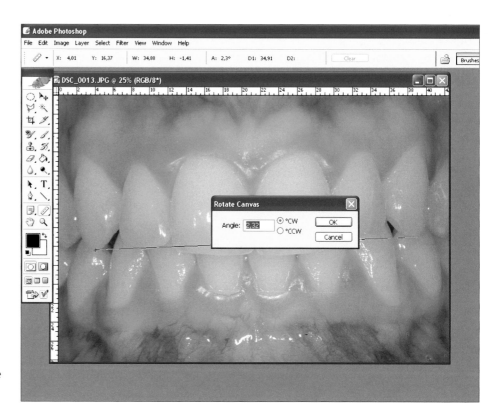

Fig. 13.2 b   Angle by which the image has to be aligned is indicated.

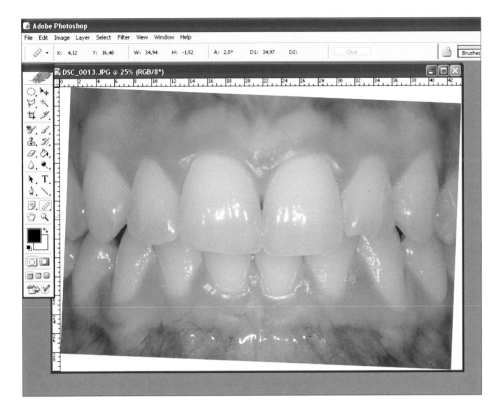

Fig. 13.2 c   *Image is rotated according to the angle found by the Measure Tool.*

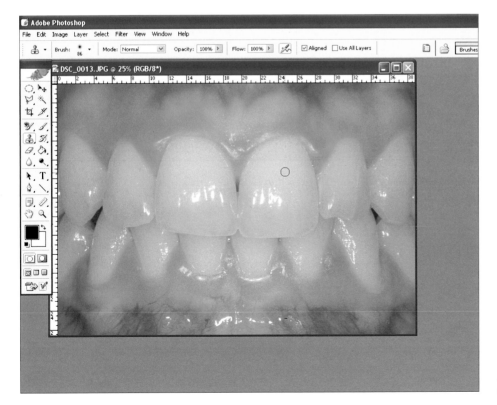

Fig. 13.2 d
Image aligned and cropped.

13.3   Brightness and contrast

Since brightness and color influence each other, brightness and contrast corrections are undertaken first before any required color corrections. Various tools are available for this in the different software programs (see Chapter 17).

Fine tuning of brightness and contrast can be achieved by the LEVELS or CURVES menu. Working with the LEVELS or CURVES menu is better in 16-bit mode (IMAGE>Mode>16 Bits/Channel). Before storing the image, it has to be transferred to 8-bit mode to reduce the file volume. Experienced Photoshop® users prefer adjustment layers for changing contrast and brightness, as this allows finer changes. Depending on the program, the image has to be switched to the 8-bit mode, because not all programs allow the use of adjustment layers in 12-bit mode.

A very useful tool is the Shadow/Highlight tool, which is new in Photoshop® CS: IMAGE>Adjustments>Shadow/Highlight (Fig. 13.3).

13.4   Color correction

Undesirable color casts can originate for many reasons. Such color casts can be eliminated in various ways using the IMAGE – Adjustments submenus. A simple solution is found in the submenu VARIATIONS, which allows color, brightness and saturation to be changed using small preview images. This could be the first choice for the inexperienced Photoshop® user (Fig. 13.4). Other options are "color balance," "selective color correction," and "color tone/saturation" and more. New in Photoshop® CS is the Photo Filter tool, offering an array of color filters.

13.5   Removing dust spots

Sometimes there are dust particles on the image sensor of the camera, resulting in small black spots in the image. These have to be removed as they can be very disturbing. To better find them, the image has to be brought to 100% magnification. The spots are removed with the Clone Tool and the Healing Brush.

For more details, see Chapter 16.

13.6   Sharpening

Sharpening of digital images is almost always necessary due to the interpolation process during image generation. This is true for images taken with the camera as well as for scanned images. Degree and method of sharpening depend on the type of image (many details or large color areas) and the purpose (offset printing, ink jet printer). As a rule, images which are to be printed by an inkjet or dye sublimation printer should be sharpened visually from the screen image. Images for offset printing can be more intensely sharpened. More details are given in Chapter 17.

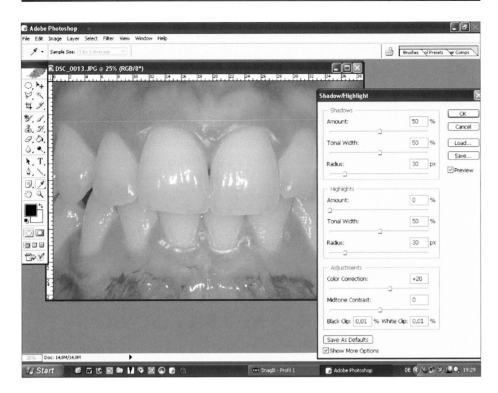

Fig. 13.3   Shadow/Highlight box is opened – a versatile tool of Photoshop®.

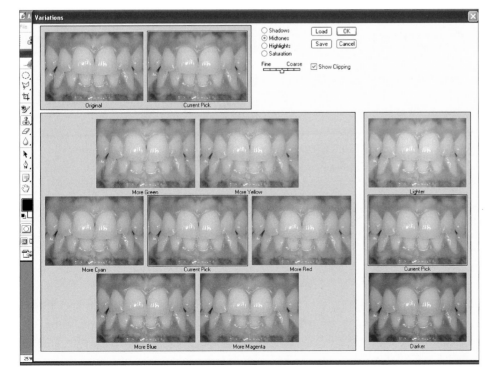

Fig. 13.4   "Variations" is a very good possibility to improve the colors of an image. This is especially useful for the beginner.

For these reasons, many image archives do not sharpen images at all.

An alternative approach is to sharpen the image on a separate layer. A duplicate layer is created, named "Sharpening layer". Then the image is sharpened cautiously using the Unsharp Mask (USM) in most cases.

It is better not to sharpen an image at this point than to "oversharpen" it, as this can destroy the image.

These basic adjustments can be performed rather quickly with routine shots. If there are more important pictures, these adjustments should be performed using a copy of the original. The valuable originals and the raw files must be stored separately.

More details concerning image editing are provided in Chapter 17.

Workflow III: Image archiving 14

Archiving digital data is today often referred to as "Digital Asset Management". An asset is only an asset if you can find it. Therefore, asset management is one of the key steps in the digital workflow. Without proper archiving, the whole endeavor can be useless, as sometimes a picture archive turns out to be a mass grave for digital data. This topic would deserve a separate book, as the demands on such an archive depend very much on the user (dental office, clinic, professional archive, number of people having access, etc.). Nevertheless, only some general recommendations are given here.

Procedure fundamentals
- Image files are renamed.
- Keywords and captions are added.
- Files are copied to another (external) hard drive (or network server). The asset management application has access to this harddrive.
- A second copy is made on a second hard drive (located anywhere else) and/or images are written on CD or DVD.

As mentioned at the end of chapter 12 it is recommended to copy the image files on a CD/DVD just as they come out of the camera and before they are edited. This copy can be used in emergency cases. It stays outside the archiving procedure.

14.1   Digital asset management applications

There is a huge variety of archiving software programs on the market. Very often good archiving software is "bundled" with the camera. These programs can be sufficient for smaller archives.

In general, it is advisable to use a program with a well-known software house behind it. Some well-known programs are:

- Portfolio (Extensis)
- Cumulus (Canto)
- Fotostation Pro (Fotoware)
- Photo Mechanic (Camera Bits)
- Iview Media Pro (iview Multimedia Ltd.)
- Photoshop® CS 2 (Adobe)

With these programs, you can be sure to get the support you need and have a program which will still be on the market in a couple of years.

For smaller archives, database modules from standard image editing software are available, for example, the album module from PhotoImpact, ACDsee, or amateur programs such as PhotoRecall or PhotoCat. There are also good Shareware and freeware programs available for image archiving (e.g., Thumbs).

Most of these applications work according the same principles. They generate a "record" of each image consisting of "fields" which contain certain information, including:

- Thumbnail image
- Filename
- Date of creating the record
- Date of image capturing and/or modifying
- Path to the directory where the original image file is stored
- IPTC and EXIF data
- Some additional information

The record does not contain the image file itself. The file stays where it is, only a path to the file is created. Therefore, the place where the original file is located must not be changed; otherwise the image cannot be retrieved by the program, as there is no path to the file.

It is strongly recommended to try different archive programs before purchasing one, as user demands differ greatly. All programs can be downloaded as a trial version for a limited period of time.

A dental office has other needs concerning archiving and management of images than does a large clinic or a major medical company. For clinics, there are special applications on the market, offering far more options than storage and retrieval of images. The Imagic company in Switzerland developed ImageAccess, a powerful image and document management system. Due to its modular structure, the program offers a variety of options from image acquisition to scientific tasks and high-end presentation possibilities (www.imagic.ch) .

14.2 Renaming the files

To avoid naming problems, it is recommendable to re-name every image file. Cameras number the image files, but at some point, there will be two different files bear-ing the same number. A simple method to avoid these problems is to add the date (format YYYYMMDD) to the file name given by the camera or given according to image content. Such a file name can look like this:

20050107_ABC_mueller_7654.jpg

The name contains: date of shooting_three-letter-code_patient name_number given by the camera and format extension. For smaller archives, the three-letter-code and the content/patient name may be superflu-ous.

Files can be batch-renamed before or after they are adjusted by image editing. This is possible with Photo-shop® or other programs (e.g., Photo Mechanic, Irfan-View). In Photoshop® CS you find the batch-rename function (file browser open) when clicking on FILE>Au-tomate and then BATCH. Then the Batch Rename Menu opens. By clicking on "Destination" you can find a destination folder. Storage in the same folder is possi-ble as well. The file can be renamed using up to six cat-egories (Fig. 14.1).

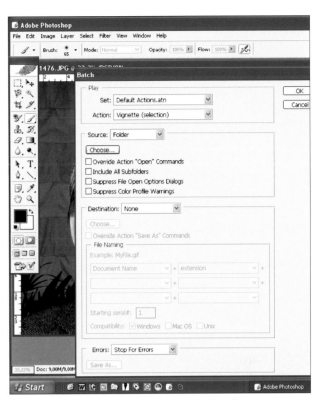

Fig. 14.1 Batch renaming is possible with Photoshop® CS.

Such a file name has numerous advantages:

- Every image has a unique name.
- The original folder on the (external) hard disk can be found easily, if the images are stored on this drive in dated folders (one per day or one per month, accord-ing to the number of pictures).
- Image retrieval is easy even without asset management program, if the date of shooting is known.
- Images in folders are sorted automatically in a chronological order.

Alternatively, asset management programs like Fotostation®, or image browsers like Irfanview® or Photo Mechanics® can be used to rename the files. Renaming can be done after editing the pictures or directly after image transfer to the PC.

14.3 Adding information

There is an old saying that one picture is worth a thousand words. This is only true if the picture contains some words: captions and keywords. These are the key to a good archive.

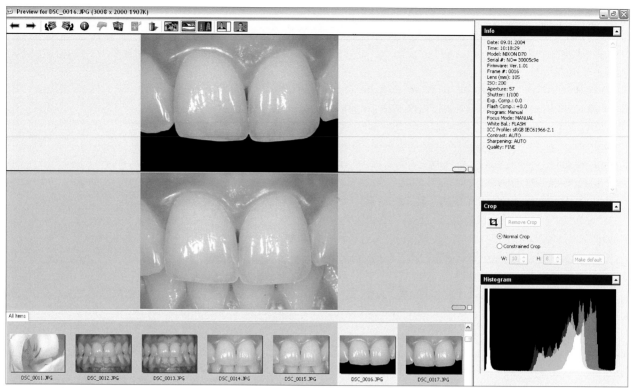

Fig. 14.2   Photo Mechanics is a versatile program speeding up the workflow. EXIF data can be looked up in the window top right.

14.3.1   EXIF information

Digital cameras store the EXIF (exchangeable image file format) information along with the image data automatically. This EXIF information is meta data (literally "data about data"), concerning technical aspects such as date and time of exposure, focal length of lens, aperture, camera settings, etc. They can be viewed in most archiving programs (Fig. 14.2). If not, there are EXIF viewer programs, which can be downloaded from the Internet as freeware (e.g., PhotoStudio, ExifReader).

Photoshop® users find the file information in the FILE menu.

These automatically recorded data should not be confused with IPTC data.

Fig. 14.3   EXIF and IPTC data become part of the data file.

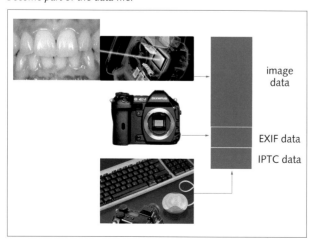

14.3.2 IPTC information

Unlike EXIF data, IPTC (International Press Telecommunications Council) information has to be added manually (Fig. 14.3). The International Press Telecommunications Council was established to safeguard the telecommunication interests of the world's press. Now its activities are primarily focussed on developing and publishing industry standards for the interchange of news data.

IPTC data is a worldwide standard for the descriptions, keywords, and copyright information of digital photos that most image editing and image archiving programs can use (Fig. 14.4). The IPTC standard saves the descriptive information together with the actual image data.

Adobe Photoshop®, for example, has a separate menu item (File Information in the File menu) for IPTC entries, through which texts can be written directly into the files (Fig. 14.5). Among other things, the texts can include certain keywords (see below), photo rights, the name of the author and possibly copyright notices, as well as links to web sites. Many viewer programs (e.g., IrfanView), available free for private use, are also capable of displaying the IPTC information and so does the already mentioned ExifReader, which can be downloaded for free.

Captions of the image and keywords are part of these IPTC data.

Important advantages of captioning the images are:

- Captions can help find the images.
- Copyright data are at hand, as these data are attached directly to the file.
- Subjects and image content can be identified easily.

What is put into a caption has to be considered carefully. It is, for example, not recommended to type the bank address into an IPTC field. If later the town Berlin is searched and the bank of the photographer is the Bank of Berlin, there will be much confusion.

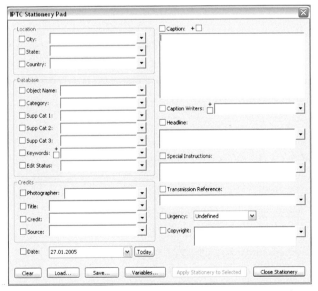

Fig. 14.4   A lot of data can be added as IPTC information in Photo Mechanics.

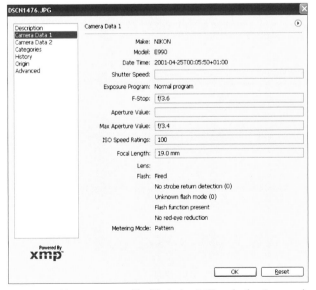

Fig. 14.5   Many programs like Photoshop® CS and other image editing programs allow checking and adding IPTC data.

XMP metadata

Initiated by Adobe Systems Inc., another meta-data platform was created (XMP = Extensible Metadata Platform). The goal is to provide an extensive platform for public and private meta-data, which can be used for both Digital Rights Management and Digital Asset Management.

14.3.3 Keywords

The key to an archive is the keyword. Most asset management applications work on the basis of keywords. The keywords necessary to retrieve the images can be added as IPTC entries in Photoshop® or as image description/keywords using an archiving program like FotoStation. Important keywords can be: treatment, diagnosis etc. Good archiving programs allow you to assign several keywords to a photo and should offer the convenient option of selecting these from a list of predefined terms. Defining the keywords is as critical as it was in an index card catalogue. Otherwise, you run the risk of drowning in a flood of keywords.

To keep control over the data entered into the system, a fixed keyword list must be created, also termed a "controlled vocabulary". This is especially important if more than one person enters keywords.

A controlled vocabulary has the following advantages:
- Searching is easier.
- No keyword chaos.
- Saves time.
- No guessing about keywords.

Beside this, category names can be added. It is advisable to give the whole system a structure by defining categories and subcategories. A simple example:
- Images
    - New Images
  - Private
      - Holidays
      - Children
      - …
  - Practice
      - Oral mucosa
      - Implants
      - Esthetic dentistry
      - Perio
      - …
  - Publications
      - JADA
      - Perio
      - …

One of the major archiving programs is Canto Cumulus. This program emulates a hierarchical folder structure. The user has to define category folders. When acquiring images into the database, the thumbnail has to be dragged and dropped onto these folders. By double clicking on that folder, the program displays all the images in that category, simply and effectively.

The complexity of the whole system depends on different details:
- volume of the archive.
- complexity of the archive.
- how many people have access?
- which kind of material is archived?
- is the system based on a PC network?
- etc.

At this point, the image files are edited (or not), the files are renamed, and keywords are added. Now the files can be transferred to the target directory. The directory NEW Images (entrance directory) can be emptied afterwards.

You will find more detailed information in the Internet provided by different professionals (e.g., Ken Bennett, Wake Forest University). It is worth thoroughly thinking through the preparation of such an archiving system and doing a bit of research in the Internet before using a trial version for tests. Digital asset management saves not just time but also money.

14.4 Storage medium and file format

Up to now, we have edited and renamed the files and added keywords and image captions as meta-data. Now it is time to store the image files. Primary concerns are storage media and file format. As mentioned before, the Adobe RGB color space is recommended, as it is larger than the sRGB. The CMYK color model is smaller and discards colors which it cannot display. Lab format too is only of limited suitability.

For standard practice, it is recommended that the JPEG file format be used for archiving pictures, as file size is much smaller compared with TIFF format. Today JPEG, too, can be regarded as industry standard. File size is much smaller, but it is a lossy file compression method. Loss of information can be neglected as long as the highest quality level is selected and the image is stored only once instead of several times ("Don't JPEG a JPEG!").

If extensive image editing procedures have been performed, the files should be saved using TIFF format, as this format allows saving the layers together with the image. If storage space does not play an important role and prints of highest quality are desired, TIFF format could be used. If RAW format shots have been taken, the RAW files should be kept as well, as these files are the "digital negatives". If digital image integrity is an issue, because images have to be used as evidence, an unaltered archive image has to be kept in the original format.

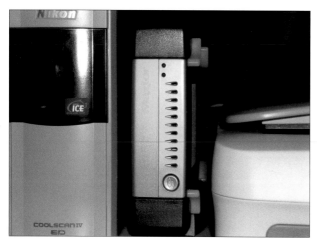

Fig. 14.6
External hard drives are ideal for backing up the image data.

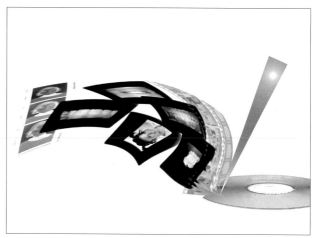

Fig. 14.7   *Digital images and digital data from scanned pictures should be stored as a copy on a CD or DVD.*

The storage medium of choice for many applications will be a network server. For a small dental office, an external hard disk (e.g., Maxtor) is very convenient (Fig. 14.6). Their volume is up to 300 GB or more, they are fast (Firewire, USB 2.0) and are accessed by the computer just like the other drives without complicated installation procedures. The asset management application can be installed in a way that it is linked to that external hard drive.

Data security asks for a backup of image data, as it does in other applications. The file should be stored in two locations: one copy on the office PC, the second on the external drive. The copy for the office PC can be stored in a folder which is named using the date of its first image. Every week or month, or at least when the folder reaches a volume of about 680 MB, images are copied from this folder onto a high quality CD with a capacity of 700 MB (Fig. 14.7). Then this folder can be deleted and replaced by a new one. Another option is to use DVDs for this purpose (capacity 4.7 GB and more). At the moment, there are still some compatibility problems.

BACKGROUND

CD-ROM

The dimensions of a CD (compact disk) are: 12 cm in diameter, 1.2 mm thick, center hole 15 mm diameter. There are two main types of CDs on the market: read-only (CD-ROM) and writable (CD-R). If large numbers of copies are needed, the read-only type is used. These disks are stamped from molds. Information is coded in a spiral track of pits, which are impressed on one side. Pits are tiny indentations about 0.12 m deep, 0.6 m broad and between 0.9 m and 3.3 m long. On one track, there are about 2 billion pits carrying the information. The total length of the track is almost 3 miles (~ 4.5 km). The distance between the neighboring windings of the track is about 1.6 µm.

The two surfaces of "lands" and "pits" are a record of the binary "1s" and "0s" used to store information. The smooth area between two pits is called "land". The spiral starts in the center of the CD. Pits and lands are covered by an ultra-thin metallic reflective layer (aluminum). As this sputtered metal film is extremely delicate, it has to be protected by a lacquer layer. This protective layer and the clear polycarbonate substrate layer underneath protect the metal layer from being damaged (Fig. 14.8).

A writable CD has a similar structure. Pits are not formed by a mold, but they are burned on by a laser beam. A third type of CD is the CD-RW (CD Re-Writable).

The reading laser beam of approximately 780 nm wavelength is guided along the length of the track. Its focus spot is about 1 µm in diameter. The laser light is reflected from the smooth land surface into a light sensing detector. When the beam hits the pits, its reflection is interrupted. The interruptions are decoded into data, music or pictures. In other words, every time the laser spot moves from land to pit and vice versa there is a change in light intensity. This transition is interpreted as 1. No transition means 0 (Fig. 14.9). The length of each land represents the number of 0s. These changes produce the signal, which represent the data stored on the CD.

As the reading beam is focused on the pits and lands on the upper side of the disk substrate, scratches on the lower surface of the CD are tolerated without causing data errors during the reading process. These scratches are simply out of focus, unless they are really deep. Besides the physical reason for this scratch tolerance, there is a second line of defense: special software which is able to deal with data errors.

CD writers are specified using three numbers (e.g., 48 x 12 x 40). The first number indicates the speed at which a CD drive will record data onto a CD-R. The second number ("12" in the above example) indicates the speed at which the CD drive will rewrite data onto a CD-RW. The last number ("40" in the above example) indicates the speed at which the drive will read data from a compact disk.

A single CD-ROM has the capacity of 700 MB, enough to store about 300,000 pages. The lifetime of a CD-R, predicted by manufacturers, is between 100 and 200 years under ideal storing conditions.

The capacity of the current technology, 700 MB and the Data Transfer Rate of about 150 kilobytes per second, is not sufficient for the storage of movie-length, high-quality video presentations. For this purpose, DVDs (Digital Versatile Disk) must be used, which allow a video compression according to the MPEG2 standard

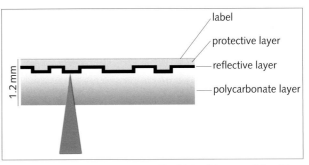

Fig. 14.8   Diagram of the different layers of a CD.

Fig. 14.9   Transitions from land to pit and vice versa cause a change in light intensity which is interpreted as "1".

and which have a data capacity of 4.7 gigabytes (one layer) or 8.5 gigabytes (two layer). Due to standard difficulties, DVDs are not yet the first choice for image archiving.

By this procedure, which can of course be modified according to individual demands, it is guaranteed that images are in two different locations.

The external hard drive (in a clinic or major practice, a directory of a network server would be used) is only used for images. It can be accessed rapidly by the archiving program. Original files are kept there; only copies are used for further applications. Besides this, we have data backup using CD-Rs, which are stored in a different place. To increase safety, a second CD-R copy can be made.

The CDs should be checked from time to time. In addition, some authors recommend that two or three sets of images be written on different CDs from different manufacturers to prevent data loss due to fabrication defects. Based on cautious estimates of CD-R media life, images should be copied onto new CDs periodically.

If CD compatibility becomes an issue, images would be copied to the new standard archival medium. If (or, rather, when) technology reaches a point at which TIFF compatibility is questionable, images can be converted to the new industry standard image format.

Offline archive

Alternatively, the archive can be managed as an "offline archive" using CD-Rs. These CD-ROMs should be numbered and not labelled with text (instead of "periodontitis", it should be marked with a key number). The image CD is then downloaded into an archive program, which generates thumbnail images kept in the archive image record. Images can be retrieved using the keywords as described above or visually using the thumbnails. To access the image data file, the offline archive shows on which CD the image file is stored.

Step-by-step procedure

1. Image transfer into the subdirectory "NEW IMAGES" on the hard disk.
2. Archive program (e.g., FotoStation) is opened, then album (subdirectory) NEW IMAGES is opened. All new pictures appear as "thumbnails" on the screen like slides on a slide viewer.
3. Image editing program (e.g., Photoshop®) is opened.
4. Photoshop®: If necessary images are edited after importing them into Photoshop® using the drag and drop function.
5. Archive program or Photoshop®: image files are renamed and keywords are added, as well as comments or descriptions. These can be assigned either to entire groups of pictures (e.g., patient's name) or to individual photos (e.g., diagnosis).
6. Archive program: Image data files are moved to the final subdirectory of the PC (or network server). A copy of this subdirectory is made on an external harddrive. The asset management program is linked to this PC subdirectory or to the external drive.

7. After moving the image files to the target directory, the subdirectory NEW IM-
   AGES is now empty again.

A weekly/monthly/as-needed copy (or two copies) onto a CD-R or DVD medium is
made of the PC directory, which should be stored at another place.

14.5   Digital longevity

Destruction of compiled information has a long history. Destruction can be performed
intentionally (e.g., by burning down libraries as in Alexandria or Cordoba, by burning books as during the Hitler regime, etc.), or it can happen accidentally or as "col-
lateral damage".

  If these catastrophes do not happen, we are able to decipher (we can try, at least)
what was written down hundreds of years ago. We can even admire paintings created by Stone Age artists more than 30,000 years ago. Unlike these pieces of analog information, digital information is fated not to survive, unless somebody takes
action to make it persist. In other words, pro-active preservation is needed.

  Everybody can read the official document of Charles V's donation of Malta to the
Hospitaler monks, written five hundred years ago and now kept in the museum of
Valetta. To read digital information requires a certain computing environment (application software, operating system, hardware platform, storage devices and special drivers). Image file formats will create even more problems (TIFF, MPEG versions
etc.) than ASCII-based text. The situation becomes worse if digital information is
compressed in order to reduce storage costs or if the information is protected by en-
cryption schemes.

  Much information does not consist of one single file, but is a composition of different files, which are reassembled at viewing time. In this context, the importance
of meta-data cannot be overestimated.

The problem of digital longevity can be divided into two sub-problems:
- Lifespan of the medium.
- Obsolescence of the format.

In the early days of CD-ROM technology, the lifespan of CD-ROMs was very limited. One of the problems was oxidation of the thin metal layer of the CDs. Today,
CD-R and CD-ROM are manufactured according to ISO standards.

  CD-ROM with a gold dye recording layer is guaranteed by Mitsui for 200 years,
while both the Kodak and the Mitsui were 98% readable in multiple reader/media
combinations after simulated aging tests.

  The major problem seems to be obsolescence. The Commission on Preservation
and Access defined the key technical approaches for keeping digital information alive:
- Refreshing
- Migration
- Emulation

Refreshing means to move a file on a regular basis from one physical storage medium to another. This avoids physical decay (of the CD-ROM) and obsolescence. Migration means moving files from older file encoding formats to contemporary formats. The goal is to limit the danger of not being able to read a wide variety of file formats used a couple of years ago.

Emulation tries to solve a similar problem addressed by migration. Unlike the migration approach, emulation is focused on the applications software. Emulation means to generate software that mimics every type of application that has been written before in order to make files run in a contemporary computing environment.

Digital photography has innumerable advantages. One of the major disadvantages (if not the biggest) is the problem of preserving the bits and keeping the file formats accessible. This is a huge problem for libraries and national institutions, but also for the individual dental practice.

Based on the recommendations given above and the considerations of this chapter, an archiving system has to be installed that guarantees physical preservation of the storage media and accessibility of the files to be stored.

Workflow IV: Data output 15

15.1   Displaying photos on-screen

15.1.1   Showing pictures on the PC screen

The fastest way to display images is on the PC screen. This can be useful for patient information. There are special programs for nearly all DSLR cameras allowing immediate data transport into a PC/Mac using a cable. Another choice is to transfer the data via the storage medium.

15.1.2   E-mailing digital photos

Within the last few years, e-mailing has become very popular. E-mailing photos to the dental lab or medical colleagues is very simple. There are other ways to send pictures via Internet (e.g., Instant messenger), but e-mailing is the method of choice.

In order to shorten transfer time, image size must first be reduced. This can be done more or less automatically. Many programs offer functions to send images via e-mail (e.g., Photoshop Elements®) (Fig. 15.1). Photoshop® allows preparing an action which reduces image size. In addition, archiving software programs reduce the data file automatically. Fotostation® offers a function called "special actions". An image file is selected, and by pressing a button, a copy of the data file is reduced to the desired size (Fig. 15.2).

Which file size is the best for e-mailing images? This depends on the purpose. If the images will not be printed, but only displayed on a monitor, then a size of 1024x768 pixels is recommended. This is the resolution most monitors have today. A 1024x768 pixel image can be displayed in full-screen format.

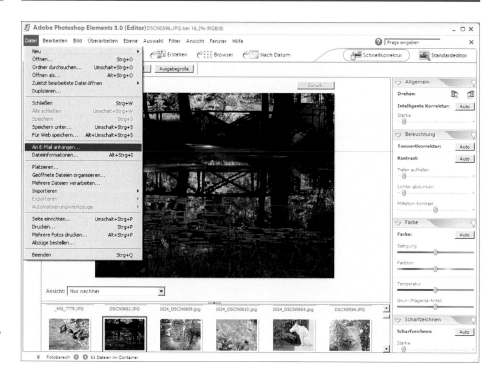

Fig. 15.1   Many programs have an option for sending images as an e-mail.

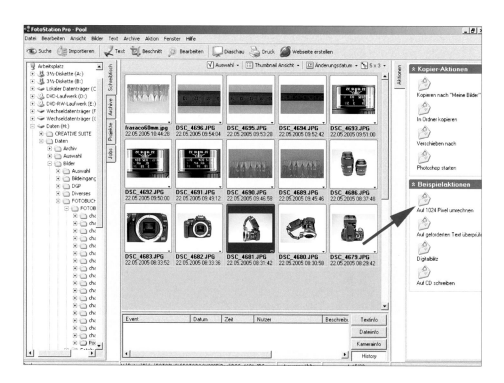

Fig. 15.2   Programs like Foto-station® or Photoshop® allow a reduction of image size by a short key.

Stored as a JPEG file with medium to high quality compression, the data size is rather small and can be attached to an e-mail easily. Instead of attaching the image file, it can be inserted into the text body as well.

Resizing an image step-by-step

- Copy of an image is opened in Photoshop®: CTRL+O (Fig. 15.3).
- Image size menu is opened: IMAGE>Image size>OK. The menu permits typing in the pixel size of the smaller image directly, in this case, 1024 x 768 pixels (Fig. 15.4). Pixel dimensions of the image are indicated above (before resizing 14.1 MB, after resizing 2.25 MB). It is important to check the "constrain proportions box" in order to avoid distortions.
- After clicking OK, the image appears with its new dimensions (Fig. 15.5). It is stored as a JPEG with medium to high quality (degree 7 to 9). An image with a size of 14.1 MB has been reduced to only 124 KB without visible loss of quality.

The same procedure applied in this context for an e-mail attachment can be used to reduce image size before embedding an image in a PowerPoint® presentation or a slide show (see below).

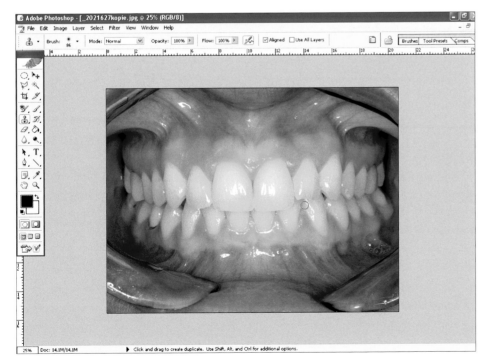

Fig. 15.3
Image is opened in Photoshop®.

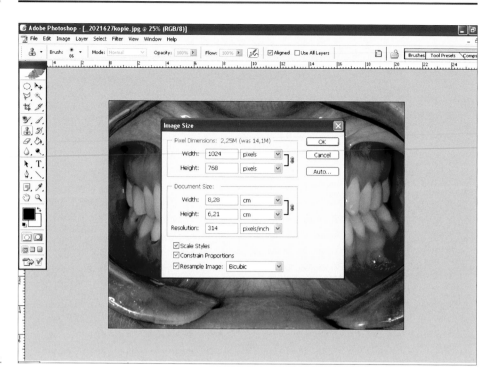

Fig. 15.4
Image width is set to 1024 pixels.

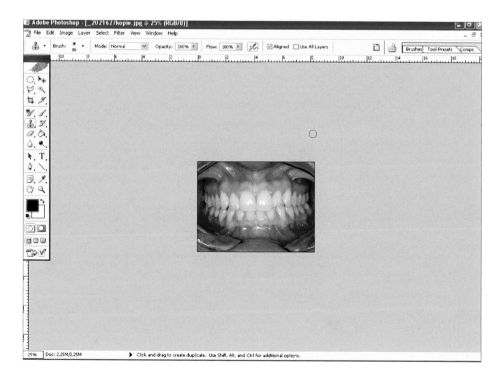

Fig. 15.5
Image is resized to 1024 pixels.

15.1.3   Embedding images in PowerPoint® presentations

PowerPoint® presentations have more or less replaced conventional slide presentations for teaching. PowerPoint® presentations can be used for patient information as well. As this type of presentation is a world-wide standard, it is discussed more in detail in Chapter 18.

15.1.4   Slide shows

Generations of people have suffered through boring post-vacation slide shows. Today, putting together a slide show with digital photographs is far easier and the result can be a fascinating event. In the dental office, slide shows can be used for patient information, e.g., for introducing the dental office team and the specialities offered by the dentist and his or her co-workers.

There are many programs on the market, freeware, shareware, and professional types. Nearly all image editing and archiving programs also offer a slide-show function.

Some examples are:
- ProShow Gold
- Photoshop® Album
- PowerPoint®
- IrfanView®
- PhotoImpact®
- Photoshop Elements®
- Windows Media Player

The procedure is similar for all programs.

Step 1: All the images to be included in the slide show must be imported in a special subdirectory. The selected images are displayed as thumbnails in a browsing window of the program.

Step 2: Images are pulled onto a time-line by drag and drop. The order of the selected images can be changed easily (Fig. 15.6).

Step 3: Image effects, transitions, and text must be added. A preview function allows these effects to be checked (Fig. 15.7).

Step 4: Music can be added. This is an important function as background sound and music give a very professional impression.

Step 5: The finished show must be stored on the PC or written on a CD/DVD.

Step 6: The show can be displayed by beamer projection, on a TV screen, on another PC, or it can be posted to a Web site.

The advantage of sophisticated programs like ProShow Gold (Photodex®) and others is they offer numerous transitions and effects. The disadvantage is the temptation to use all these effects within a single show. This has to be avoided. The secret

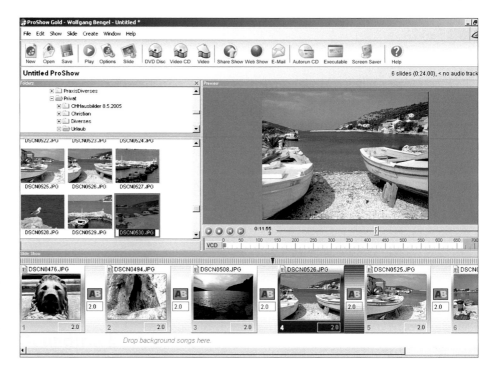

Fig. 15.6   Typical arrangement of windows of a slide-show program: image pool, sequence of images, transitions, time line and control window. The order of images can be changed easily just by dragging them to the new position.

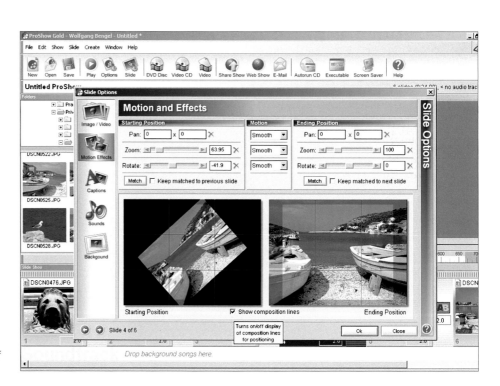

Fig. 15.7   Slide shows allow motion and zoom effects which give the show the appearance of a movie.

of a good slide show is to use these options sparingly. Otherwise, the audience will feel queasy after the show.

Some hints for selecting a program:

- Which file formats can be used?
- Can the order of the selected images be changed easily?
- Are transitions selectable?
- Which sound data format can be used?
- Can your own soundtrack recorded by microphone be added?
- Can images be zoomed?
- Does the program resize the selected images?
- Which output formats are offered?

Some hints for creating a show:

- Give some thought to the story you want to tell.
- Keep it simple and short, maximum 15 to 20 minutes.
- Start and end with your best pictures.
- Select only high quality pictures for the show.
- Reduce variety of transitions.
- Zoom and pan slowly.
- Pace the show, one image should be visible for about 5 to 10 seconds.
- Select music carefully, it should match the show.

After a short time, very impressive slide shows can be created with rather simple-to-use programs.

15.2   Printing images

Modern possibilities of printing have moved the darkroom into the office. What in the past was sometimes a nightmare of unpleasant-smelling chemicals, frustrating attempts to produce a high-quality print, and spending hours in a dark room has changed dramatically. Although the digital darkroom of today has its pitfalls, routine work can be done more or less on the side. The goal is a photo-realistic or photo-quality print.

For our purposes, two types of printers can produce photo-quality prints:

- Ink-jet printers
- Dye sublimation printers

15.2.1   Ink-jet printers

It is said that a researcher started the development of ink-jet printers (bubble-jet technology) when he accidentally touched a syringe needle filled with ink with a hot soldering iron. The heat forced a drop of ink out of the needle.

Two techniques are used: thermal technology and piezo-electric technology. Ink-jet printers operate exactly as their name implies: Ink is sprayed onto the printing substrate in small droplets of color. When one strip of paper is covered with enough ink to form that portion of the image, the paper is advanced and the print head can continue to deposit ink until it has covered the entire sheet of paper.

Different colors are generated by spraying tiny dots one on top and/or partly beside the other. As the human eye is not able to resolve the ink dots, the impression of a mixed color is generated. Most digital printers use a combination of four or six colors to print full-color images: yellow, magenta, cyan, and black (plus light cyan and light magenta).

It is advisable to select a printer with individual ink tanks. Dental photographs often show a color dominance (e.g., red). That means that the different colors are not used up equally. If all different colors are in one tank, this can be very expensive in the long run.

While digital cameras use pixels to measure image resolution, printer resolution is based on the number of dots per inch (dpi) the printer lays down on paper. The higher the dpi, the smaller the dot, and the harder it is to discern one dot from another with normal viewing. Printer resolutions vary from 300 to 1400 dpi and higher.

The terms printer and image resolution are very often a source of confusion. A 1400 dpi printer is able to spray 1400 ink dots per inch. But not every dot represents a pixel. A pixel is represented by a number of ink dots sprayed on top or beside each other, only visible with a strong magnifying glass or with a microscope.

The resolution of an image which is going to be printed by an ink-jet printer should be about 200 dpi. This resolution can be set using the image editing program (see below). When a high-quality printer and special paper are used, a photorealistic image can be achieved.

The print size depends on the file-size and the printing resolution. A file with 1478 x 1280 pixels printed at 163 dpi will have a dimension of about 9 x 7.8 inches (1478 : 163 = 9.01; 1280 : 163 = 7.85).

15.2.2   Dye sublimation printers

Comparable or even better results can be achieved with thermal dye sublimation printers, which, however, are still relatively expensive. Prints produced on these exhibit absolute photo quality. The technology is based on a heat transfer process using thousands of tiny heating elements that come in contact with a "donor ribbon," releasing a gaseous dye that is transferred to the paper. Resolution for images to be printed out by dye sublimation printers should be 300 dpi.

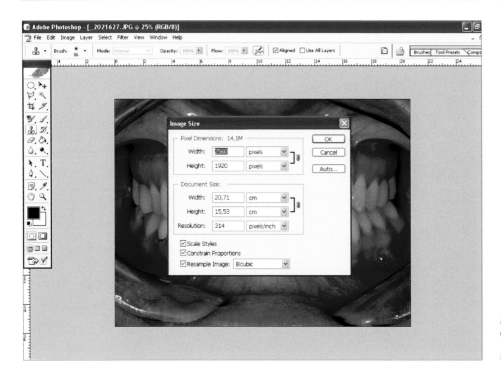

Fig. 15.8   Image Size box is opened in Photoshop®. Under "Document Size" image resolution can be checked.

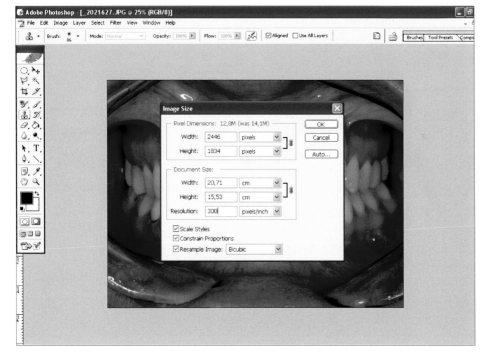

Fig. 15.9   Offset printing needs an image resolution of 300 dpi.

15.2.3   Offset printing

Books and journals are printed using the offset technology. If images for publications are sent to the publishing house, a resolution of 300 dpi is the right value. That means, the file size of an image should be big enough that the image can be printed in its final size at a resolution of 300 dpi. Images with fine line drawings should have a resolution of 600 to 800 dpi. Prepress problems such as color separation etc. will not to be discussed in this context, as these problems are normally managed by the publishing house and not by the dentist or scientist submitting a paper for publication.

15.2.4   Thermo autochrome

Thermo autochrome is a relatively new printer technology that uses heat-sensitive pigment layers incorporated directly into the paper. The three color layers—cyan, magenta, and yellow—are each sensitive to a different temperature. The printer selectively heats areas of the paper, one color at a time, to activate and then fix the pigments with ultraviolet light.

Step-by-step procedure to change the dpi value of an image:
1. Image editing software (e.g., Photoshop®) is open.
2. Image file is opened: FILE > Open > image is selected, file name double clicked. Alternatively: Browser of archive program is open and image is "dragged" into Photoshop®.
3. Image size is determined: IMAGE > Image size. Resolution can be checked. In this example (Fig. 15.8), resolution is 314 pixels per inch.
4. New resolution is entered: 300 dpi as for offset printing (Fig. 15.9). If the layout dimensions of the final images are known, in this menu the document size can also be entered using the final image size when printed.

15.3   Presenting images in PowerPoint® presentations

PowerPoint presentations and presentations using similar programs have replaced the slide presentation. This is discussed more in detail in Chapter 18.

15.4 Presenting images in individually printed photo books

At the inception of digital photography, one of the most cited arguments against digital images was: "I do not need images on a screen. I need printed images, like pictures in a photo album." Digital photography has generated a completely new type of photo album, the individually printed photo book.

These booklets can be used not only as a gift after a holiday or a special event, but also for introducing the office team and the whole spectrum of treatment options and specialties to the new patient.

There are many special companies offering this service:
www.mypublisher.com/deluxeBooks;
www.shutterfly.com/photobooks/info.jsp;
www.snapfish.com/helpphotobooks
www.fotobuch.de
www.fotobuch24.de
www.fotoquelle.de/download/fotobuch.
www.fujifilmnet.ch/Buch/BuchInfo.asp

…

The procedure is generally the same.
- The layout software is downloaded from the Internet and installed.
- Images are selected and stored in a special subdirectory.
- Using the layout software images are arranged in the book.
- Text is added, as well as a cover image.
- Then the whole file is sent to the photo book company via Internet or after writing the file on a CD.
- Seven to 10 days later, the individually printed photo book is ready.

Special problems in digital photography

16

16.1   Neutral color rendition/using a gray card

Color rendition has always been a difficult task in photography. Many factors influence correct color reproduction. A main factor is the color temperature of the incoming light. Beside this, properties of the object to be photographed are important, and of course properties of the camera itself (white balance, sensor technology, software).

The best way to find out how colors are influenced is to take a photograph of a reference object of known color and to compare the result with the real colors of the object. This can be done using a gray card or a color reference card. A gray card is a

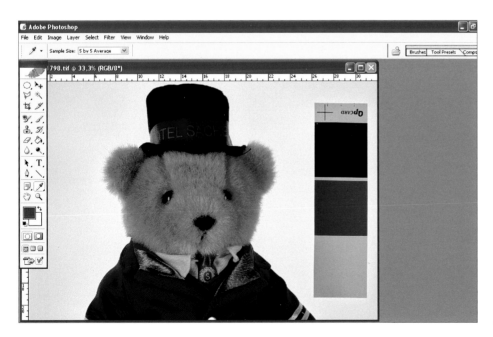

Fig. 16.1   Image including a gray card is loaded.

piece of gray cardboard or plastic which reflects 18% of the incident light. This is exactly the standard reference value against which all photo light meters are calibrated. Therefore, the main purpose of a gray card is to help meter the light precisely. In addition, a gray card is truly neutral. That means the RGB values are equal. Therefore, a gray card can be used to neutralize colors.

In section 16.3, a suggestion is made on how to use a mini gray card in clinical photography. The following refers to extraoral photography.

1. Select an appropriate white balance setting of your camera (see below).
2. Take a picture of your object including the gray card. This is the reference image.

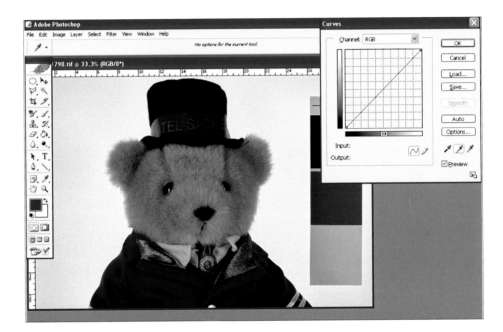

Fig. 16.2   Gray eyedropper is selected from the curves menu.

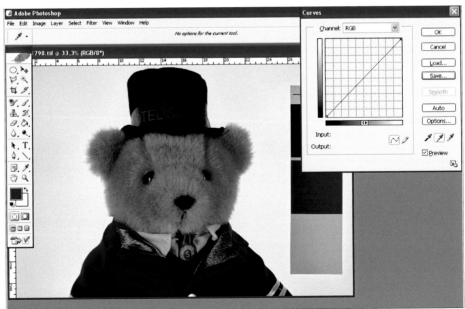

Fig. 16.3   Changes by using the eyedropper to neutralize the image can be saved.

3. Remove the gray card and expose an image of your object or a series of images under the same lighting conditions.
4. Load the image with the gray card in Photoshop® (Fig. 16.1).
5. Select the eyedropper tool by pressing "I". Click right and select sample size: 5 by 5 average.
6. Open "curves.menu": Ctrl.+ m. Select gray eyedropper (the middle one) (Fig. 16.2).
7. Move eyedropper over the gray card and click: the image is set to neutral. That means the R, G, and B values will have the same value in the gray field.

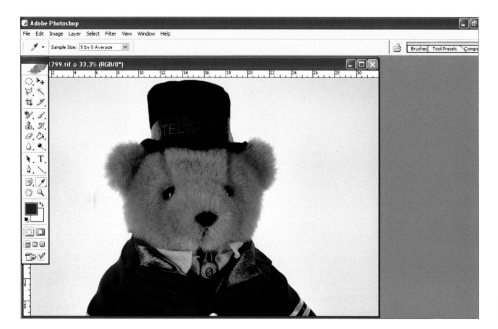

Fig. 16.4   Image without gray card is loaded.

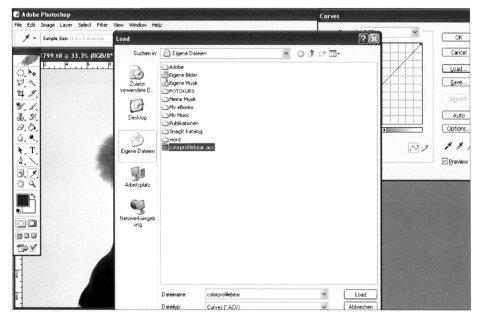

Fig. 16.5
Correction profile is loaded.

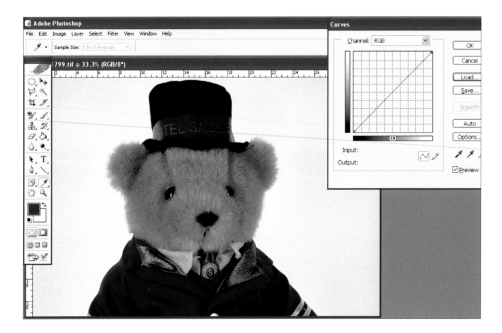

Fig. 16.6   Corrections are applied to the image.

8. Save the correction by clicking "Save" in the curves dialog (Fig. 16.3).

9. Open the next image without gray card included (Fig. 16.4).

10. Open curves dialog by: IMAGE > adjust > curves or Ctrl.+ m and click "Load", "load-menu" opens (Fig. 16.5).

11. Select the correction profile you saved before and click "Load" again: the image is color corrected in the same way (Fig. 16.6).

12. Repeat this with all further images you took in the same session under the same lighting conditions.

For the beginner this may look complicated, but it is a fast and easy method. In the same way (without gray card), color corrections can also be performed automatically with clinical photographs.

Gray cards are available from different companies: e.g., Kodak, Macbeth, Fotowand, Qpcard (16.7 and 16.8). The Qpcard 101 is very good: it is a gray card with a black and a white part. The gray field can be used for color neutralization, the other parts for the black and the white point setting (Fig. 16.9 a-b and 16.10 a-c). The Qpcard 201 is a color reference card with 27 color fields: white, black, 5 gray tones, and 20 colors. It can be used together with a small computer program for automatic color correction.

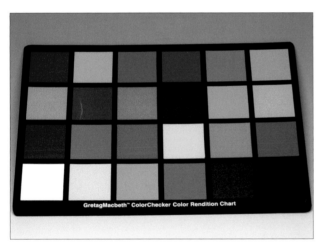

Fig. 16.7   Color checker from Gretag Macbeth®.

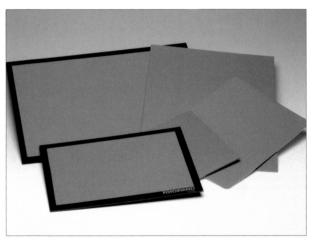

Fig. 16.8   Choice of gray cards from different manufacturers.

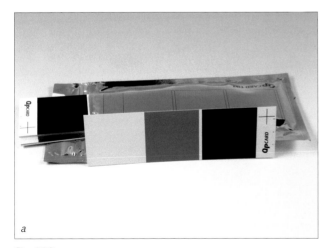

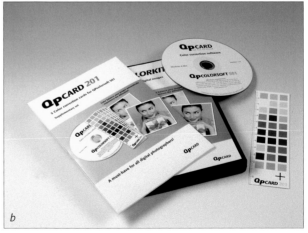

Fig. 16.9
The QPcard can be used as a gray card and for setting the black and white point (a). The QPcard color can be used for optimizing colors (b).

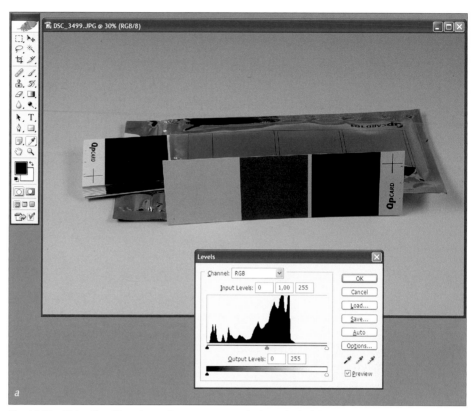

Fig. 16.10   Using the QPcard: Levels menu is opened (a). With the black eyedropper, the black field of the card is clicked (b). After clicking on the white field of the QPcard with the white eyedropper (c).

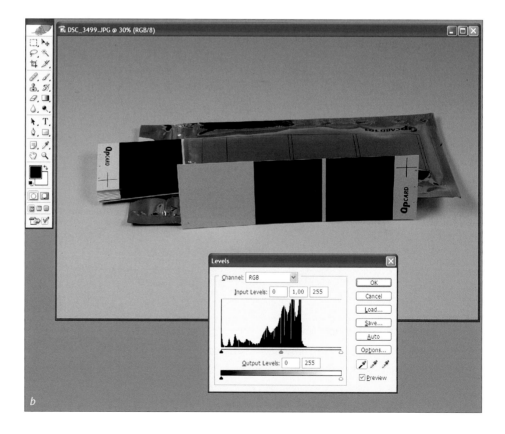

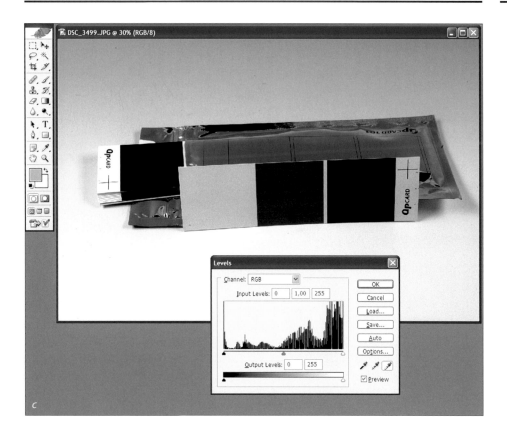

16.2   White balance setting

When we read a book, its paper always appears white to us, even completely different lighting conditions. This is due to the so-called color adaptation of our brain. We see the paper white, because we know that it is white. When we move from the bright, blue-tinted sunlight to the dim, yellow-tinted indoor lighting, our eye automatically adjusts to the different color of light and changes our perception accordingly.

A digital camera "sees" and records the paper as it is, depending on the illumination. Bright daylight gives a blue cast, incandescent lighting a yellow, and fluorescent lighting a green one (Fig. 16.11 a-f).

If you expect to get accurate colors in your photographs, your digital camera must be told what "color" of light is illuminating the subject. This is called "white balancing": you show the camera something that should look neutral (white or gray card) and use that as a reference point, so that all the other colors in the scene will be reproduced naturally.

The AUTO-White Balance function a camera offers is nothing more than a guess, which sometimes comes surprisingly close. But according to the experience of many digital photographers, it is not the best choice in most situations. Customized white balance settings are better, such as "cloudy" or electronic flash. Beside this, good cameras offer the possibility of fine-tuning the WB setting in steps of 100 K.

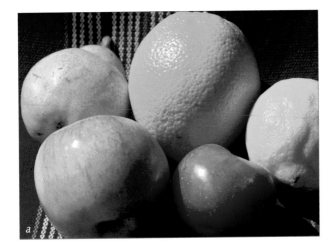
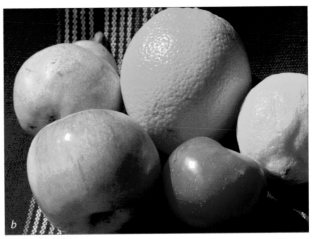
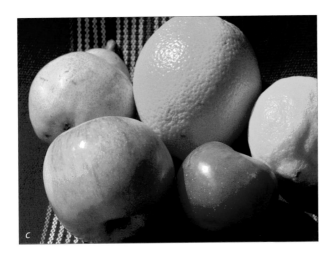
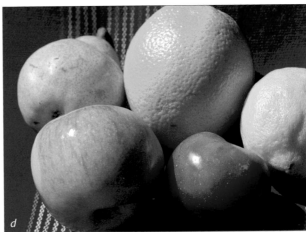
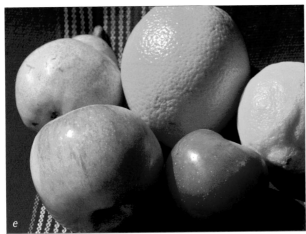
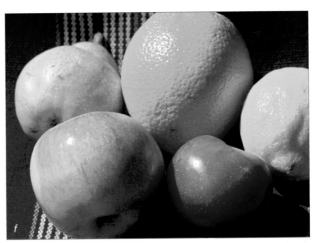

Fig. 16.11   The fruit basket was shot in bright sunlight with different white balance settings of the camera: sunlight (a), shadow (b), clouds (c), tungsten light (d), neon light (e) and electronic flash (f). Distinct differences are visible.

For clinical work with electronic flash, the "flash" setting is appropriate.

When shooting RAW files, the white balance setting can be performed as part of the conversion process.

If you work under unusual lighting conditions and if you want accurate colors, where the hues don't shift from shot to shot, there's no substitute for setting the white balance yourself manually anytime the lighting conditions change. Especially under mixed lighting conditions, or to compensate for light sources with a strong color cast, a manually performed white balance is recommended.

The necessary steps to white balance a digital camera differ from one camera to the next. Details have to be looked up in the operating instructions. The procedure in principle is as follows:

1   Take a white piece of paper or a neutral gray card.
2   Point the camera at it.
3   Perform the necessary settings of the camera.
4   Press the white balance button of the camera.

As an example, the procedure for the Nikon D1X is described below.

Step 1: In the shooting menu, White Bal is highlighted,
the multi-selector is pressed.

Step 2: WB is highlighted, multi-selector is pressed to the right.

Step 3: Set is highlighted, multi-selector is pressed to the right.
Message "Please release the shutter" appears.

Step 4: A white or gray object (often the backside of a gray card is white for this purpose) is placed so that it fills the viewfinder.

Step 5: The shutter release button is pressed all the way down. This meters the color temperature as the value for the white balancing. This value is stored in the camera memory. No image will be recorded.

Step 6: The measured value can be stored as one of three "Preset values" in order to speed up this procedure when shooting under the same lighting conditions.

As digital cameras have a tendency toward cool color rendition, "warm cards" (cards with a light bluish color) are recommended for "normal" applications. The result: color rendition of the camera is a little bit warmer, skin tones and landscapes look more pleasing. This is not recommended for medical documentation.

16.3 Assessment of tooth color/brightness

For many years, attempts have been made to use photography to improve communication between dentists and dental technicians. Up to now, no method has been described which could replace shade selection by the dentist and/or the dental technician by using dental photographs alone. Other methods are used to assess tooth color shade and tooth brightness. Nevertheless, an image provides the dental technician with a lot of valuable information concerning tooth morphology, surface texture, color distribution, luster, and other properties. To obtain a high-quality clinical image and numerical values that make it possible to determine the tooth color, a digital image is generated and loaded into image editing software. This software provides numerical values of color and brightness of the image (or parts of it).

The question is, how reliable can a digital camera be and which factors influence color rendition and image brightness in photography? In photography, color rendition and image brightness are influenced mainly by the light, the camera technology, and the various image output devices. In this context light and camera technology are of major interest.

Influence of light

Photography means "writing/drawing with light". One of the most important properties of light is its color temperature (color of light radiated by a "black body", expressed in °Kelvin). Unlike our brain, which adapts to different color temperatures and always "sees" a white sheet of paper as white, even when lit by a yellowish light source, a camera sees the color temperature as it is: neutral at 6000 °K, yellowish at 2800 to 4000 °K, and bluish at temperatures between 7000 and 9000 °K.

Color temperature of daylight changes depending on the time of the day, the season, the weather, and the direction a window is facing. Therefore, daylight affects color rendition of an image, causing a certain color cast. This is the reason why color shade selection in the dental office should not be performed under daylight. Room illumination affects color rendition as well. Very often "daylight" fluorescent tubes are used, trying to imitate daylight. Normally they do not have a continuous spectrum and are not perfectly neutral.

The dental operating lamp is another source for a color cast. Here, halogen bulbs are often used, which have a color temperature between 3000 and 3400 °K, causing a yellowish cast.

Light reflected from the clothing of the patient (as well as from assistant and dentist), the walls, and the ceiling can cause a weak color cast. Therefore, neutral tones are recommended for the operating room.

The color temperature of the flash light itself is very important. Powerful flash lights with short flash duration time tend to be somewhat more bluish compared to weak flash systems. In addition, color temperature depends on the mixture of gases in the tube. The type of flash is important as well, as it determines the lighting angle. A ring flash with axial light direction causes a different color rendition than a side (point or a twin) flash. The amount of light fired by a flash and thus the image brightness also depend on the charge of the flash capacitor. Often, the capacitor is not recharged completely when the flash ready LED indicates that the flash is ready to fire again. It is advisable to wait another three or four seconds.

The influence of these factors cannot be avoided completely, but can be minimized by the following measures:

- Daylight should be blocked out.
- Neutral colors for ceiling, walls and clothing.
- Use of a powerful flash.
- Aperture should be closed at least to stop 16 or 22.
- Flash condensator should be given time to recharge completely.

Influence of camera technology

Lens

Every lens has its own color characteristic. This depends on the type of glass used for the lens elements and the coating on their surfaces to prevent flare. As this characteristic does not change from one exposure to the next and as it has only a very weak influence, the color characteristic is not really a problem for our purposes.

Moreover, the lens has an indirect influence on color rendition. Its focal length determines – together with the chosen magnification ratio – the working distance and consequently the lighting angle, if a flash system is used which is fixed to the lens.

Camera alignment/patient position

In this context, camera alignment must be mentioned, although it is not a technical property of the camera, but a question of its handling. It is important to align the camera in a repeatable way. The optical axis of the camera should always be oriented according to the anatomical planes of the patient. It should be perpendicular to the patient's frontal plane and go over into the occlusal plane without an angle. Only in this way can repeatable results be expected concerning the inclination of the camera in relation to the front teeth. To facilitate alignment, the use of a grid screen is strongly recommended. Some researchers recommend the use of a chin rest to stabilize the patient position.

Exposure mode

Modern cameras offer different exposure modes. In addition to a manual exposure mode, in which we can preset aperture and exposure time manually, three automatic modes are usually available: aperture priority (aperture is preselected, camera sets the exposure time automatically; symbol A), shutter priority (aperture is set by the camera after the shutter speed was set; symbol S), and program mode (both parameters are set by the camera; symbol P). In dental photography, the manual and the aperture priority modes are used.

The chief problem is that the camera does not "know" whether an object is very dark, very bright, or is somewhere inbetween. Therefore, the exposure system of the camera always tries to generate a picture with a medium brightness value, corresponding with a medium gray tone. The consequence is that very bright objects (e.g., a white cast) are reproduced too dark, while dark objects are reproduced too bright. In these cases, an exposure compensation has to be used to adjust exposure. For bright objects, light has to be added; if the object is dark, light has to be reduced. Therefore, an automatic exposure mode cannot be used for obtaining reproducible results when tooth brightness is assessed.

To make it more complicated, the different light metering characteristics of a camera (spot, center weighted, and matrix metering) also influence image brightness. In dental photography, spot and center weighted systems often result in images which are too dark, as the white teeth are often in the image center. An exposure compensation (plus correction) has to be used in these cases. Matrix systems take different image segments into account individually for light metering. Normally, the center and the lower segments are taken into account more than the upper image parts. This works well for general photography, but can lead to wrong exposures in dental photography.

To obtain reproducible results, a manual exposure mode and a manual flash mode (without TTL flash metering) must be used.

Camera sensor

In a digital camera, the image of an object is projected onto the surface of the sensor. As this sensor consists of millions of single photo elements, the image is split into millions of picture elements (pixels). Brightness is recorded for each single pixel and then transformed into an electric signal. Color is generated by internal data processing, as photo diodes are color blind. Therefore, color rendition and image brightness depend highly on the type of sensor, the filters used for generating color information, the computer algorithms, the white balance settings, and other influencing factors.

In order to attain reproducible results in terms of color rendition and image brightness when using a digital camera, the following guidelines must be followed:

- Work in the same surroundings.
- Use the same equipment (digital SLR camera with macro-lens and electronic flash).
- Choose the same magnification ratio (e.g., 1:1).
- Select a manual exposure (no automatic exposure mode); that means always preset the same aperture.
- Select the manual flash mode (no TTL flash metering).
- Select a fixed white balance (no automatic white balance).
- Select the same image resolution.
- Select the same file type (TIFF or JPEG with same degree of image compression).
- Set a low ISO value (e.g., ISO 100 or 125).
- Put a black background behind the teeth in order to avoid differences of the semi-transparent tooth due to the tongue position of the patient.
- Use a standardized camera alignment.

Even if all these rules are obeyed, there will be differences causing a color cast and a variability in image brightness. These are mostly due to a certain technical variability of the camera system (aperture opening, flash function etc.). Hence, a method must be employed which permits fine-tuning of color rendition and image brightness.

Procedure to obtain comparable results

If a certain variability of the images cannot be avoided completely, even if maximum efforts for standardization have been made, one has to find a method to eliminate differences as far as possible. In professional photography, a gray card is used for these purposes.

A gray card is a piece of cardboard or plastic with a surface which has a reflectance value of 18%. A gray card is a neutral target. That means the red, blue, and green values are equal. The idea is to put something in the picture that has a known value, in other words, that we know to be pure gray and then let the software make sure that that object really is gray. In this manner, a color cast of the whole picture will be eliminated.

Because normal gray cards available in photographic stores are too large to include in a 1:1 shot, only a small piece of gray card, punched out using an office holepunch, is fixed above a tooth with a small amount of vaseline.

A world industry standard of image editing software is the Adobe Photoshop® program, which is used to neutralize the image and meter the colors.

Step-by-step-procedure to obtain comparable photographic results

Step 1: Open the Info box.

> After starting the Photoshop® program, the Information menu is opened, which gives us the color information of each single pixel. WINDOW > Info (or F8).

Step 2: Open the image data file.

> The image to be analyzed is opened by Ctrl + O or FILE > Open and then navigate through the files until you reach the image data file, then double-click (Fig. 16.12).

Step 3: Blur the gray card.

> As the surface of most gray cards is not completely homogeneous, there will be small color differences in close-up shots of their surface. Therefore, we have to blur the gray card.
>
> Click M to select the marquee tool and select the central part of the gray card (Fig. 16.13).
>
> Choose FILTER > blur > Gaussian blur and apply this filter to the selected area in order to even the gray card image. Radius 8, Terminate by OK.
> Deselect the section by SELECT > deselect or Ctrl.+D.

Step 4: Eliminate a color cast.

> To eliminate an overall color cast, we open the LEVELS dialog by Ctrl. + L (or IMAGE > ADJUST > LEVELS). A histogram appears and three

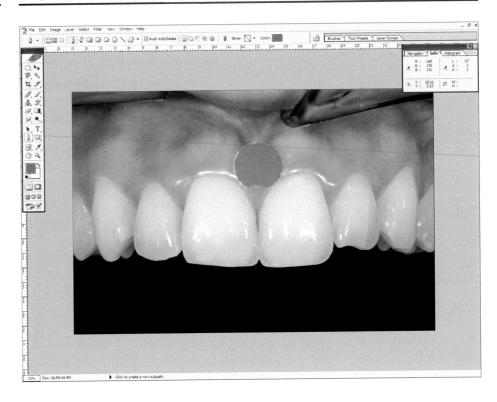

Fig. 16.12   Image with gray card included is opened in Photoshop®.

eyedropper tools. The middle one is the gray one (Fig. 16.14). It is selected and moved over the piece of gray card included in the picture.

By clicking again, the global color cast of the image is eliminated.

This can be controlled by checking the INFORMATION panel: The R, G, and B values, which were slightly different before, have the same value now. The Lab values are changed as well: a and b are set to 0, the L value does not change (Fig. 16.15).

Terminate this step by OK.

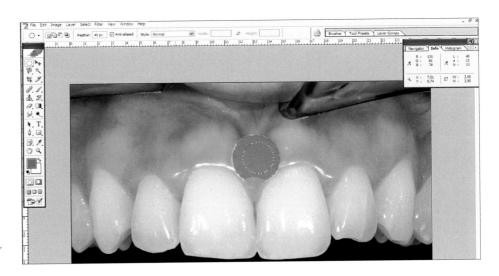

Fig. 16.13   The central part of the gray card is selected in order to blur this area.

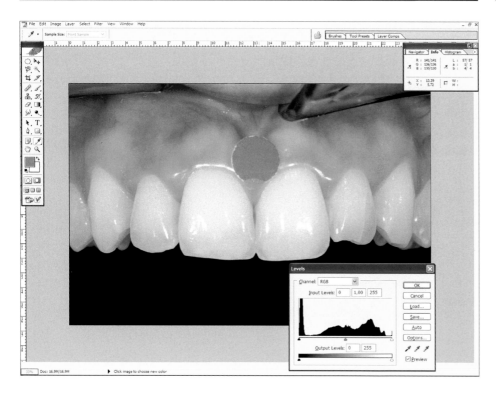

Fig. 16.14
Levels dialog is open.

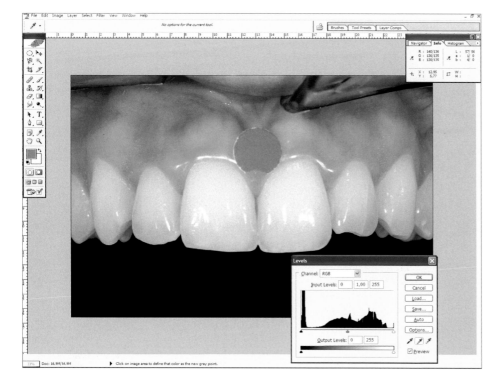

Fig. 16.15   Image is set to neutral by clicking with the gray eyedropper on the piece of gray card.

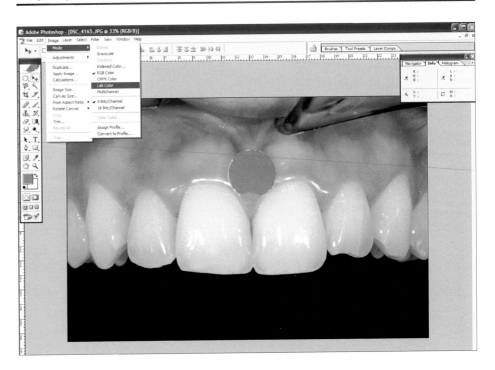

Fig. 16.16   *Changing the color mode from RGB to Lab.*

Step 5: Change the color space
In this step, the color space is changed from RGB to Lab. This is necessary if L*a*b* values are to be recorded using the Photoshop® histogram. Furthermore, it has the advantage that Lab values can be compared with results of electronic devices which also use the Lab values.
If these data are only used for patient information and a comparison with other data is not planned, this step is not necessary: IMAGE > Mode > Lab Color (Fig. 16.16).

Step 6: Fine-tune image brightness
To acquire images with a comparable brightness, image brightness is set to a medium value. The brightness of an image is expressed by the L value. By IMAGE > Adjustments > Brightness/Contrast, the overall image brightness can be changed. The brightness level is adjusted to an L value of 54. By this, brightness of the whole image is set to a fixed value, which then can be compared with image brightness of other images (Fig. 16.17).

Step 7: Select the area to be measured
The tooth to be measured is selected by using the magnetic lasso. After this, the selected tooth is surrounded by a broken line on the monitor. That means that all measurements refer only to the image content within this line. To select the magnetic lasso, click on the magnetic lasso icon in the tool bar or type L. Move the lasso over the margin of the area to be selected and start by clicking. As you drag the lasso icon slowly along the edge of your area or object, the tool drops fastening points to anchor the selection. If a point is not placed correctly, it can be eliminated by DELETE and placed directly by clicking.

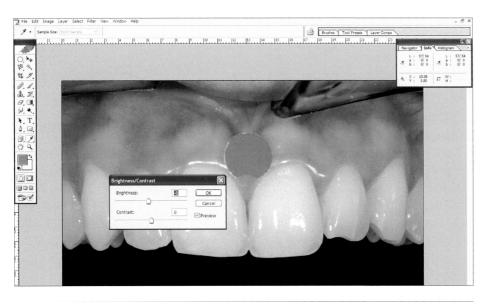

Fig. 16.17
Fine-tuning image brightness.

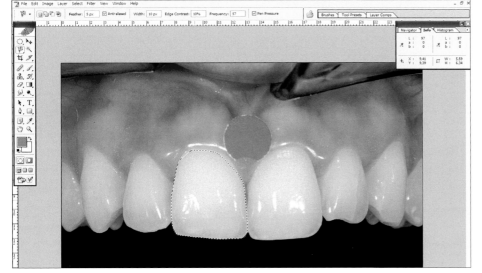

Fig. 16.18
Area to be measured is selected.

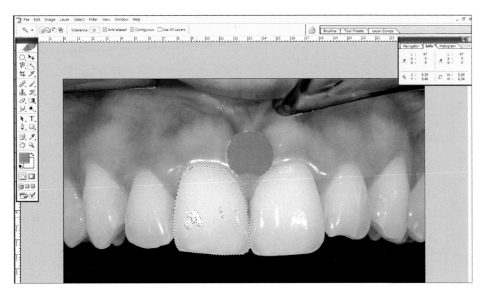

Fig. 16.19
Reflections are excluded.

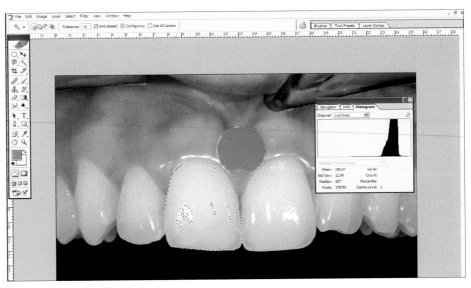

Fig. 16.20   Histogram is opened, lightness can be measured.

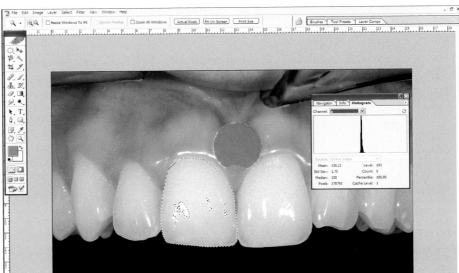

Fig. 16.21
a-value is measured.

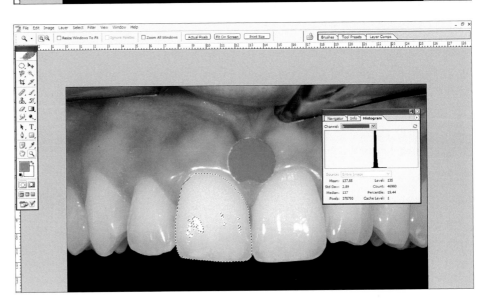

Fig. 16.22
b-value is measured.

When you reach the starting point again, doubleclick: a broken line appears ("marching ants"). The area is selected (Fig. 16.18).

Step 8: Exclude reflections

Reflections on the tooth surface must be excluded, as they may differ from shot to shot and have a great influence on the result. This can be done easily by use of the "magic wand" + ALT. To select the magic wand, click on the magic wand icon in the tool bar or type W. Move the cursor over the reflections within the selected area, press ALT (the magic wand icon appears), and click. By repeating this procedure, all reflections can be excluded (Fig. 16.19). Tolerance level is set to 20.

Alternatively, the masking mode can be used to modify the selected area.

Step 9: Determine the Lab, a and b values

L, a and b values of the selected area are determined.

Up to Photoshop® Version 7.0, the histogram is opened by IMAGE>Histogram. In Photoshop® CS (vs. 8.0) click WINDOW>Histogram. Then click the arrow button under the white cross in the right upper box angle and select "expanded view". Select "show statistics" and then Lightness channel. Write down the L values. In the same way, a and b values are determined. The Photoshop® histogram gives information about the mean L, a and b values, their median, the standard deviation and the number of pixels which were taken into account (Fig. 16.20 to 16.22).

To transform the Photoshop® Lab values into the CIELab values, one has to consider that the range of these values is different in the two systems. In Photoshop®, the range of the L(PM) value (= Photoshop® Mean Value of L) is from 0 to 255. The CIELab L* values range from 0 to 100.

A transformation can be done by the formula:

$L* = L(PM) \times 100/255$.

In the same way, the a and b values are transformed. The Photoshop® values reach from 0 to 255, the CIELab values from +120 to +120. The transformation formula is:

$a* = (a(PM) - 128) \times 240/255$ (a(PM) = Photoshop® mean value of a)

$b* = (b(PM) - 128) \times 240/255$ (b(PM) = Photoshop® mean value of b)

Compared with electronic devices such as spectrophotometers and colorimeters, the use of digital photography for the assessment of tooth color and the outcome of bleaching procedures has the advantage that there are not only numerical data which can be evaluated, but also an image. This is valuable to provide a clinical impression. In some cases, it might be more important for the dental technician than the numerical data.

16.4 Cleaning the camera sensor

As in conventional photography, dust can be a major problem in digital photography as well (Fig. 16.23). If there are dust particles on the sensor, there will be spots and smudges on the digital images, especially visible on those pictures shot with the lens stopped down.

To be more precise, the dust does not sit on the sensor but on the surfaces in front of it (e.g., dichroic mirror, low pass filter). Because this surface is charged, it attracts the dust particles. These particles may enter the camera body when lenses are changed. Therefore, it is good practice when changing lenses to hold the camera so that the body front is directed at the floor.

Dust particles may also be the result of internal mechanical abrasion processes of moving parts. Most digital SLR cameras have their own strategy for fighting dust. The Sigma SD10 has encapsulated the sensor completely by a dust protector (Fig. 16.24). This is helpful, but it does not guarantee that there will never be dust on the sensor. Moving mechanical parts inside the camera can also be a source of dust. In this case, the dust protector can be taken out in order to access the sensor. Olympus created a "vibrating" sensor for the E-1, which removes dust particles by an ultrasonic vibration of the sensor. The particles shaken off the chip surface are then trapped by a small piece of adhesive tape.

The best way to check the sensor is to stop down the lens to f/22 and take a shot of an evenly illuminated bright object like white paper or blue sky. Open the resulting image in Photoshop® and enhance image contrast (AutoLevels).

Dust can be removed by different means. Don't use abrasive tools or liquids, as this runs the risk of ruining the sensor. Do not rub the sensor surface. This is a sure way to damage the sensor. Follow the instructions of the camera's operating manual. Normally there is a setting which keeps your camera set to BULB. Use a magnifying glass and ensure good illumination. Try to remove dust with regular Q-tips first. You don't need

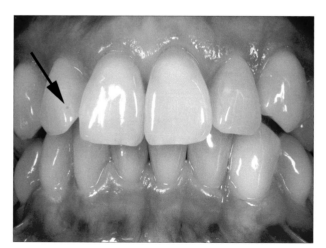

Fig. 16.23   Dust spots are a major problem in digital photography. This single spot could be removed quickly by the healing brush tool.

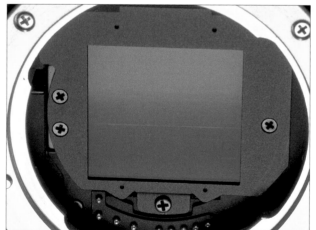

Fig. 16.24   In the Sigma SD-10, the sensor is protected by a glass filter covering the camera opening.

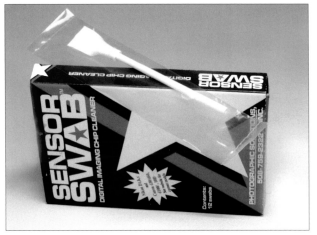

Fig. 16.25   The Sensorswab from Photographic Solutions is specially designed to clean the digital sensor.

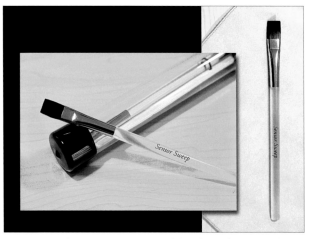

Fig. 16.26   The Sensor Sweep is a soft brush which attracts dust particles (Illustration: Copper Hill Company).

to touch the sensor surface. Often dust particles "jump" to the Q-tip due electrostatic forces. Another possibility is to use a Sensor Swab (Photographic Solutions, Fig. 16.25).

For more details of sensor cleaning, visit www.phase.com/copperhill/ccd_cleaning. The Copper Hill Company offers different sets of items for this purpose, including soft brushes (Sensor Sweep) (Fig.16.26). Other types of sensor brushes with different sizes for different sensors are offered by a company called VisibleDust (www.visibledust.com).

Adhesive tape is not recommended. There is always the danger of adhesive left on the sensor surface, which will ruin the most expensive part of the camera. The same can be true for the so-called SpeckGrabber (Kinetronics Corporation). This tool might be interesting for rather big particles which are visible. But normally dust cannot be seen even through a magnifying glass.

A questionable method is the use of carbon dioxide gas to blow the dust away. This method does not remove the dust. It only moves it from one point to the next. Don't use the compressed air of the dental unit, unless you are sure that it is oil free.

Take care of the lens surfaces as well. Under certain conditions, dust particles on the lens surface can create dark spots on the image as well, especially when shooting with the aperture closed down (Fig. 16.27).

A completely different way to solve the problem is a software solution offered by Nikon. The Nikon Capture software has a feature called Image Dust Off. The software attempts to map out a sensor dust pattern with help from the user and a reference image. It then applies a correction to all images in a batch process. This is, of course, not a real solution to this problem. The problem should be addressed at the source (i.e., the mirror chamber) instead of afterwards in the software.

If every recommended method fails, get the sensor cleaned professionally. If there are only few dust particles visible, Photoshop® will help to "clean" the image.

Fig. 16.27   Especially when closing down the aperture, dust particles on the lens surface can also cause dark spots on the image. In this case, dust on the back side of the lens caused a dark spot.

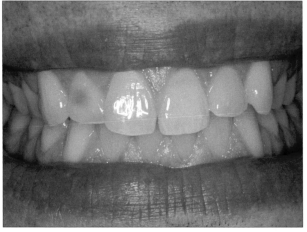

16.5 Integrity of digital images

Medical documentation is very often based on images. Therefore it is important to maintain the integrity of the image file.

Image manipulation has been a problem since the beginning of photography in the 1850s. Digital imaging has added a new technology which can be used by almost anyone to fake photographs; however, digital imaging offers a new possibility to detect manipulation.

Everybody has to find out for him- or herself the value images have as proof or documentation. In forensics, there may be other standards necessary than in the "normal" dental practice. It does not make much sense for a dental practice to follow a protocol according to the guidelines created by the Scientific Working Group on Imaging Technologies (SWGIT) of the FBI. But it makes sense to know these guidelines (www.fbi.gov/hg/lab/fsc/backissu/oct1999/swgit1.htm), which state that it is essential to maintain an archive image. That means an exact copy of the image recorded by the camera onto its original media. This unaltered image can be compared with the final image in order to find out if the image content or image quality has been altered.

If image adjustments are necessary, all image changes should be tracked. In Adobe Photoshop® CS, an image creator can automatically record an audit trail by invoking the History Log feature in the Preferences pane. Using this feature, every tool can be recorded along with its settings. The recordings can be added to the metadata and reviewed later.

Some companies offer special software solutions allowing the detection of even the smallest image change. Canon offers a Data Verification Kit for the EOS 1Ds and the Mark II model. This kit includes the software, a Secure Mobile (SM) card reader, and a dedicated memory card.

RAW files are virtually unalterable without leaving traces experts can detect. For medical purposes, this may be a simple solution. For forensic matters, using RAW files may not be safe enough as the processing information does not become part of the archive file. For dental purposes, it may be sufficient to keep the original archive files together with the information on which adjustments have been performed. If a RAW format was used, all information on any image adjustments must also be kept.

Image editing – useful Photoshop® procedures

17

Image editing measures can be divided into those which improve image quality and those which change their content. Changing image content is not allowed in medical documentation. It has become common at conferences for the lecturer to declare that he or she has not manipulated the images. Although this was naturally possible to do before the age of digital imaging, it is now far simpler.

Due to their technical characteristics, it is necessary to make some enhancements to digital images. These can be done using practically any of the image editing software programs on the market.

In this chapter a short overview is given over some standard procedures which might be of interest for the dental photographer.

17.1   Image editing programs

There are numerous image editing programs on the market which are updated regularly. Therefore, it is not possible to present a complete overview of all programs and their features in one single book. The program mainly referred to in this context is Adobe Photoshop®.

Adobe Photoshop® is the industry standard of professional image editing software programs. It allows improvements to be done quickly and automatically and has huge possibilities not reached by other programs. Although a "normal" user will never make full use of the program, it is recommended, as it has a clear and logical structure. It is not necessary to use the latest version, which is rather expensive. For our purposes an older version will do as well.

Adobe Photoshop® Elements® is the little brother of Photoshop®. Many options have been taken from the standard program. This program will be sufficient for most non-professional users.

PhotoImpact XL (Ulead) is a versatile editing program for beginners and advanced users. It runs only on Windows platforms.

Paint Shop Pro (Jasc) is one of the most professional programs on the market with many options (only for Windows).

Corel Graphic Suite/PhotoPaint offers many options for professional use. Available for Windows, Mac, and Linux.

Roxio Photosuite is a program which promises fast results, particularly for the beginner.

The Gimp is a very versatile freeware program, first made for Linux, now also running under Windows and Mac.

Basic image editing procedures can be also be carried out with most image browser/archiving programs. The features offered may be sufficient for the beginner. A recommendation for beginners: Don't try to learn more than one editing software program at a time, you'll only waste your time. Concentrate on one single program.

The procedures described below are divided into three groups:
- Image editing procedures to enhance images.
- Image editing procedures to change image content.
- Advanced procedures.

17.2   Some preparations

17.2.1   Program set-up

Photoshop® is a powerful tool offering more possibilities than you might need. Therefore it is possible to "personalize" the program surface for different tasks. You can set up and save custom work areas, called workspaces.

The right way to start is to begin with the default settings. After acquiring some experience, the user realizes that certain groupings of palettes work best when performing specific tasks. The default setting is shown in Fig. 17.01.

The Window menu displays a list of all palettes. Check marks indicate which palettes are currently open (Fig. 17.02). Once you have determined which palettes you want open, you then want to save your workspace. To save a workspace, select Window > Workspace > Save Workspace with everything in the desired position. A dialog box appears and asks you to name this workspace. Give it a name that describes what this workspace will be used for. Descriptive names work much better than using a naming structure such as "Workspace 1," or "Workspace 2." Instead use a naming convention that helps you easily identify the workspace, such as "Masking" or "Color Correction."

In the same way, workspaces can be deleted: Windows > Workspace > Delete Workspace. There is also an option to delete "All" workspaces and a possibility to return to the situation when starting Photoshop® (Reset).

In order to maximize working space the palettes can be docked to the "Palette Well" – a docking area in the top right of the screen. To do this, a click on the top right triangle opens a menu box with the different options. One of them is "Dock to Palette Well" (Fig. 17.3).

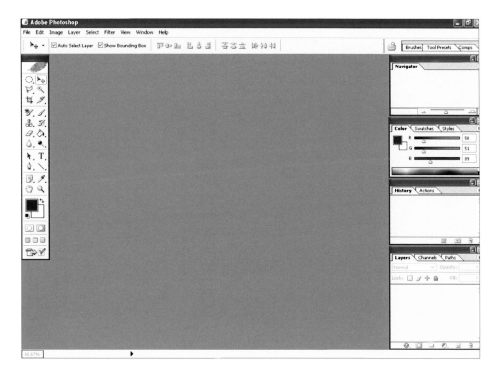

Fig. 17.01
Default settings of PhotoshopCS®.

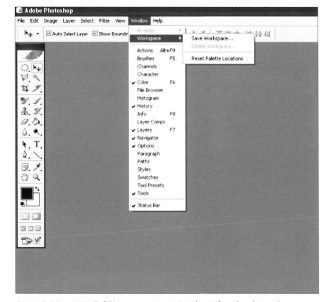

Fig. 17.02 WINDOW menu open. Look at the check marks.

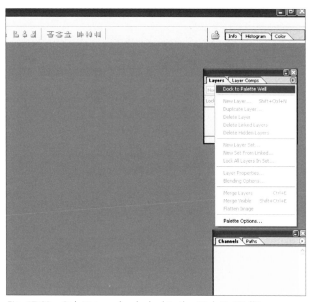

Fig. 17.03 Palettes can be docked to the "Palette Well".

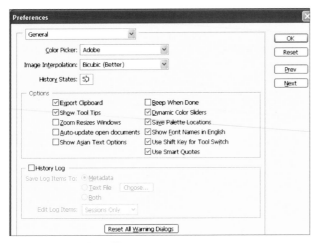

Fig. 17.04   Number of history states set to 50.

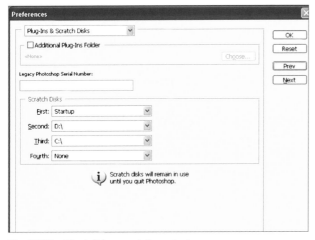

Fig. 17.05   Hard disk space is important.

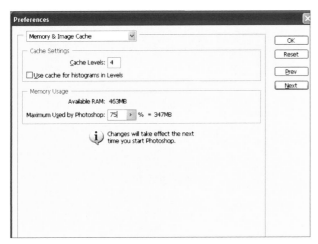

Fig. 17.06   Memory usage is set to 75% or minimum 200 MB.

To speed the work with Photoshop® it is advisable to keep in mind short keys:

- F5 opens and closes the brushes box with the Brush Presets.
- F6 opens and closes the color slider.
- F7 opens and closes the Layers palette.
- F8 opens and closes the Info palette.
- F9 opens and closes the Actions palette.

There are many keyboard shortcuts used in Photoshop®. They can be looked up and edited under EDIT>Keyboard Shortcuts (or Alt+Shift+Ctrl.+K). By pressing Ctrl. + K (or EDIT > Preferences>General) some individual adjustments can be made.

The number of history states should be changed from 20 to 50 (or higher). This is the number of working steps which can be revoked (Fig. 17.04). After pressing NEXT, the File Handling menu box opens. Under "Maximize PSD File Compatibility" the option "Ask" or "Never" should be checked.

After pressing NEXT, several times the menu box "Plug-Ins & Scratch Disks" opens. Here Photoshop® is given additional hard disk space (Fig. 17.05). Another NEXT click opens the Memory & Image Cache box. Memory usage is set to 75% or a minimum of 200 MB (Fig. 17.06). Again, press NEXT and deactivate "Allow background processing", if the box is checked.

For advanced users, it makes sense to work with two monitors, one to work on the actual image, the other for the palettes and tools. For this option a dual (or triple) graphic card is necessary.

17.2.2 Calibrating the monitor

When editing an image, the monitor image is the only view you have. The quality of image retouching greatly depends on how accurately the monitor displays it. There is a wide range of tools available. There are expensive hardware and software packages which measure color directly off the screen. Some monitors include calibration software that can be used to set up the monitor in the first place, and then automatically update it as the phosphor age.

Adobe Gamma calibrator

This program comes as part of Adobe Photoshop® from version 5.0 onwards. Adobe Gamma eliminates unwanted color casts from the monitor and ensures the best display possible for the work environment (Fig. 17.07). In addition, Adobe Gamma characterizes the monitor by means of an ICC profile, which is a file that includes a description of the characteristics of it. This profile can be used by any application that uses ICC profiles to compensate for a monitor's color-display limitations.

To calibrate the monitor and create an ICC profile in Adobe Gamma:

1. Choose Start> Settings> Control Panel.
2. Double-click Adobe Gamma.
3. Select Step By Step Wizard, and then click Next.
4. In the Description text box, type a name for the profile. Type a name you will easily identify, such as the monitor name and the date.
5. Click Next, and then follow the on-screen instructions. Before you save the settings, you can use the Before and After buttons to see how the changes you made affect the monitor's display.

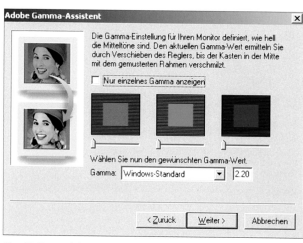

Fig. 17.07   Adobe Gamma Assistant.

Colorimeter tools

Another very popular way to calibrate the monitor is to use a colorimeter like the Spyder2 device from ColorVision (Fig. 17.08). Without having the knowledge of color theory or color management, the user is able to calibrate his or her monitor within a few minutes. The Spyder2 tool can be used for calibration of CRT and LCD monitors and for laptop monitors as well.

Monitor calibration should be repeated from time to time as color rendition changes.

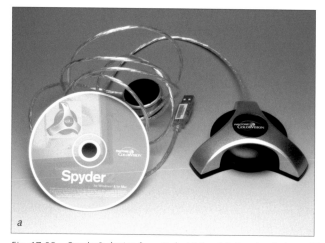

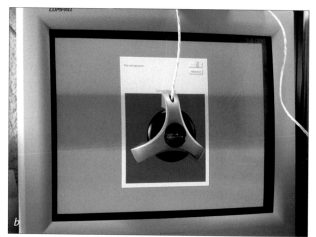

Fig. 17.08   Spyder2 device from ColorVision (a). Spyder during calibration process (b).

17.2.3   Basic procedures

Loading an image

There are different ways to load an image:

- Using the Photoshop® built-in browser, the image is selected and then doubleclicked.
- Using another image browser program (e.g., Fotostation), the monitor image of the program can be reduced to a small image line on the right. The image is selected and dragged into the Photoshop® program.
- Select FILE>open and navigate to the image to be opened.

Saving an image

To save a Photoshop® file, select one of the different save options found in the File menu.

- Save: The Save option is used after an image has already been named and saved. Using the Save option integrates and saves any changes made since the image was last saved. The Save option is available via keyboard shortcut (Ctrl-S for Windows) or the File Menu: FILE>Save.
- Save As: The Save As option is used to save a new image that has not been saved before, or an image that has been saved previously but needs to be saved under a different name (keyboard shortcut: SHIFT+Ctrl.+S).

17.3   Image editing procedures to enhance images

Much image information is generated by interpolation processes after the moment the image is captured. This is one of the main reasons for the fact that all digital images have to be edited. For routine shots, you can preset your camera appropriately so that a part of the work is done automatically. However, if the aim is a high-quality image, it is advisable to edit the image afterwards or, even better, to shoot raw files and do the whole editing work afterwards.

In the daily routine, the JPEG file format is recommended. This has the advantage of small file size without losing too much of image information. As JPEG is a "lossy" file format, which discards image information every time the file is saved, JPEG files must be avoided for intensive multiple-step image editing, in which it is necessary to repeatedly save interim results. For these cases, it is better to transform the initial image into a TIFF file, do the editing, and save the final result as JPEG again, if hard disk space is a consideration.

If images are changed considerably by the editing process, it is generally advisable to work on a copy of the original image.

The following standard procedures may be necessary to improve the image:

- Aligning and cropping the image.
- Adjusting brightness and contrast.
- Adjusting color.
- Sharpening the image.

As one of these points influences the other, the order of these measurements should not be changed.

17.3.1 Aligning and cropping the image

Sometimes an image is not completely symmetrical and a little bit oblique (Fig. 17.09). It is loaded into Photoshop® (Fig. 17.10) and the crop tool (press C) is selected. With this tool, a selection of the image is made. As changes will be rather small, the whole image is selected first. The image is now surrounded by a rectangle with handles at each side. The center of the image is indicated by small cross hairs. By moving the handle on the right side towards the center of the image, the cross hairs also move. When the cross hairs meet the contact point of the central incisors, the image is symmetrical. The part of the image outside the rectangle appears darker. By double-clicking the image within the frame, the image is cropped.

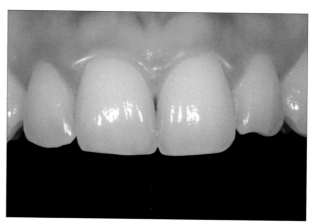

Fig. 17.09
Image is slightly oblique.

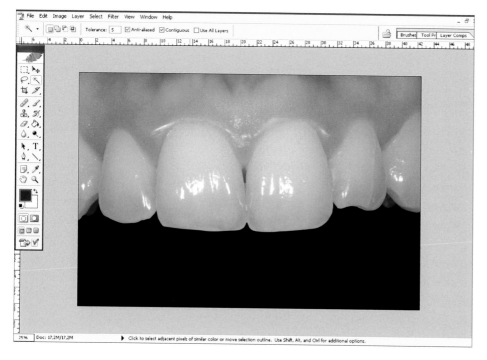

Fig. 17.10
Image loaded into Photoshop®.

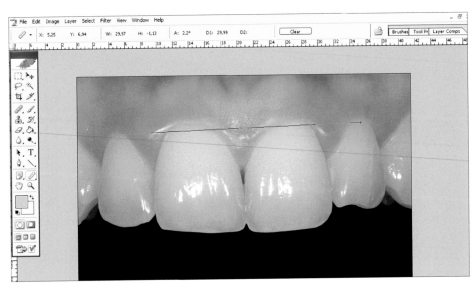

Fig. 17.11   Line is drawn between two points which should be at equal levels.

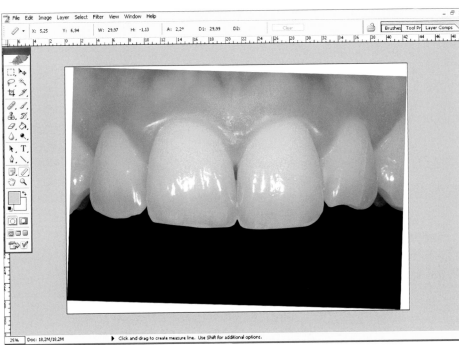

Fig. 17.12   Image is rotated.

Now it has to be aligned. If an image has to be aligned and cropped, it is better to align first.

It is quite easy to find the proper aligning angle.

- Select the eyedropper (press I). The tool icon contains a small black triangle indicating that there are some options hidden behind this icon. By clicking on this triangle and holding it a second, three options can be selected.
- Select the Measure Tool.
- Click on the highest point of the gingival margin of the tooth #7 and draw a line to the corresponding point of tooth #10 (Fig. 17.11).

- Select IMAGE > Rotate canvas > Arbitrary. The proper angle is indicated in a pop-up window. Press OK, the image is rotated by the indicated angle (Fig.17.12).
- To remove the white triangles generated by turning the image, the crop tool has to be used again. The final result is shown in Fig. 17.13.

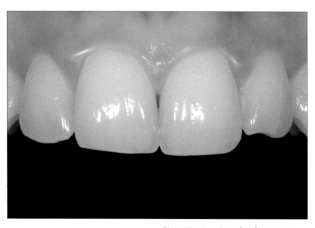

Fig. 17.13   Result after rotating.

17.3.2 Adjusting brightness and contrast – tonal range

Image brightness and color reproduction influence each other. Therefore, brightness and contrast are adjusted first, then the color is optimized. There are several ways to adjust brightness.

Adjusting the tonal range with the histogram in the Levels dialog

- The image is opened in Photoshop®. The Levels dialog is opened by IMAGE > Adjustments > Levels (or Ctrl. + L). The histogram appears (Fig. 17.14). A histogram shows how pixels of an image are distributed. What looks like a mountain is nothing other than a row of 256 bar graphs standing one beside the other and indicating how many pixels of a certain brightness are in the image. On the left are the dark ones, beginning with black (=0), on the right are the bright ones, ending with white (=255).

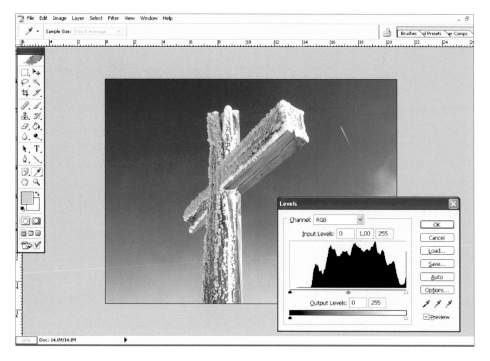

Fig. 17.14   Levels box open to adjust tonal range.

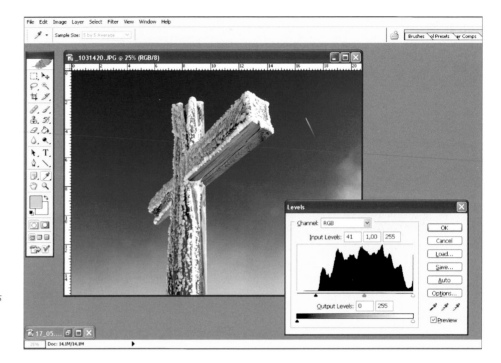

Fig. 17.15   Left (black) slider is moved towards the bar graphs. In this case a little bit to far in order to demonstrate the effect move clearly.

- Three triangular sliders are arranged beneath the bar graphs: on the left the black one, on the right the white one, and in the middle the gray one. By moving the sliders, the tonal range of an image is adjusted. The black slider is moved to the point where the "mountain" begins (right direction). By doing this, anything to the left of it in the histogram will be turned pure black. The white slider is moved to the point where the "mountain" ends (if possible). By moving the two sliders, the gray one is moved as well. It can also be moved

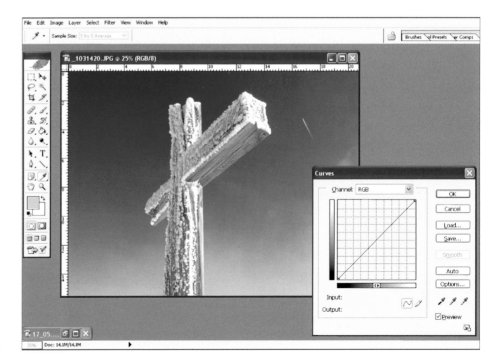

Fig. 17.16   Curves box is open.

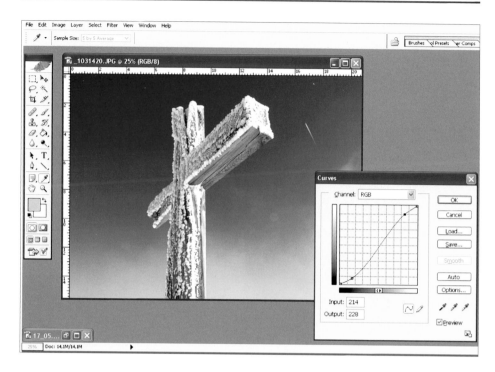

Fig. 17.17   *In most cases, an S-shaped curve gives good results.*

separately to increase or decrease overall image brightness. Figure 17.15 shows the result after moving the left slider to the right. The image shows a little bit more contrast, the sky is darker than before.

Fine-tuning of colors is possible as well with this tool, as changes are not only applicable to the whole RGB image, but also to each color channel separately.

Adjusting the tonal range using the Curves dialog

A second option to adjust the tonal range is the Curves dialog.

- The image is opened, the Curves dialog is opened by IMAGE > Adjustments > Curves (or Ctrl. + M). The Curves dialog box appears, which shows two tonal scales (input and output). The middle of the diagram displays the curve which is a straight line in the beginning (Fig. 17.16). By moving the cursor on the curve and clicking on this point, a point of the curve is selected.
- Bending the whole curve to the right makes the image darker, bending it to the left makes it brighter (click on the middle point and drag it to one side).
- By setting two points and bending the curve into a S-shaped figure, contrast is enhanced (Fig. 17.17).

The Curves dialog provides the best control over an image's tonal quality, as lights and shadows can be changed separately. As with the Levels dialog, color corrections are possible by applying the corrections only to one of the three color channels (see below). Applying target values to the shadow and highlight pixels is possible in the Curves and the Levels dialog as well.

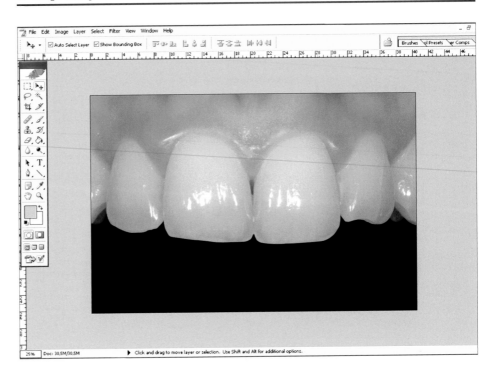

Fig. 17.18
Image with slightly reddish cast.

Adjusting the tonal range and correction of color using the Curves dialog

- An image with a reddish color cast is opened in Photoshop® (Fig. 17.18).
- Curves dialog is opened. The red channel is selected. The color cast is reduced by bending the curve to the right (Fig. 17.19).

There are numerous other ways to correct the color of images (see below).

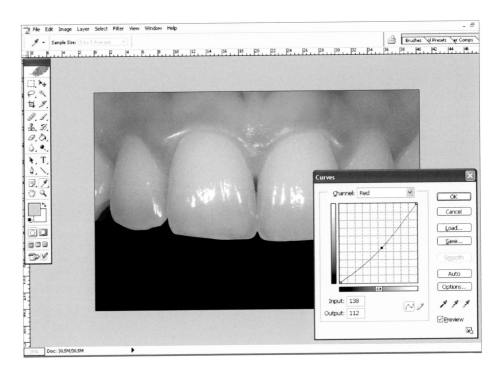

Fig. 17.19   *Removing the reddish cast by bending the curve to the right. This change is applied only to the RED channel.*

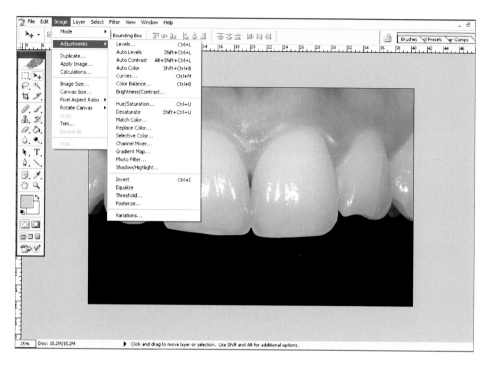

Fig. 17.20   There are many options for changing colors in Photoshop®.

17.3.3 Adjusting color

Photoshop® offers a wide variety of methods to change the color. Most of them can be found in the IMAGE > Adjustments menu (Fig. 17.20). For the beginner, the Variations dialog is a fast way to achieve good results in a more intuitive manner.

The automatic functions (auto levels, auto contrast, auto color) do not work very well when applied to intraoral images, as these images usually have a color dominance which leads to "overcorrected" results with ugly color casts.

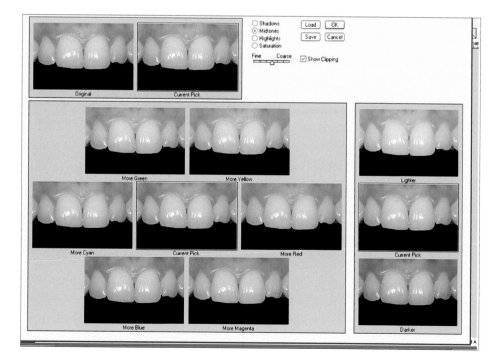

Fig. 17.21   For the beginner "VARIATIONS" is a good option for correcting colors.

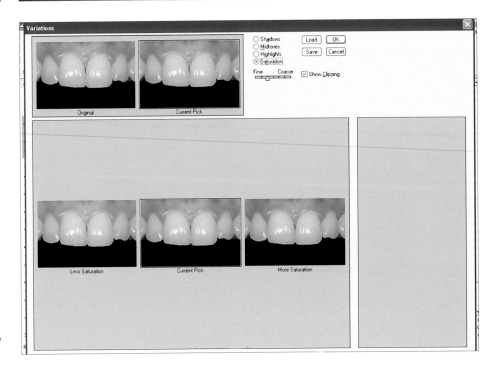

Fig. 17.22   "VARIATIONS" can change the saturation as well.

Variations

A fast and intuitive way to obtain correct colors is the Variations dialog, provided the monitor is adjusted properly. Open the image, select IMAGE > Adjustments > Variations (Fig. 17.21). There are different fields showing different variations of the image. The large field at bottom left is nothing other than a color wheel, displaying the original in the middle and a more yellow, red, magenta, blue, cyan and green variation. The right field shows the current choice in the middle and a brighter plus a dark-

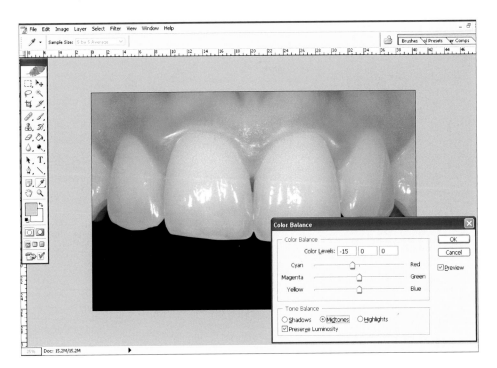

Fig. 17.23   "Color Balance" is an easy-to-use tool for removing color imbalances.

er variation. The field at the top left shows the original together with the current choice.

The degree of the changes can be adjusted from fine to coarse and the changes can be applied on Midtones, Highlights and Shadows.

By clicking on one of the variation fields, this image becomes the current choice. The advantage of this method is that the user can achieve good results without knowing sophisticated details of more complicated methods.

Sometimes it is sufficient to reduce color saturation. In this case, the Saturation box must be checked (Fig. 17.22).

Color balance

Another very good and easy method is applying the Color Balance function: IMAGE > Adjustments > Color Balance or press Ctrl. + B (Fig. 17.23). With the Preview box checked, you can move the sliders towards the indicated directions. Results are shown directly on the screen. Again, changes are applicable to the dark, middle and bright areas of the image.

Photo filter

A new way to influence color reproduction is by using the Photo Filter option (Photoshop® CS): IMAGE > Adjustments > Photo Filter. A variety of Photo Filters is offered, imitating the effect of colored filters used in conventional photography.

The filter is selected, its density adjusted and the Preserve Luminosity box is checked (otherwise image brightness changes due to the filter effect). In this example, only the left half of the picture was selected to show the difference between be-

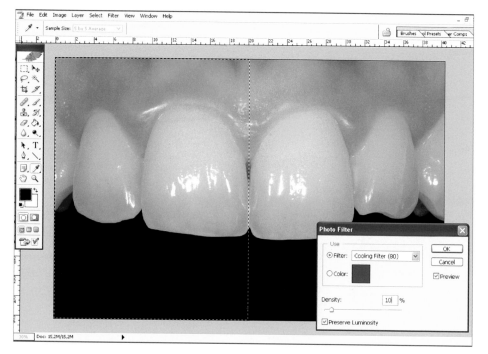

Fig. 17.24   A new option in Photoshop® is the Photo Filter function.

fore and after (Fig. 17.24). To remove a yellowish cast, a blue filter with a low density was applied. The "Underwater" filter is also a good choice in many cases.

17.3.4   Sharpening the image

Digital images very often appear slightly fuzzy due to the interpolation process when generating the image. This has to be compensated by sharpening. Sharpening should always be the last operation. In this context, sharpening does not mean improving fuzzy images due to poor focusing or camera shake. Sharpening means enhancing contrast along the margins of image structures. This can partly be done by the camera. A medium value should be the preset of choice when setting up the camera.

The degree of sharpening depends on the image content. Pictures with a lot of details need more sharpening. If the same degree of sharpening is applied to a portrait or a blue sky, the skin or sky may look rather coarse afterwards.

Furthermore, different purposes demand different sharpening. Images for offset printing may be sharpened a little bit more than images only displayed on a monitor. The only general recommendation that can be made is: as a standard procedure, sharpen only moderately.

Extensive image archives normally do not sharpen their images before they are stored. In this way, they are free for all options and not limited in their creativity. If images are stored as JPEG files after pre-sharpening them, compression and sharpening could possibly combine and cause blotchy pictures.

The most frequently used method for sharpening an image is the Unsharp Mask. The term "Unsharp masking" is a holdover from conventional photographic processes used to increase contrast along areas where the tones abruptly shifted.

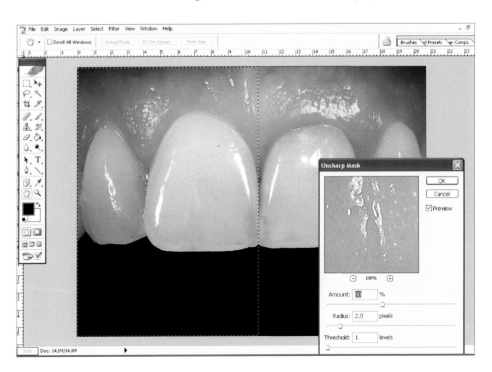

Fig. 17.25   Unsharp Mask – a classical tool for image sharpening.

- Select FILTER > Sharpen > Unsharp Mask.
- A box opens where different adjustments can be made (Fig. 17.25).
- Amount: Sharpening means adding contrast to edges, that means adding density along the dark edge and subtracting density along the light edge in an area of contrast. By adjusting the "Amount", the degree of the sharpening can be adjusted.
- Radius: defines how "broad" the effect of sharpening is. It defines the area that will be affected. If the image shows a lot of detail, a low number should be preferred. For a standard screen resolution, a radius setting of 0.5 works well. For a standard printing resolution, the radius should be increased to 1.5. Images with low tonal differences and without fine detail (e.g., sky, skin) can be improved by increasing the setting to about 3 or even more.
- Threshold: defines what level of contrast to sharpen. A zero setting means that everything is sharpened. For sharpening skin, the number must be higher (>6) unless every pore is important.

The settings shown in Fig. 17.25 are a good choice for "average images". This setting allows the image to be sharpened twice. The second sharpening is done by applying the same filter again (Ctrl. + F).

A basic setting for print is: amount = 125, radius = 1.5, threshold = 3.

The left half of the image in Fig.17.25 shows the situation after sharpening.

Here are some recommendations from Photoshop® expert Scott Kelby on how to adjust "Amount", "Radius", and "Threshold" for different objects.

Object	Amount	Radius	Threshold
"soft objects": babies, flowers, rainbows etc	150%	1	10
Portraits	75%	2	3
Technical objects, landscapes	225%	0.5	0
Objects with well defined edges, objects out of focus	65%	4	3
All-purpose sharpening	85%	1	4
Web graphics	400%	0.3	0

17.4 Image editing procedures to change image content

17.4.1 Changing images in selected areas

Selections can be made by using different tools. A selection is an image area (or more than one) to which all the editing procedures are applied. Figure 17.26 shows an image with the lateral regions too dark. The goal is to increase image brightness only within these areas. A selection using the Rectangular Marquee Tool (press M) is

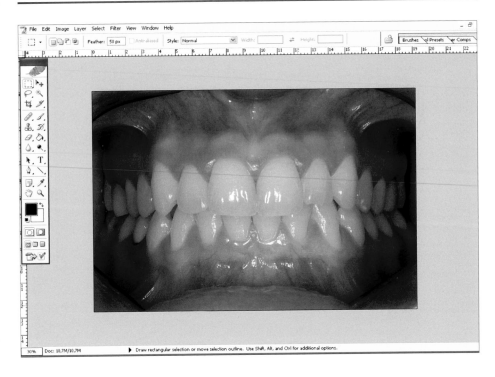

Fig. 17.26   Lateral parts of this image need more brightness.

made. A second selection is added by pressing and holding the Shift key before the Marquee Tool is used (Fig. 17.27). In order not to see the outline of the selected and changed areas, a feather of 50 pixels is set. That means the transition from changed to unchanged areas is not visible. To increase brightness in the selected areas, the Levels dialog is opened (Ctr. + L) and the middle slider (the gray one) is moved to the left side. The result shows an image with lighter premolar and molar areas (Fig. 17.28).

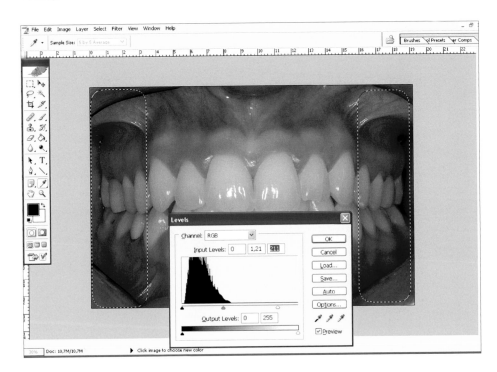

*Fig. 17.27
Lateral areas are selected.*

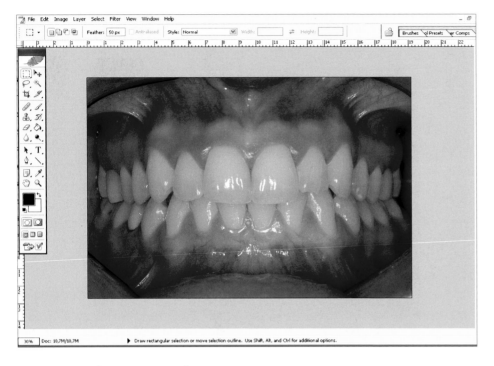

Fig. 17.28   Now lateral parts have the proper brightness.

17.4.2   Changing colors

An extensive variety of options is offered by Photoshop® for changing colors.

Hue/saturation

- To change the color of the eye, the image is loaded, the eye selected using the Lasso tool (press L) with a feather of 3 pixels (Fig. 17.29).

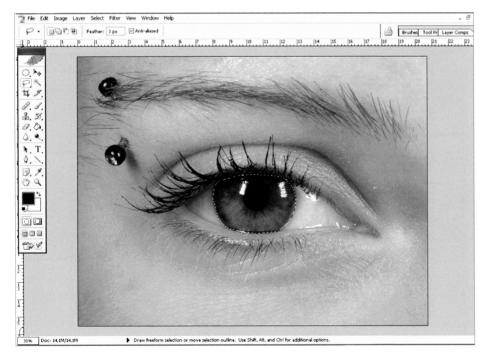

*Fig. 17.29
Part of the image is selected.*

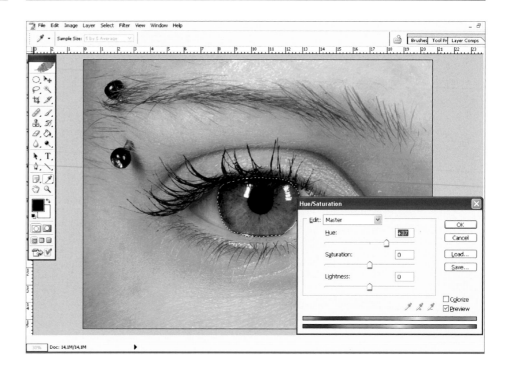

Fig. 17.30   Moving the slider changes the color.

- The Hue/Saturation menu is opened: IMAGES > Adjustments > Hue/Saturation (or Ctrl. + U).
- By moving the Hue slider to one side, color is changed (Fig. 17.30)
- Click OK and Ctrl. + D to deselect the selection and store the image (Fig. 17.31).

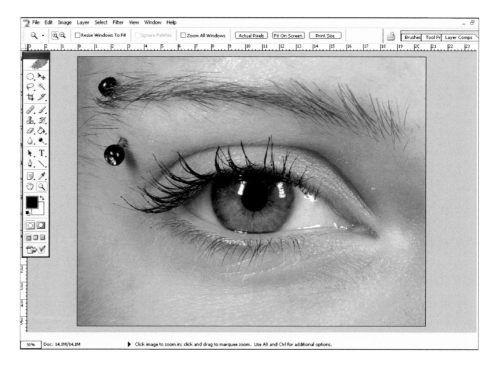

Fig. 17.31   Result: green eyes.

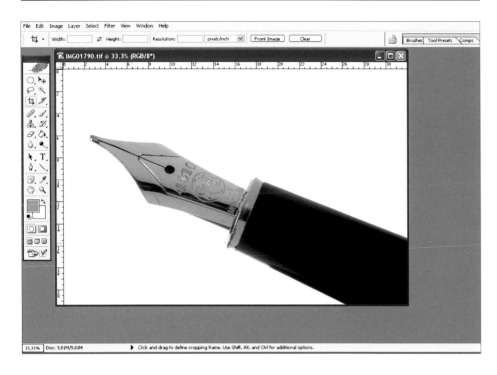

Fig. 17.32 Image is loaded.

Replace color

The white background of an image has to be changed to gray to match this background with others.

- Image is loaded (Fig. 17.32).
- The Replace color menu is opened: IMAGE>Adjustments>Replace color. The color to be replaced (in this case the background) is selected by clicking with the left pipette on the background. The selection area shows the selected parts as white (Fig. 17.33).

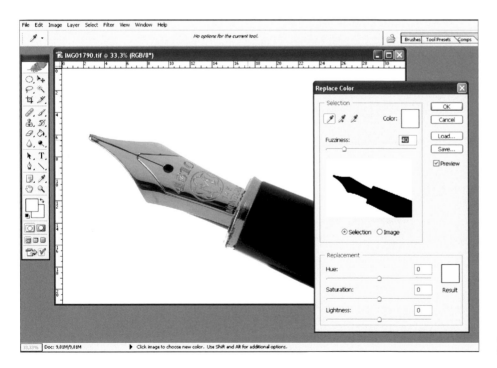

Fig. 17.33 Part of the image to be changed is selected.

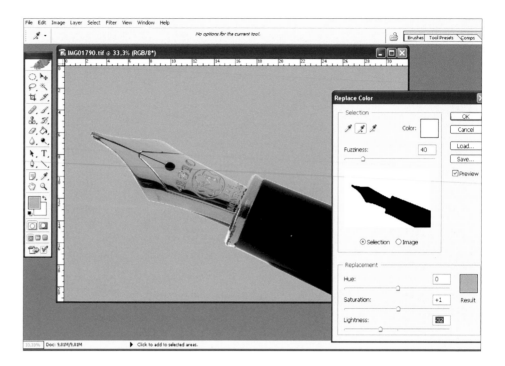

Fig. 17.34
Result: color is replaced.

- Lightness is reduced to obtain the gray background (Fig. 17.34).

Color balance

- An image of the tongue is too red (Fig. 17.35).
- The Color Balance is opened (Ctrl. + B).
- The cyan-red slider is moved to the left, reducing the red (Fig. 17.36).

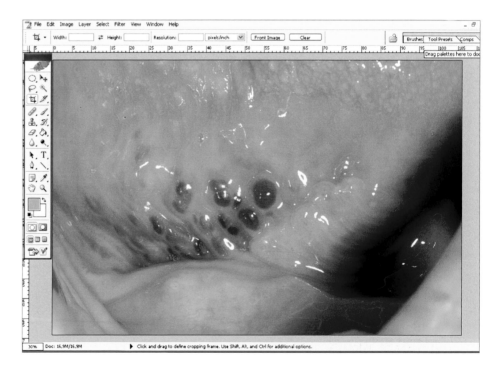

Fig. 17.35   Tongue is too red.

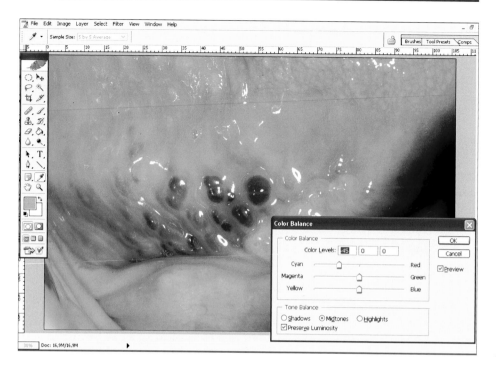

Fig. 17.36   *Cyan-red slider is moved to the left.*

Removing a color cast by reducing saturation

- An image with a reddish color cast is loaded (Fig. 17.37).
- The Hue/Saturation slider is moved to the left reducing the reddish cast. IM-AGE>Adjustments>Hue/Saturation (Fig. 17.38).

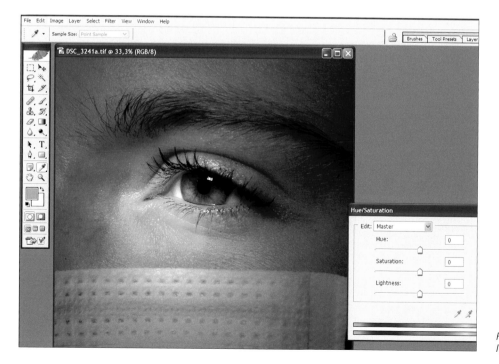

Fig. 17.37
Image with a reddish color cast.

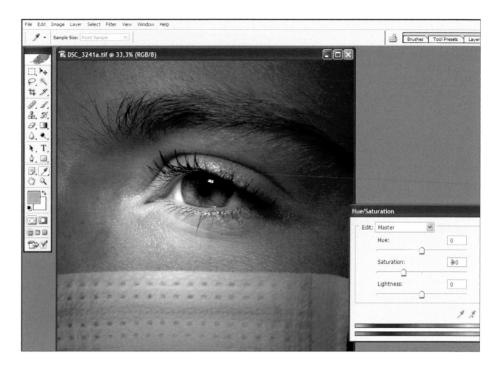

Fig. 17.38   Saturation is reduced, the color cast is eliminated.

Eliminating a color cast by using the Curves menu

- An image with a reddish color cast is opened. The Curves menu is selected (Ctrl. + M). The RED channel is selected (Fig. 17.39).
- The curve is moved to the right. The red cast disappears (Fig. 17.40).

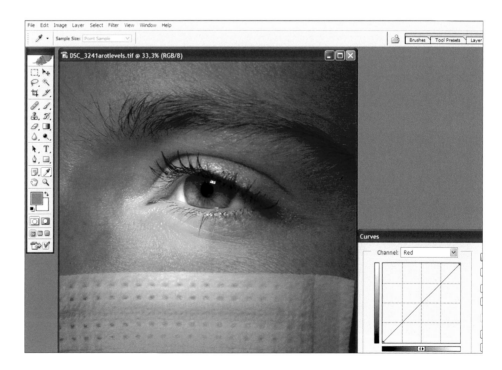

Fig. 17.39   Removing a color cast with the Curves dialog. RED channel is selected.

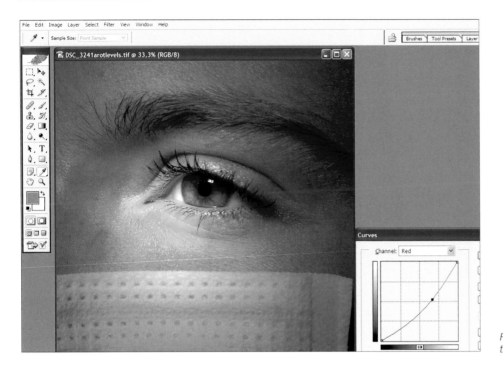

Fig. 17.40   Bending the curve to the right removes the cast.

Eliminating a color cast by using the Levels menu

- An image with a reddish color cast is opened. The Levels menu is selected (Ctrl. + L). The RED channel is selected (Fig. 17.41).
- With the RED channel selected the middle slider is moved to the right. The red cast disappears (Fig. 17.42).

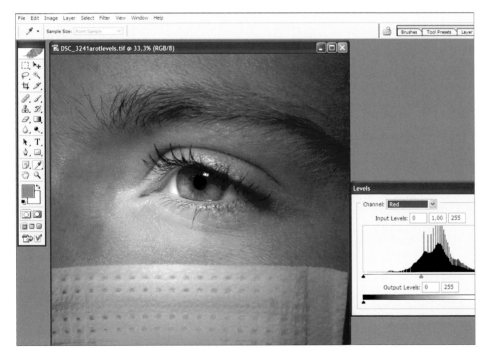

Fig. 17.41   Image with red color cast; Levels menu open, RED channel selected.

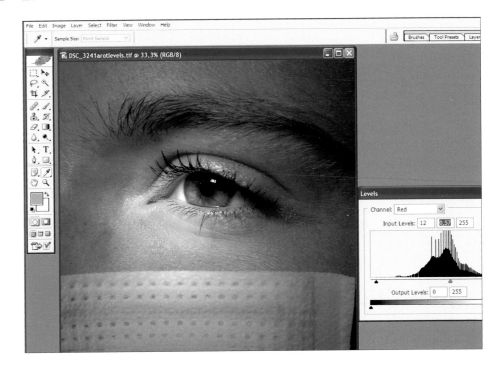

Fig. 17.42   Middle slider moved to the right. Color cast eliminated.

Selective color changes

- An image with a black background is opened. The color of the background has to be changed Selective Color menu is selected (IMAGE > Adjustments > Selective Color). The BLACK colors are selected (Fig. 17.43).
- Sliders are moved to change only the black colors (Fig. 17.44).

Black and white from color

Sometimes it makes sense to use black and white images. Modern photographic sensors always record color. There are different ways to take out the color of an image. Some cameras offer special features for this.

Photoshop® has different procedures, some of them are listed below:

- IMAGE > Mode > Grayscale
- IMAGE > Adjustments > Desaturate
- IMAGE > Adjustments > Channel Mixer

One of the most individual methods is using the Channel Mixer.

- A colored image is opened (Fig. 17.45).
- Channel Mixer is selected: IMAGE > Adjustments > Channel Mixer. The Monochrome box is checked. The red Source Channel is automatically set to 100 % (Fig. 17.46).
- By changing the Source Channel settings, a black and white image is generated with variable tones. (Fig. 17.47).

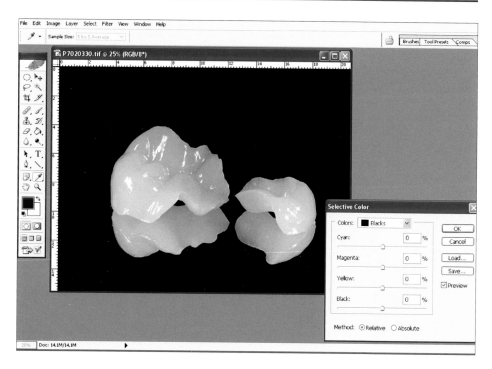

Fig. 17.43   Selective color menu opened, blacks are selected.

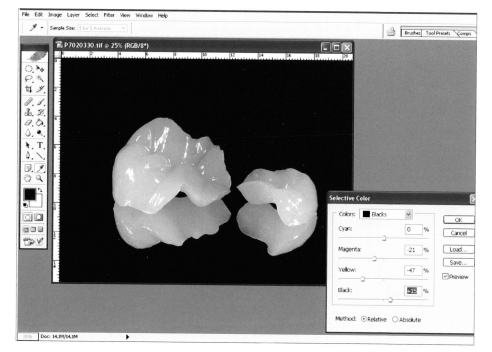

Fig. 17.44   Moving the sliders changes the selected colors.

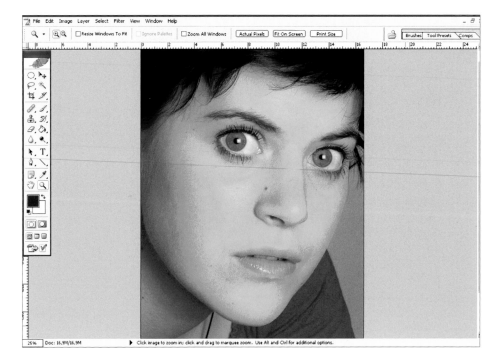

Fig. 17.45   Black and white from color: Image is opened.

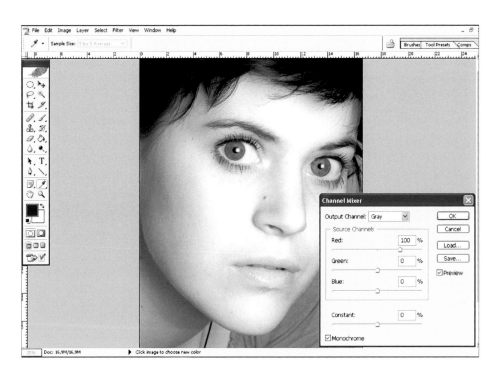

Fig. 17.46   Channel mixer is opened, "Monochrome" check box is checked.

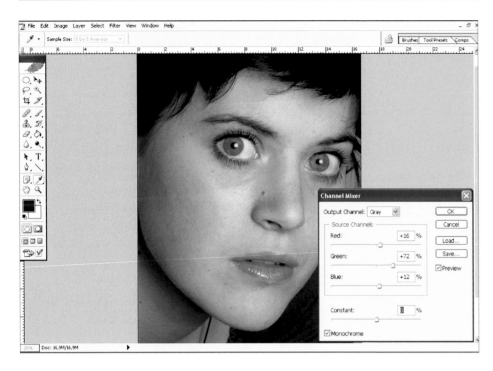

Fig. 17.47   *Moving the red, green, blue sliders gives different tones.*

17.4.3   Selective sharpening

Basic functions of sharpening using the Unsharp Mask were discussed above. Sometimes results are better when only parts of the image are sharpened. The idea is to keep the skin softer and to sharpen only eyes and lips.

- Image is opened in Photoshop®. With the Elliptical Marquee Tool (press M), eyes and mouth are selected. Press Shift and hold down while adding a second and third selection. A smooth transition is guaranteed with feather 30 pixels (Fig. 17.48).

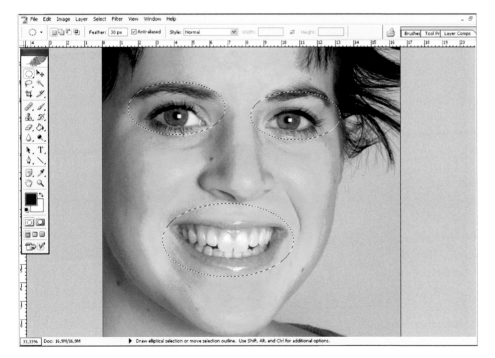

Fig. 17.48   *Selective sharpening. Areas to be sharpened are selected.*

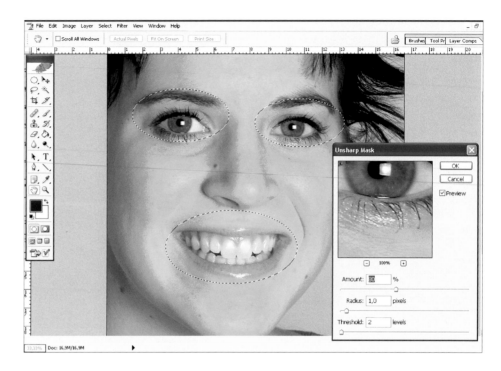

Fig. 17.49   Sharpening with the Unsharp Mask.

- Unsharp Mask is applied: FILTER > Sharpen > Unsharp Mask (Fig. 17.49). Amount: 80%, Radius: 1.0, Threshold: 2.0.
- Press OK, deselect (Ctrl. + D) and save the changed picture.

17.4.4   Optimizing a portrait using layers

Layers are an important feature in modern image editing programs. Layers allow working on details of an image without influencing the rest of the image.

Layers can be compared with transparent plastic sheets. Each of them contains a part of the image. If these sheets are positioned exactly each on top of the others, the whole image can be seen. To work on a detail, the layer containing this part of the image is selected.

- Image is opened. Sharpening reveals all imperfections of the skin, all blemishes and pores (Fig. 17.50).
- Layers menu is opened: WINDOW > Layers (or press F7).
- By dragging the layer on the "Create a new layer" icon (second from right), the layer is duplicated. Alternatively, click right and select "Duplicate Layer". The copy of the background layer is now active (indicated by blue color) (Fig. 17.51).
- Now the copy of the background layer is blurred using the Gaussian Blur: FILTER > Blur > Gaussian Blur. A high radius of 8 pixels is set (Fig. 17.52).
- Opacity is reduced to about 60% by moving the opacity slider to the left (Fig. 17.53). Now we have a composite image: a normal one below and a blurred one, partially transparent on top.

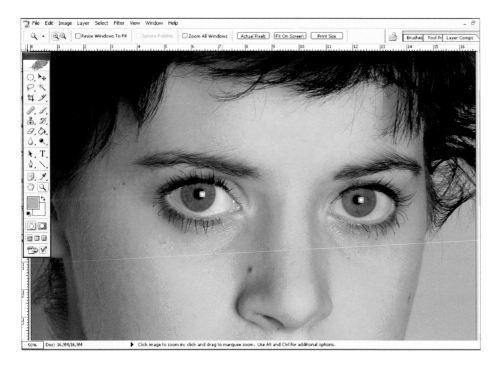

Fig. 17.50   Image is opened.

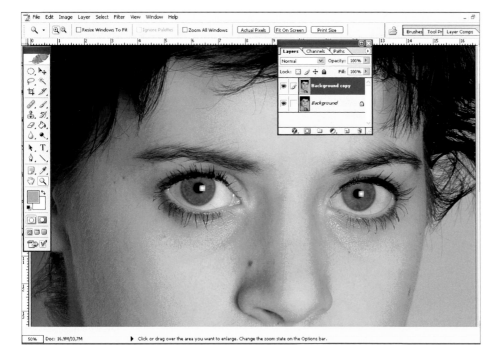

Fig. 17.51   Layer is duplicated.

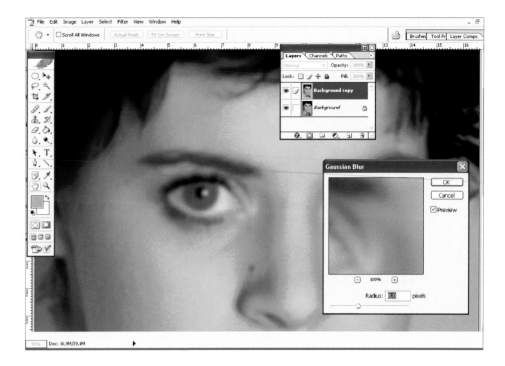

Fig. 17.52
Copy layer is blurred.

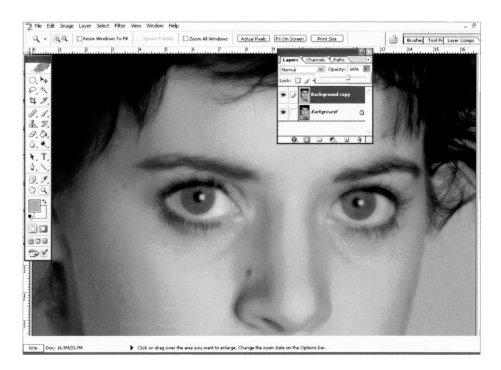

Fig. 17.53
Opacity is reduced (60%).

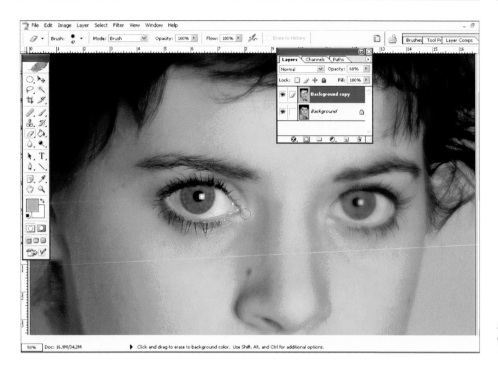

Fig. 17.54 Areas to be sharpened are treated with the Eraser Tool.

- The Eraser Tool (press E) is selected and an appropriate tool size is selected. The tool is moved over the parts of the face which should not be blurred: especially eyes and lips. The Eraser removes the effect of blurring, eyes and lips show more details again. In Fig. 17.54, the girl's right eye has already been treated with the eraser, the left one is still blurred.
- To reduce all layers to a single one, the image is flattened: LAYER > Flatten image and save. Figure 17.55 shows the before and after situation.

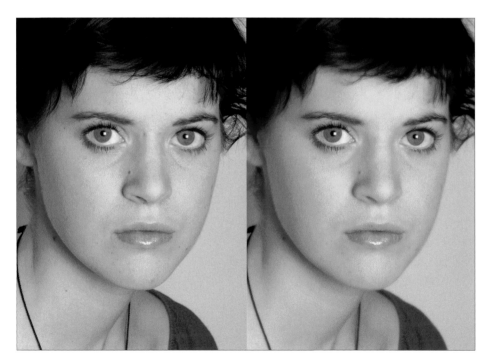

Fig. 17.55 Before (left) and after situation after enhancing the portrait.

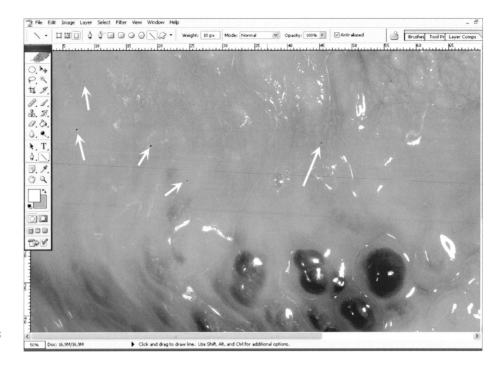

Fig. 17.56   Multiple dust spots
on the image.

17.4.5   Removing dust spots

Dust is a real problem in digital photography, just as it was before in conventional photography. There are numerous recommendations to prevent dust particles from entering the camera and being caught by the sensor surface. Dust particles are very tiny, but the single sensor element is even smaller. The result: disturbing black spots, especially visible on bright and uniform backgrounds, e.g., sky, tooth surface etc.

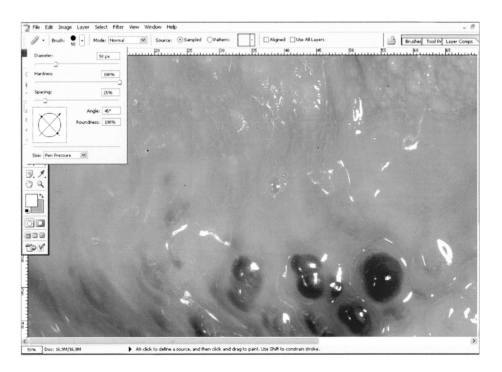

Fig. 17.57
Healing brush tool selected.

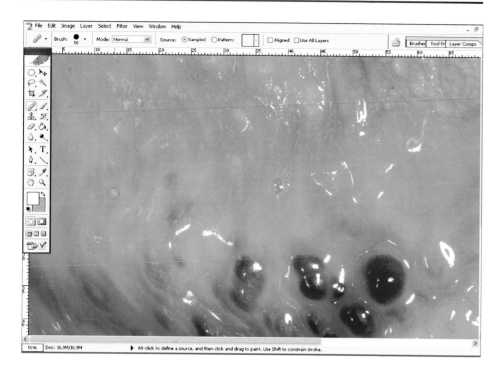

Fig. 17.58
Dust spots are eliminated.

There are different methods to remove dust spots from the image. A very simple one is using the Healing Brush Tool (press J).

- Image is loaded and displayed with an appropriate magnification. Some of the spots are indicated by arrows in this example (Fig. 17.56).
- Healing Brush Tool is selected (press J) and option menu is opened to adjust the tool size (Fig. 17.57).
- Move the tool beside a spot, define the source with ALT + Click, move the tool over the spot and click again. The spot is eliminated. Repeat this with all black dust spots (Fig. 17.58).

With the same technique, imperfections on the skin, blemishes and acne spots can be removed. Unlike the Clone Tool, the Healing Brush also matches the texture, lighting, transparency, etc. of the sampled pixels to the source pixels. As a result, the repaired pixels blend seamlessly into the rest of the image.

17.5   Dental imaging

In North America and the United Kingdom, the term "imaging" is used to describe all procedures which result in an image regardless of whether the systems used to produce these are conventional or digital. In dental practice, "imaging" refers more specifically to the simulation of the results of treatment on a monitor. The technical requirements for this are a camera, a PC, and an imaging program.

There are special imaging programs on the market, but whoever does not need dental imaging on a permanent basis can use commercial image processing programs, which do not offer as many special features but are far less expensive (e.g.,

PhotoImpact, Corel PhotoPaint, Photoshop® or Photoshop® Elements). If the user does not need the latest version of the software, these programs can be purchased for under $100. The more complex professional programs such as Photoshop® (Adobe) are more expensive and are suited to the more ambitious user because of their many features.

Sources of images include:

- Intraoral video camera with PC connection.
- Digital photographic camera.
- Conventional photograph which must be available on a PC in digitized form.

The purpose of this overview is to give some simple examples of simulations possible with every image editing program on the market. Changes which are frequently simulated are:

- Closing gaps between teeth.
- Changing color of teeth.
- Changing tooth shape and gumline.
- Changing existing fillings.
- Changing angle of teeth.

Fig. 17.59   The patient should be informed that imaging only means a simulation of a possible result.

This can be achieved by changing the available components of the image, for example, through compression, distortion, rotation, moving, etc.

In principle, the mouse or – even better – a graphic pen is used to mark and select the area to be changed. This area is then duplicated and changed or moved to a different location. With a little bit of practice, good results can be achieved quickly even with commercial image editing programs. Another possibility is to build up a database from which details can be removed and inserted into the image which is to be altered.

Imaging is time-consuming. It is a responsible activity which demands knowledge of the subject, esthetic skills, and a feel for psychology. It cannot be trusted to an external dental technician but should be done by the dentist him- or herself or specially trained personnel under direct supervision. Otherwise, there is the risk that unrealistic proposals for treatment are suggested which subsequently prove untenable. This would lead to much disappointment and trouble after treatment. In any case, the patient must be made aware – if possible, in writing – that the results of dental imaging are no guarantee of treatment, and only approximate a possible result (Fig. 17.59).

Dental Practice of Drs. Beatrix and Wolfgang Bengel
Darmstädter Str. 190a
64625 Bensheim
Tel.: 06251 - 76095 - email: wbengel@gmx.de

TREATMENT SIMULATION

Patient: N.N.
Date: X.X.04

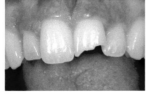 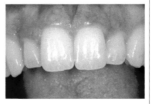

initial situation   treatment proposal

Dear Mrs. N.N.,

The result of treatment shown here is a computer simulation. This can only be an approximation of later treatment and only serves as point of reference.
Anatomical an technical issues may dictate changes from this.

Best regards

W. Bengel

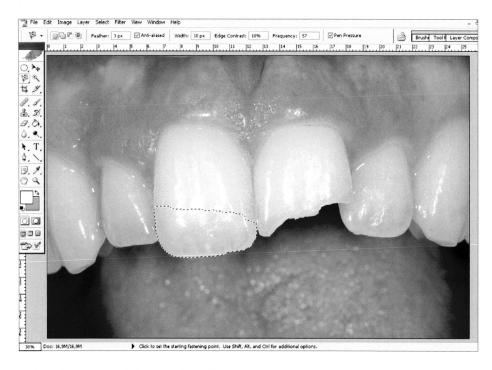

Fig. 17.60 Corresponding edge
of the neighboring tooth is selected.

17.5.1 Repairing a tooth by duplicating corresponding structures

As an example, a fractured edge must be replaced.

- The Image is opened in Photoshop®. Using the Lasso Tool (press L) the corresponding edge of the neighboring tooth is selected. To get a smooth transition later, a small feather of 3 pixels is selected (Fig. 17.60).

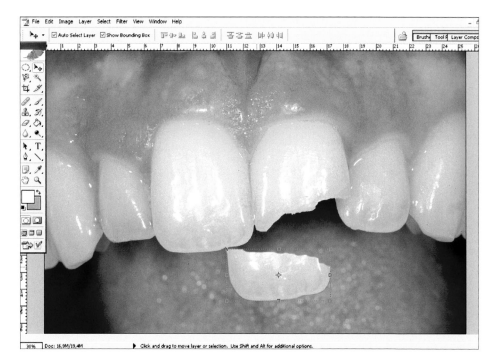

Fig. 17.61 Edge is duplicated.

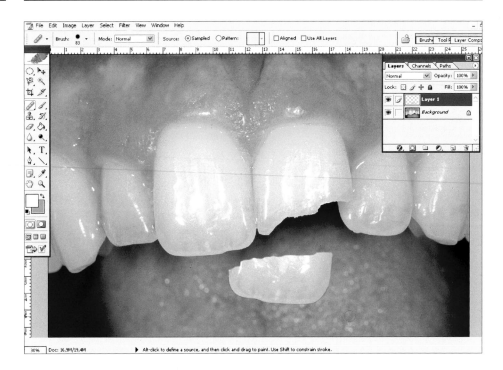

Fig. 17.62   *Edge is flipped.*

- The selected piece is duplicated: EDIT > Copy and then EDIT > Paste, or Ctrl.+C, Ctrl.+V.
- The Move Tool is selected (press V), the copied piece is dragged to the fractured tooth (Fig. 17.61).
- By EDIT > Transform > Flip Horizontal the piece is turned around (Fig. 17.62).
- With EDIT > Transform > Rotate it is rotated a little bit und moved into the proper position (Fig. 17.63).

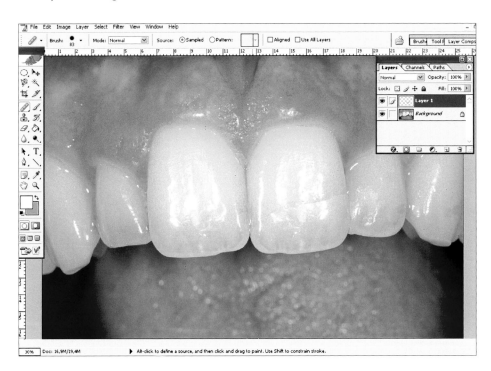

Fig. 17.63   *Edge moved into the right position.*

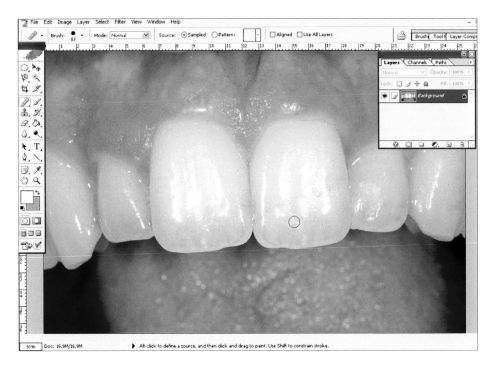

Fig. 17.64   *Transition from edge to tooth is repaired.*

- The image is flattened (LAYER > Flatten Image) and the transition is "repaired" using the Healing Brush Tool (press J). Figure 17.64 shows the result.

By copying and pasting the selected piece of tooth, a new layer was created, making it necessary to flatten the image afterwards.

17.5.2   Closing a diastema

There are several options to make teeth broader.

Option 1: Using the Clone Stamp Tool (press S)
- The tooth to be broadened is selected using the Polygonal Lasso Tool (press L). The new contour after broadening is taken into account (Fig. 17.65).
- Using the Clone Stamp Tool the lateral part of the tooth is copied. The selection guarantees that the border appears clean and smooth (Fig. 17.66).
- The same procedure is repeated with tooth #9 (Fig. 17.67)

Option 2: Using a mask
   Sometimes selecting is rather difficult. Working in the Quick Mask Mode (press Q) can help. The image is covered by a red mask, which protects the image below (Fig. 17.68). With the Eraser, the mask can be removed; using the Brush Tool the mask can be enlarged just by painting red color on the image. Finally, return to Standard Mode (press Q again).Tthe selected area is surrounded by a black and white line ("marching ants").

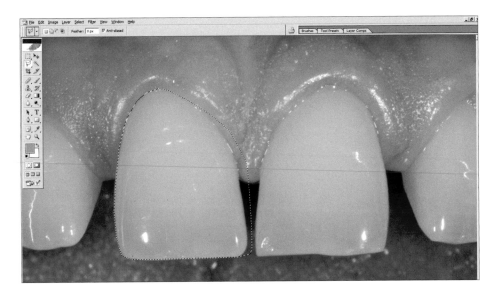

Fig. 17.65   Broader contour of the tooth is drawn using the Magnetic Lasso Tool.

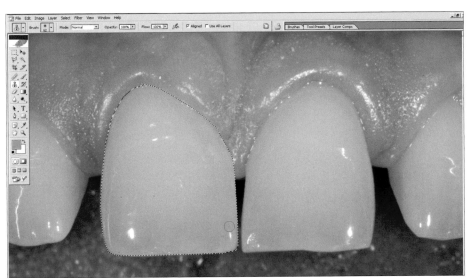

Fig. 17.66   Contour is filled using the Stamp Tool.

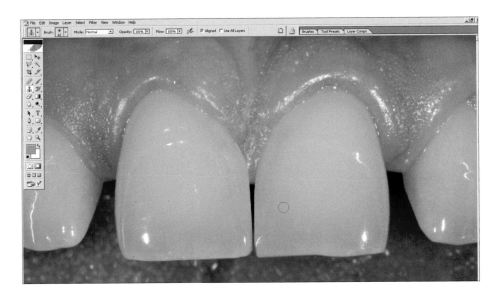

Fig. 17.67   Neighboring tooth is treated the same way.

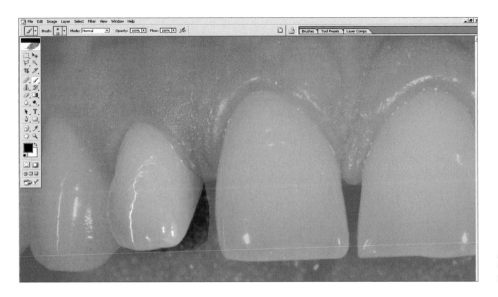

Fig. 17.68   Working in the Quick Mask Mode helps to fine-tune the selection.

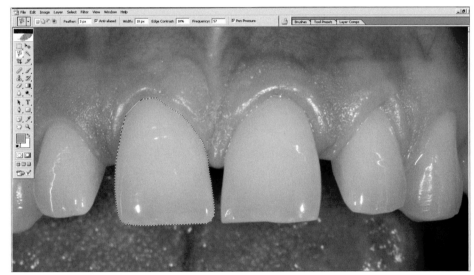

Fig. 17.69   Tooth to be transformed is selected.

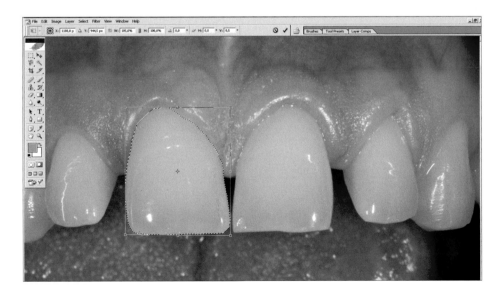

Fig. 17.70   Transformation frame is displayed.

Option 3: Using the Transformation Tool

■   The tooth to be broadened is selected by the Magnetic Lasso Tool
     (press L, Fig. 17.69).
■   By EDIT > Free Transform (or Ctrl. +T) a rectangle with handles is placed around
     the object. By dragging the handles the tooth can be modified in all directions
     (Fig. 17.70).

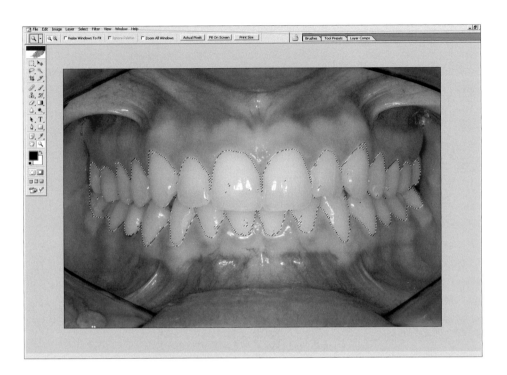

*Fig. 17.71   Teeth to be
"whitened" are selected.*

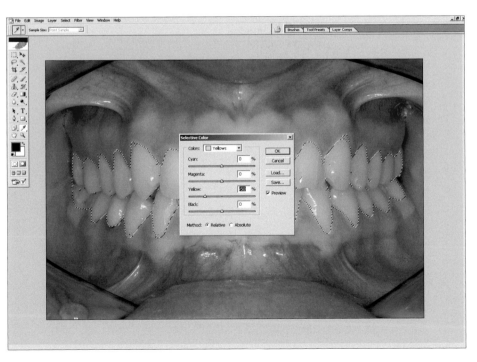

*Fig. 17.72   Yellow is reduced
selectively.*

17.5.3 Whitening teeth

Bleaching teeth means reducing the yellowness and increasing brightness.

- The image is opened in Photoshop® and a selection is made using the Polygonal Lasso Tool in combination with the Quick Mask Mode (Fig. 17.71).
- IMAGE > Adjustments > Selective Color is opened. YELLOW is selected and reduced (Fig. 17.72).
- Finally, brightness is increased: IMAGE > Adjustments > Brightness/Contrast.
- Before and after situation combined in one image (Fig. 17.73).

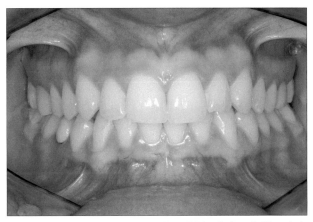

Fig. 17.73   Before (left) and after situation shows the difference.

17.5.4 Integrating images in a letter

The result of such a simulation can be printed together with an image of the initial situation. There are many more situations where it makes sense to integrate images into a letter. Very often patients cannot remember the initial situation before treatment started. This might give reason for complaints as special problems and treatment difficulties are quite often forgotten as well. A subtle marketing tool is to show the before and after situation in a letter which is added to the bill after treatment is finished. This can be done very fast.

- First, a letter with a standard text (or individual text) is prepared: FILE > New. An option box opens, "Preset" is set to A4, "Background content" = white, Resolution = 200 pixels/inch (when printed with an inkjet printer later).
- Text is added: Horizontal Type Tool is selected, font family, style, color and size are adjusted. Text is typed. The text appears on a new layer. If a standard text is used, a complete letter can be saved together with the text.
- Images to be integrated are opened. Image size has to be reduced to the dimensions necessary for the letter. Example: Document size, width: 8 cm, height is set automatically, if "Constrain proportion box" is checked. Resolution: 200 dpi. It is important that the images have the same resolution as the blank letter.
- The Move Tool (press V) is selected, moved over the first image and dragged (click and hold) into the desired position of the letter. Same procedure with the second image.
- Finally the image-letter is saved (if necessary) and printed (Fig. 17.74). Before saving the letter, the number of layers is reduced, thus reducing the file volume (LAYER > Flatten Image).

*Fig. 17.74
Images integrated into a letter.*

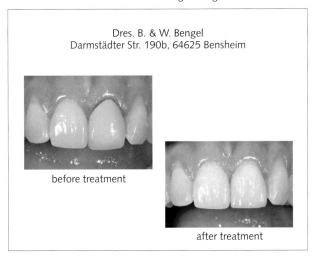

Dres. B. & W. Bengel
Darmstädter Str. 190b, 64625 Bensheim

before treatment

after treatment

17.6   Advanced procedures

Photoshop® and other editing programs offer endless possibilities for editing images and creating new compositions. Normally, this has nothing to do with photo documentation, as here the image content should not be changed, but for increasing the visual attractiveness of PowerPoint presentations, some of them might be useful.

What is here categorized as "advanced procedures" is very easy for the more experienced Photoshop® user. Some examples are listed below. It must be emphasized that this selection is highly subjective.

17.6.1   Actions

Frequently, it is necessary to repeatedly perform certain multiple-step procedures. By creating "Actions", these procedures can be run automatically.

For instance, images must often be reduced to an image size of 1024×768 pixels. This is necessary when images are sent as an e-mail attachment to the dental lab or if they are to be integrated into a PowerPoint presentation. The following example shows how an action can be created to reduce an image to 1024 pixels.

- An image is opened with a volume of more than 18 MB. Actions are selected by WINDOW>Actions or ALT + F9. The action recording windows opens (Fig. 17.75).
- "Create new action button" is activated (icon row below, second from right). Dialog box opens, action can be named, a function can be selected to trigger the action. Name "1024" is typed in and a set is selected where the action can be found. Finally the RECORD key is pressed. A red icon appears in the action box, indicating that all further steps are recorded.

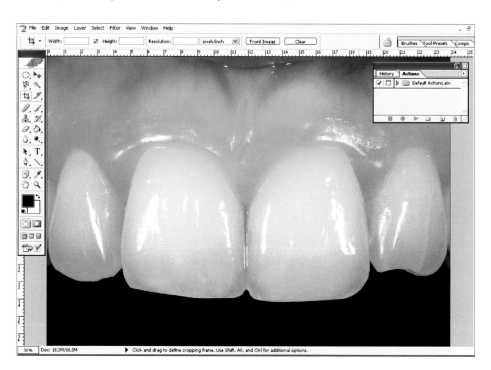

Fig. 17.75   Action Recording Window is opened.

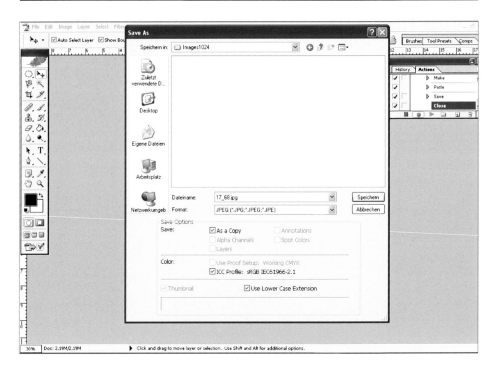

Fig. 17.76   Image saving dialog.

- The image is resized: IMAGE > Image size > 1024 is typed in the dialog box. "Constrain proportions box" is checked. Press OK.
- Image is displayed in the new size. Now it has to be saved separately, otherwise the original would be lost. FILE > Save As – the Save As box opens. Destination is selected, the image is saved (Fig. 17.76). By clicking on the far left icon, recording the action is stopped.
- To apply the action, the image is opened, action set is opened (F9) and the action is selected. By clicking on the black triangle in the icon row, the action is started: image size is reduced, image is copied in the predefined folder.

It is very useful working with actions. More details can be found in the Photoshop® reference books.

17.6.2   Removing red eyes

When people are photographed sitting in the dark, the pupils are dilated. The result is often a picture showing the reflection of the retina with its blood vessels (red eyes). Several methods exist to replace the color. Modern editing programs offer special functions for that (e.g., Photoshop® and Photoshop® Elements).
Here is a method which works quite well.

- Image is opened showing a friendly colleague with red eyes (the dog seems to have another problem, his iris is red, the pupils black). F7 opens the Layer menu (Fig. 17.77).

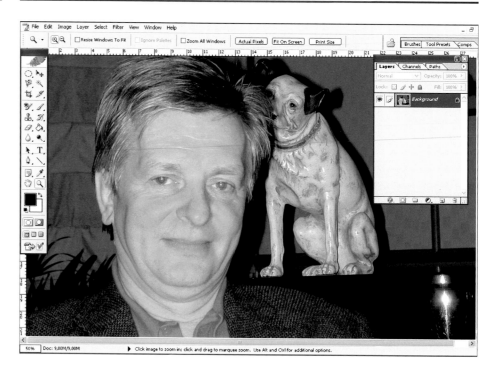

Fig. 17.77   Removing red eyes: initial situation.

- Double-clicking on the background layer in the layer palette and OK transforms the background layer into a normal one (Layer 0). Then the image is zoomed in to increase precision, and red pupils are selected with the Polygonal Lasso Tool, press Shift for the second selection (Fig. 17.78).
- IMAGE > Adjustments > Selective Colors opens the menu; RED is selected, as well as "Absolute". Black slider is moved to 100%. This step may be repeated, if necessary (Fig. 17.79).

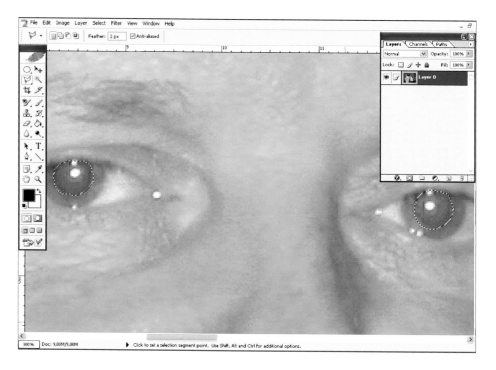

Fig. 17.78   Red pupils selected.

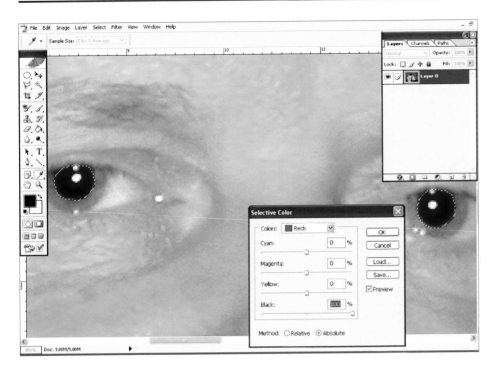

Fig. 17.79   REDS in the Selective Color selected, black slider moved to the right.

- If a reddish color cast remains, this can be removed using the Color Balance: IMAGE > Adjustments > Color Balance. The cyan-red slider is moved to the left, then OK (Fig. 17.80).
- After zooming out and deselecting the selected areas, the portrait has a very natural appearance, as the reflections in the eyes are not touched (Fig. 17.81). Now we have to see what we can do for the dog!

Most programs offer more or less automatic functions to remove the red eye effect.

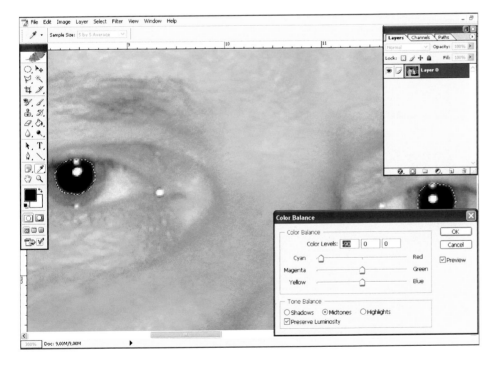

Fig. 17.80   Color Balance removes remaining red color cast.

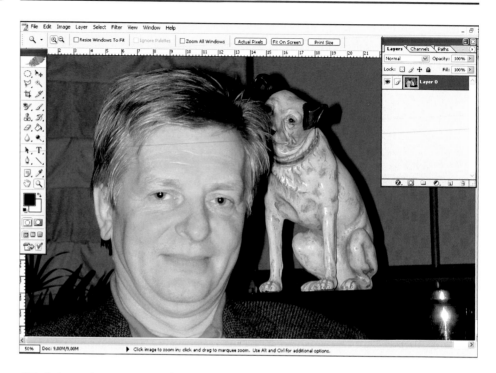

Fig. 17.81
Result after removing red eyes.

17.6.3   Creating a lighting studio setup

With Photoshop®, virtual lighting set-ups can be created. A simple example is shown below. The goal is to present an object with special illumination on a reflective underground.

Step 1:   A new document is opened. FILE > New. Appropriate size is chosen; e.g., 1024 x 768 pixels. The background layer is filled with a light blue color (Fig. 17.82) by pressing ALT+Backspace. A new blank layer above the

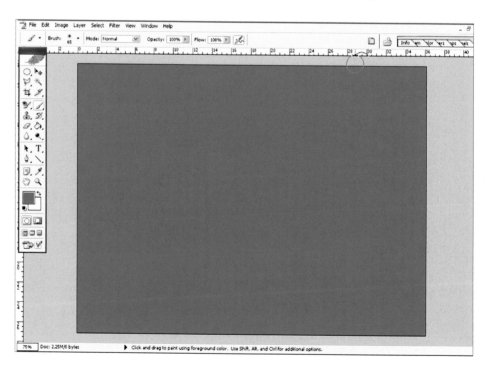

Fig. 17.82   Creating a studio
set-up starts with a light blue
background.

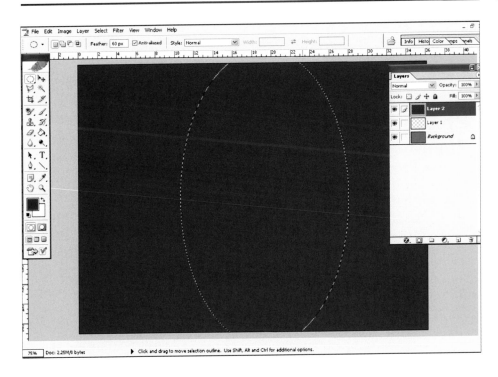

Fig. 17.83   New layer with darker blue, elliptical soft selection.

background layer is generated by clicking on the "Create a New Layer icon" at the bottom of the Layers palette.

Step 2:   For the new layer, a darker shade of blue is selected as foreground color. The layer is filled with this color again by pressing ALT + Backspace. A tall oval-shaped selection is dragged using the Elliptical Marquee tool (M). To soften the edges, a feather of 60 pixels is entered (Fig. 17.83). If working with higher resolution (300 dpi), a feather of 170 pixels is recommended.

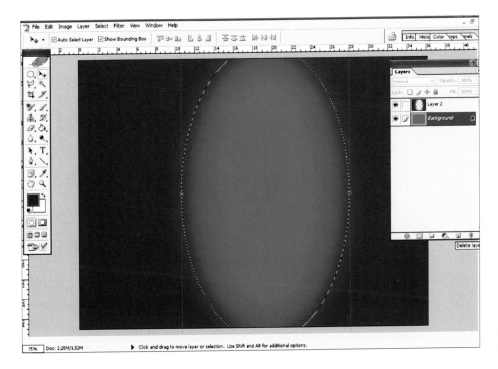

Fig. 17.84   A soft-edged hole is cut out of the dark blue layer.

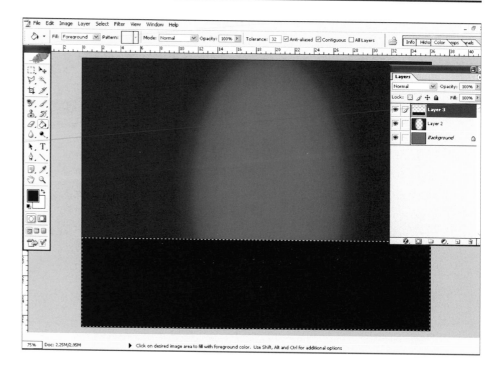

Fig. 17.85
Another layer with dark blue.

Step 3:   By pressing BACKSPACE, a soft-edged hole is made in the dark blue layer. It reveals the light blue layer beneath. This gives the impression of light shining down (Fig. 17.84). Selection is deselected by Ctrl. + D.

Step 4:   A new layer is added. With the Rectangular Marquee tool (M), a horizontal selection across the bottom quarter of the image is drawn. A dark blue color is chosen as Foreground color. The rectangular selection is filled with this tone by pressing ALT + Backspace. Selection is not yet deselected (Fig. 17.85).

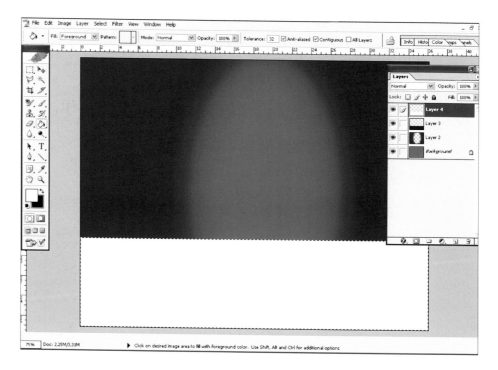

Fig. 17.86   *Layer is filled with the foreground color.*

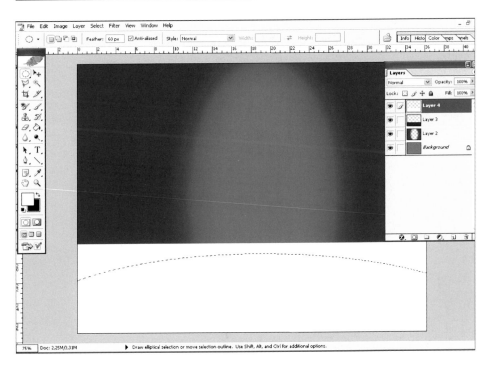

Fig. 17.87   Oval soft selection.

Step 5:   Another layer is added. Foreground color is set to white by pressing the
          letter D then X. The selection is filled with white by pressing ALT + Back-
          space (Fig. 17.86).

Step 6:   Selection is deselected (Ctrl.+D) and a wide oval is drawn over the white
          rectangle with the Marquee tool (M). The feather is again 60 pixels
          (Fig. 17.87).

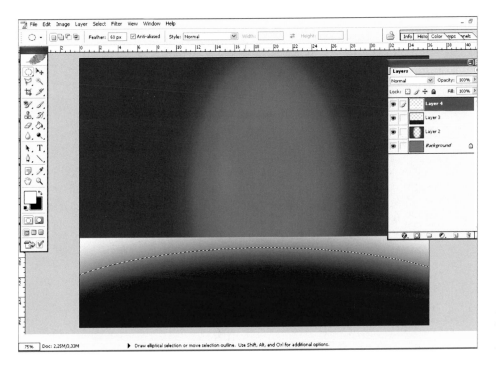

*Fig. 17.88   Again, a soft-edged
hole is punched out of the white
layer. The dark blue layer beneath appears again.*

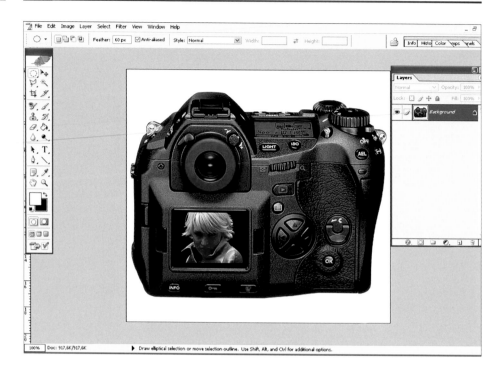

Fig. 17.89   Object to be presented is displayed.

Step 7: Press BACKSPACE to punch a soft-edged hole out of the white layer. It reveals part of the dark blue layer below. This gives the effect of falling light (Fig. 17.88).

Step 8: The photo of the object to be placed on the background is opened (Fig. 17.89). The object is selected by using the Wand for selecting the white background, then the selection is inverted by SELECT>Inverse (or Shift+Ctrl.+I).

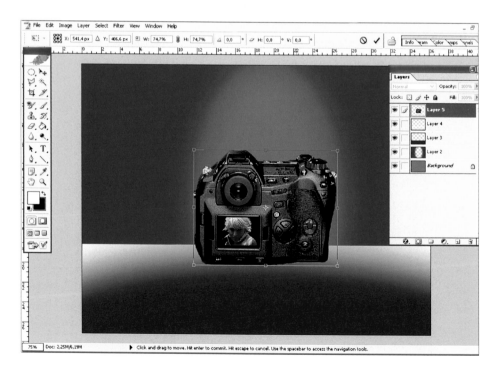

Fig. 17.90   Resizing the object with the Transformation Tool.

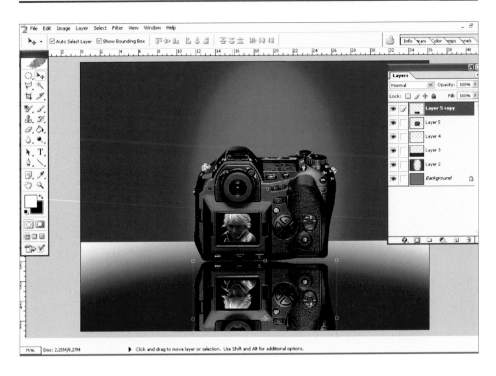

Fig. 17.91
Mirror image of the object.

Step 9:   After switching to the Move tool (V), the selected object is dragged onto
the background. If necessary, the object can be resized by EDIT > Free
Transform (or Ctrl. + T). A frame appears around the object. Holding
SHIFT and dragging one of the corner points resizes the object.
Press ENTER to lock in your transformation (Fig. 17.90).

Step 10: A reflection of the object is generated by duplicating the object layer. First
press Ctrl. + J then press Ctrl. + T to bring up Free Transform. Choose Flip

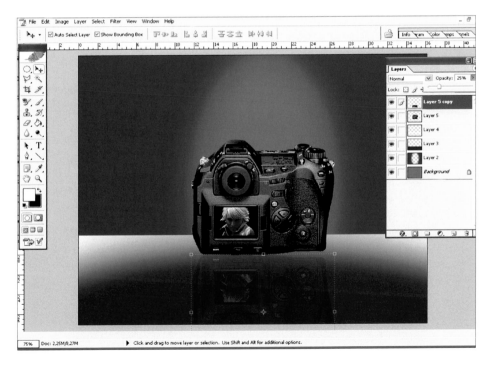

Fig. 17.92   Opacity is de-
creased to generate a natural
looking mirror image.

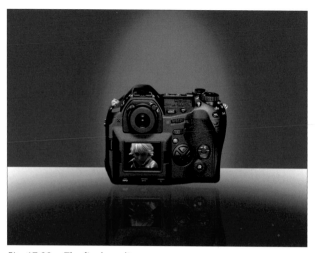

*Fig. 17.93   The final result
looks like a real photograph.*

Vertical to flip your object copy layer upside down. Press Shift and drag the object down until the contour lines of original object and its copy are in contact (Fig. 17.91).

Step 11: As the underground is not a perfect mirror, the opacity of the flipped object is reduced to 25% to give the impression of a reflection (Layers palette top right; Fig. 17.92).

The result in Fig. 17.93 gives only a vague idea of how powerful modern image editing programs are. Not more than basic knowledge is necessary to create virtual images which cannot be distinguished easily from "real" images.

17.6.4   Creating collages with layer masks

Collages are often used for covers or for the title slide in a slide presentation. There are different methods of generating a collage. The Layer Mask technique is one of the most powerful ways.

Step 1: First, the background photo is opened (Fig. 17.94).

Step 2: Then the first photo which has to be melted together with the background is opened.

Step 3: The letter "V" is pressed to activate the Move Tool in the toolbox. The second photo is moved onto the background photo. It appears on its own layer (Fig. 17.95).

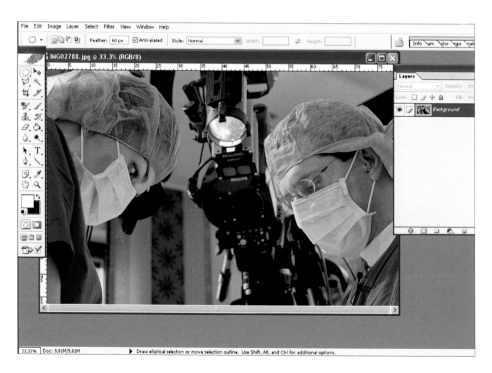

*Fig. 17.94   Creating a collage:
Background photo is opened.*

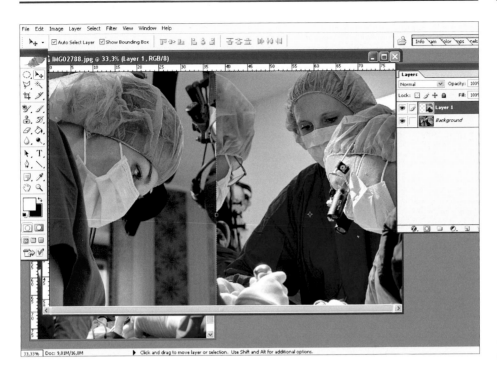

Fig. 17.95 Second photo is moved onto the background photo.

Step 4: A click on the Layer Mask Icon (second icon from left at the bottom of the layer palette) activates the mask. Pressing "G" and RETURN opens the Gradient Picker. The Black to White Gradient is chosen (first row, third from left) (Fig. 17.96).

Step 5: The Gradient Tool is clicked just beside the left edge of the top photo (in this case the right one) and dragged to the right. The starting point of this click and drag action makes the image totally transparent; at the end point

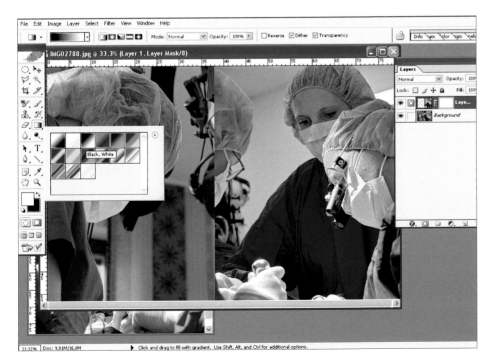

Fig. 17.96 Choosing the black and white gradient tool.

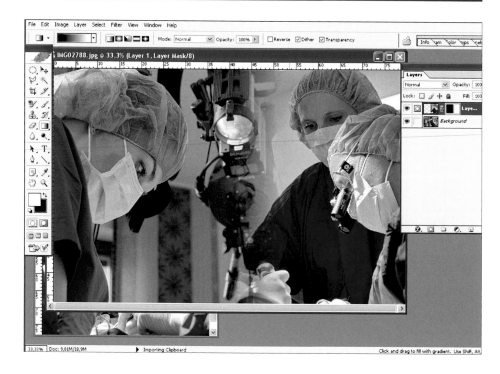

Fig. 17.97   Second photo
blends into the background.

the image has 100% opacity. When the mouse is released, the top photo
blends into the background. Both photos are melted together (Fig. 17.97).

Step 6:   A third photo which has to be integrated is opened. An appropriate area is
selected with the Marquee Tool. A soft border of 60 pixels was selected to
blend in the new element seamlessly (Fig. 17.98).

Step 7:   The selected area is copied (Ctrl. + C) into the composite photo (Ctrl. + V).
The opacity of this third picture element is reduced (Fig. 17.99).

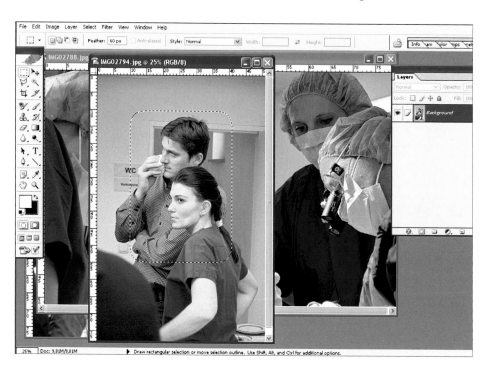

Fig. 17.98   Third photo with
soft-edged selection.

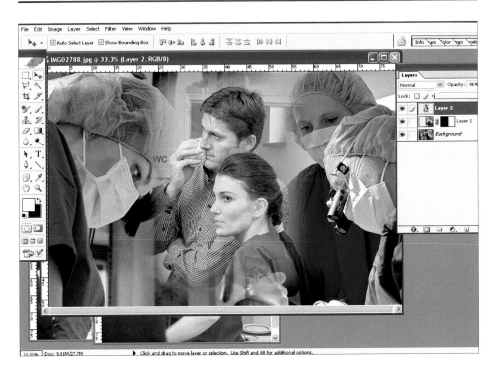

Fig. 17.99
Third photo integrated.

Step 8:   To add a title, the Marquee Tool is selected ("M"; feather 0 pixels) and a
          rectangular area at the bottom is drawn. With the color picker ("I") the
          color of the operating clothes is picked up. The rectangle is filled with this
          color (ALT + Backspace) (Fig. 17.100). If this rectangle has another opacity
          than the third picture element, it has to be placed on a separate layer.

Step 9:   Finally, the text is added ("T") (Fig. 17.101).

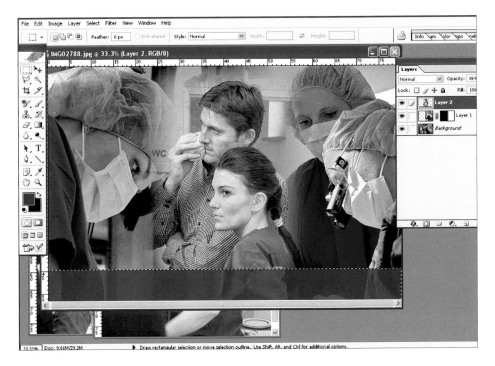

Fig. 17.100   *Opacity of third
photo is reduced.*

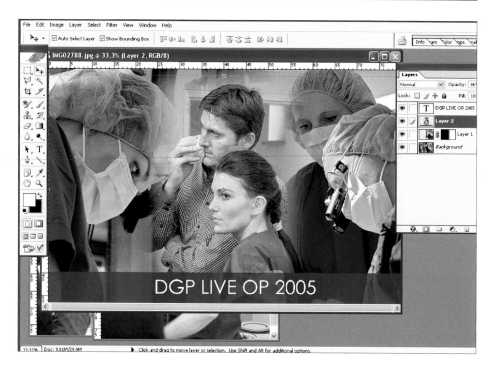

Fig. 17.101   *Text is added.*

Layer masks are a simple tool to melt images together. The only thing needed for this technique is a rough idea of how the image should look afterwards.

Blending images together is always tempting. The secret to good results is: Keep it simple.

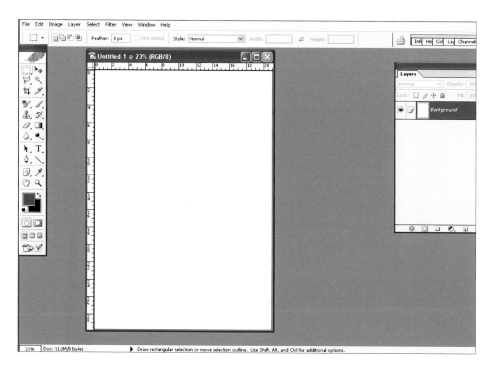

Fig. 17.102
New document generated.

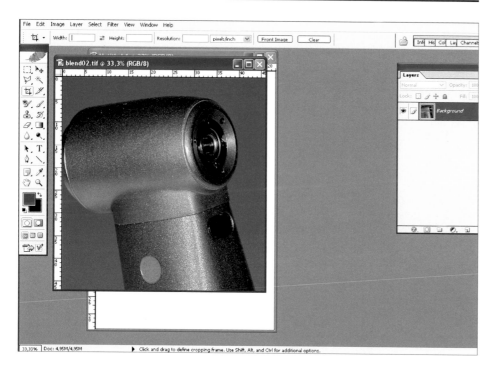

Fig. 17.103   Photo is opened.

17.6.5 Blending a photo with its background

A similar technique is used to blend a photo with its background.

Step 1: A new document is generated: Ctrl.+N, Preset: A4, Resolution 200 pixels/inch, background color: white. Finally press: OK (Fig. 17.102).

Step 2: The photograph to be blended is opened (Ctrl. + O) and an appropriate area is selected (Fig. 17.103).

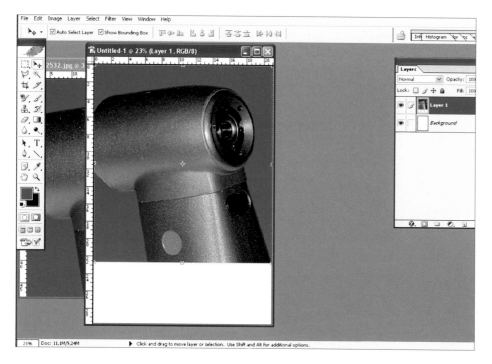

Fig. 17.104   Photo dragged onto the background.

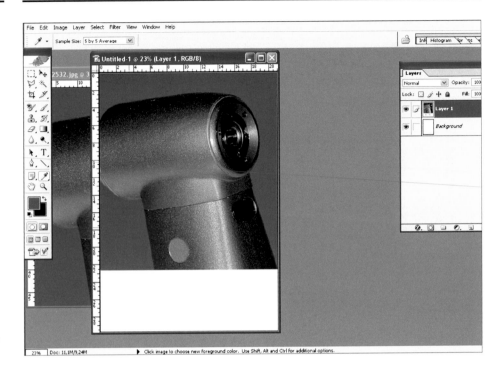

Fig. 17.105   Background color
of the photograph is selected.

Step 3: Activate the Move Tool ("V") and drag the image onto the background.
Size can be adapted by Ctrl. + T (Fig. 17.104).

Step 4: Select the color picker and pick up the background color of the photograph. Gray is now the selected color (Fig. 17.105).

Step 5: Activate the background layer in the Layers Palette by clicking on the
background layer. Then press Ctrl. + Backspace to fill the background with
the selected color (Fig. 17.106).

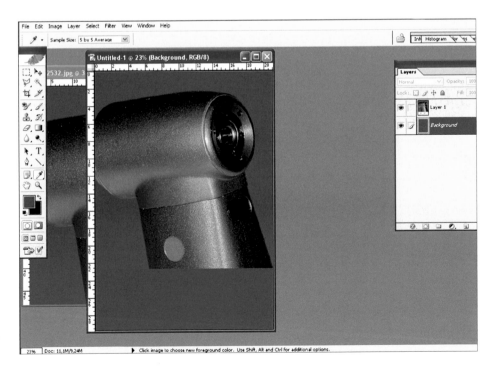

Fig. 17.106   Background is
filled with the background color
of the photo.

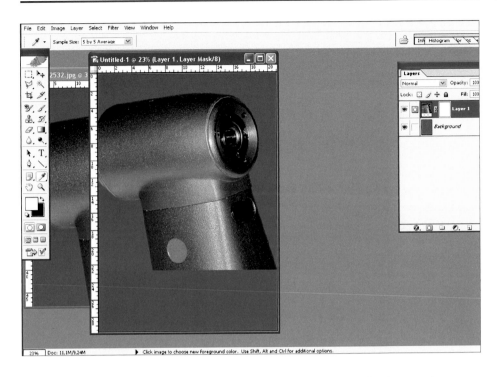

Fig. 17.107
Add layer mask icon is clicked.

Step 6: Now a Layer Mask is used to blend the photo with its background. Layer with photo is activated by clicking on it. Then the "Add Layer Mask Icon" is clicked (Fig. 17.107).

Step 7: The Gradient Tool is activated ("G") and the Black to White Gradient is selected (Fig. 17.108).

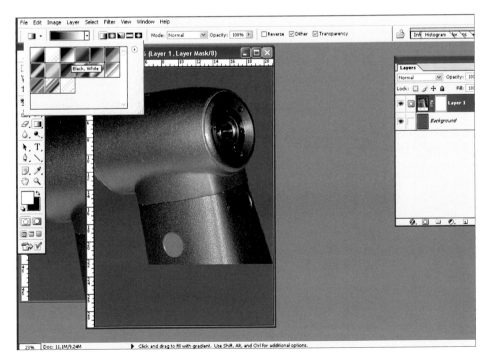

Fig. 17.108
Gradient tool activated.

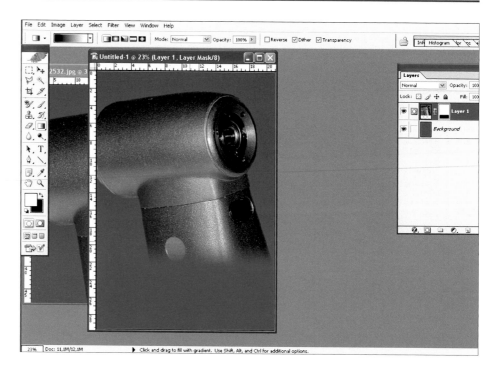

Fig. 17.109   Photo is blended into the background.

Step 8:   The cross of the Gradient Tool is placed at the lower border of the photo, then click and with the mouse button pressed down move the cross up wards. When releasing the mouse button, the photo is blended with the background (Fig. 17.109).

Step 9:   Finally, text can be added ("T"). If necessary, the opacity of the text can be reduced (Fig. 17.110).

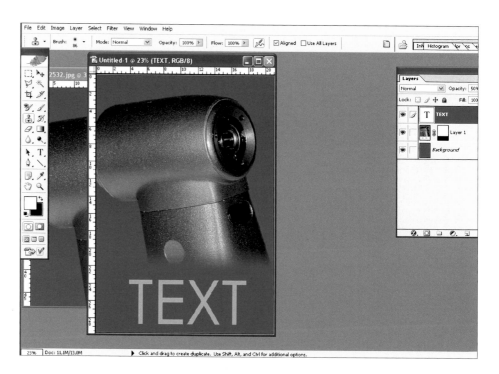

Fig. 17.110   Text can be added on a separate text layer.

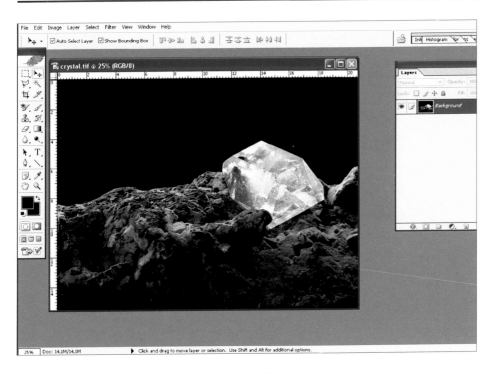

Fig. 17.111   Image is loaded.

17.6.6   Elegant transparent typing

This effect has an elegant appearance and can be used for covers or slide presentations.

Step 1: An image is loaded (Fig. 17.111).

Step 2: Type Tool is selected ("T"). Appropriate font, font size and font color (white) are selected. Text is typed (Fig. 17.112).

Step 3: By typing Ctrl. + T "Free Transform" is activated. The cursor is moved outside of one edge of the frame appearing around the text. The cursor

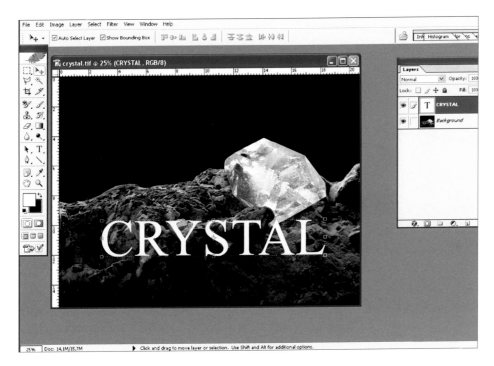

Fig. 17.112   Text is added.

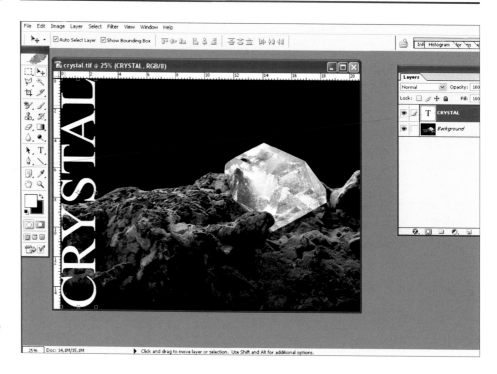

Fig. 17.113   Text is moved into the final position by "Free Transform".

takes on a double arrow shape. Click and hold, and move the cursor counterclockwise. With the Shift tab pressed down a precise vertical position of the text can be reached easily. With the cursor inside the frame, the text can be moved into the final position. Press RETURN to apply the transformation (Fig. 17.113).

Step 4: Opacity of the typing is reduced in the Layers Palette to a value of about 50% This gives the image an elegant appearance (Fig. 17.114).

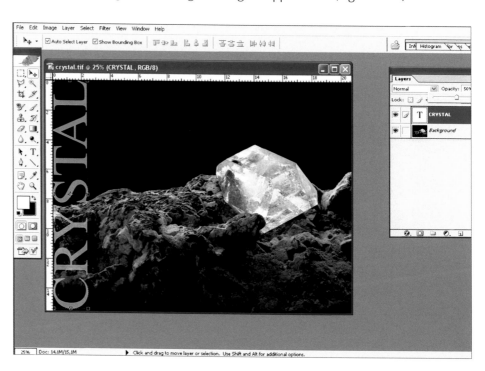

Fig. 17.114   Reducing opacity of the text gives the image an elegant appearance.

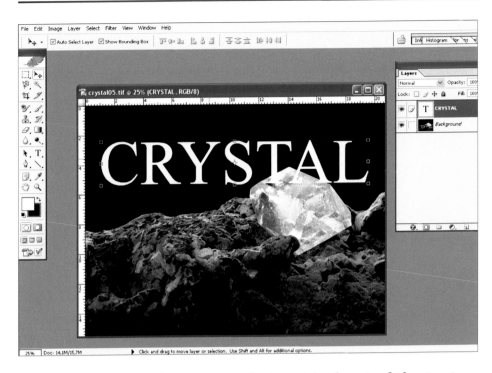

Fig. 17.115   Text is typed in front of the background image.

17.6.7   Placing a background object in front of the text

Step 1:   Image is opened. Text is typed and moved into the right position. At this stage, text is in front of background image (Fig. 17.115).

Step 2:   Background Layer is activated by clicking into the image. Magnetic Lasso Tool ("L") is activated and a piece of the crystal which will be in front later is selected. By pressing Ctrl. + J, this piece is copied onto a new layer (Fig. 17.116).

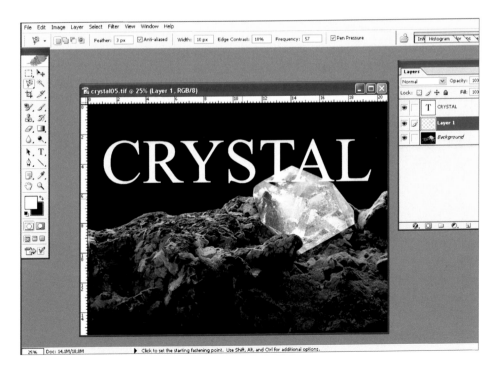

Fig. 17.116   Part of back-ground photo is duplicated onto a new layer (Layer 1).

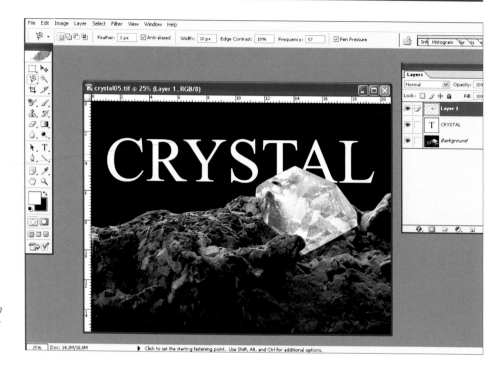

Fig. 17.117   Layer 1 moved on top of the text layer. Typing appears behind the background image.

Step 3: The Text Layer is pulled down one step, Layer 1 is on top now. By this, the text is placed behind the background image, giving the whole arrangement a three-dimensional impression (Fig. 17.117).

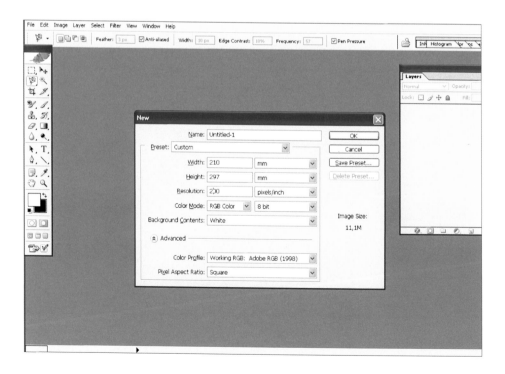

Fig. 17.118
A new document is opened.

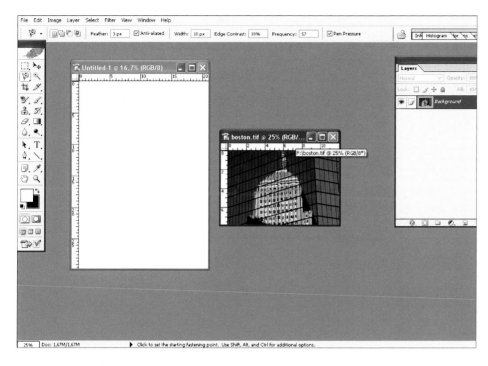

Fig. 17.119   Image is opened.

17.6.8   Polaroid effect

Placing a photograph in front of a white background with a soft shadow is a nice way to present images. Especially pictures of a patient can be treated with this classic Photoshop® effect.

Step 1:   A new DIN A4 document is opened. Ctrl.+N like in section 17.5.4.
As PRESET "A4" is selected, resolution is 200 dpi, background is white (Fig. 17.118).

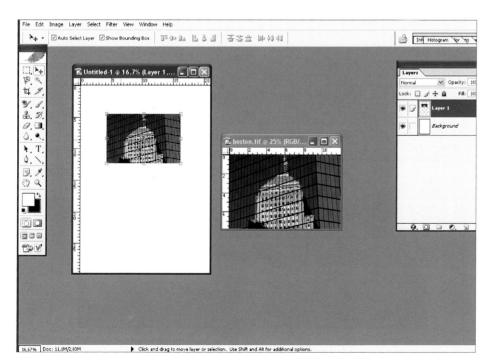

Fig. 17.120   Photograph is moved onto the background.

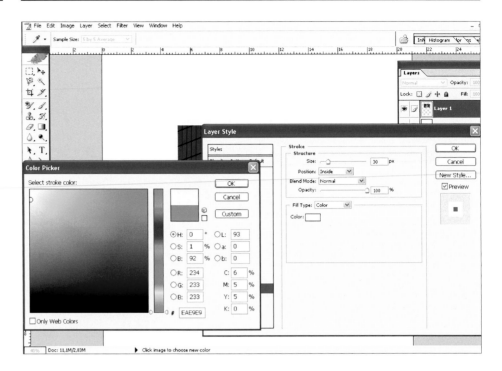

Fig. 17.121   Frame is added.

Step 2: The photograph on which the effect is to be applied is opened: Ctrl. + O.
Image size must be adapted, and resolution must be the same as for the
new document (200 dpi) (Fig. 17.119).

Step 3: Photograph is moved onto the white background ("V") (Fig. 17.120).

Step 4: Now the frame has to be added. "Add a Layer Style" icon (Layers Palette,
left icon, bottom row) is activated. Click on "Stroke". Layer Style box opens.
Size 30 pixels, position: inside. Color: select a very light gray (Fig. 17.121).

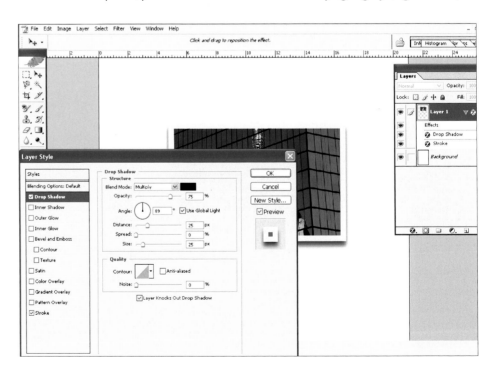

Fig. 17.122
Shadow effect is added.

Step 5: Click OK for the color selection, the frame appears around the image. Don't click OK for the Layer Style. Instead, click directly on the word "Drop shadow". Set an angle of 89, distance 25 px, size 25 px. Then click OK in the Layer Style box (Fig. 17.122).

Step 6: Image seems to float in front of the white background, casting a soft shadow (Fig. 17.123).

Effects like this one can easily be recorded with a Photoshop® action. Then, with a touch of your finger, the image floats in front of the background within a second.

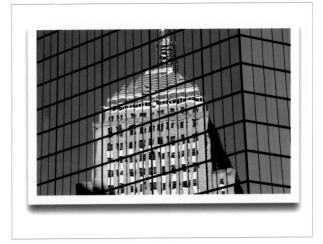

Fig. 17.123
Result: Image seems to float.

17.6.9   To insert a picture into another picture

Step 1: Open the target picture, the one into which the second picture is to be integrated (Fig. 17.124).

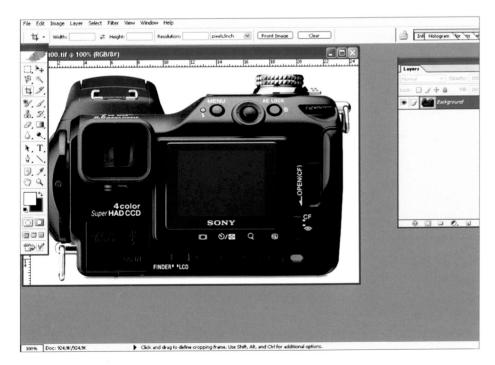

Fig. 17.124
Target picture is opened.

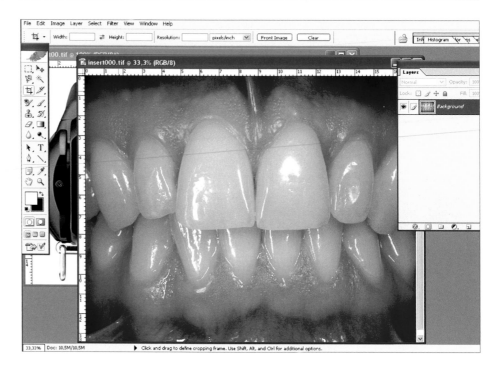

Fig. 17.125   Image to be inserted is opened.

Step 2: Open the second picture and select the whole picture by SELECT > All (or Ctrl. + A). Then press EDIT > Copy (or Ctrl. + C) (Fig. 17.125).

Step 3: Change to the original picture again. Activate the Rectangular Marquee Tool ("M") and draw a frame around the area where the second photo will appear (Fig. 17.126).

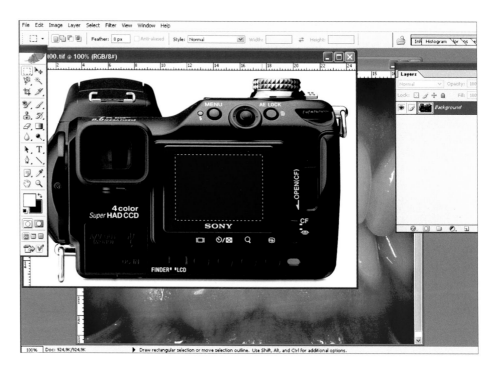

Fig. 17.126
Target area is selected.

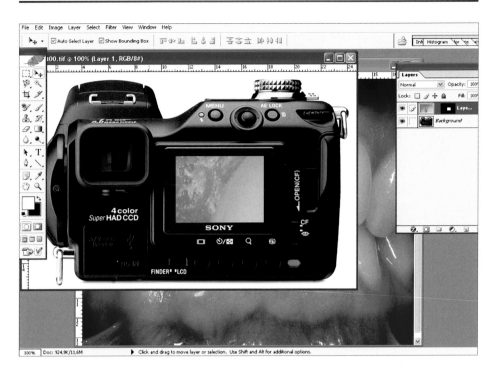

Fig. 17.127   Image is inserted. It has to be resized.

Step 4:   Press EDIT > Paste into (or Shift + Ctrl. + V). A copy of the second image is inserted into the frame. Because the image is still too large, it must be resized (Fig. 17.127).

Step 5:   Activate "Free Transform" by EDIT > Free Transform or Ctrl. + T. To reach the handles of the Marquee Frame, press Ctrl. + 0. Now the Transformation frame is completely visible (Fig. 17.128).

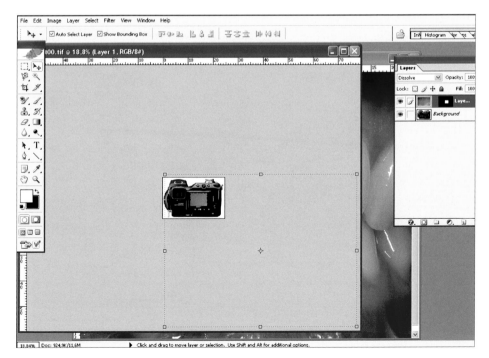

*Fig. 17.128
Resizing the inserted image.*

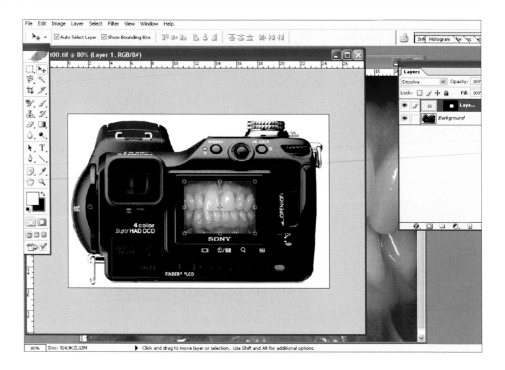

*Fig. 17.129   Inserted image
with proper dimensions.*

Step 6: Press and hold SHIFT and move one of the corner handles until the image
fits perfectly into the selected area. Then press RETURN (Fig. 17.129).

Step 7: Finally, a small shadow is added to create the impression that the image is
in the camera display and not on top of it. Click in the Layers Palette on
the icon "Add a layer style" (left one, bottom of the box), select "Stroke".
The Layer Style box opens. Select "Inner shadow", set "Distance" and
"Size" to 3 px, angle to 90 degrees. Then press OK (Fig. 17.130a).

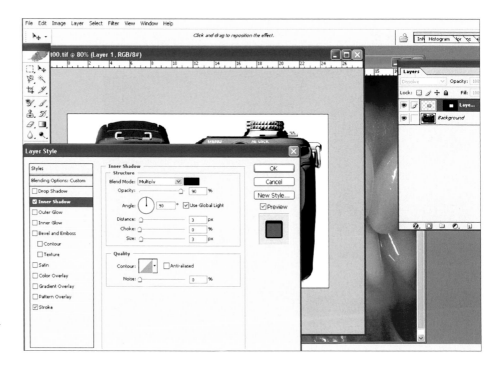

*Fig. 17.130a   To create a natu-
ral appearance, a shadow is
added.*

Now the photo is inte-
grated perfectly into the
first one (Fig. 130b).

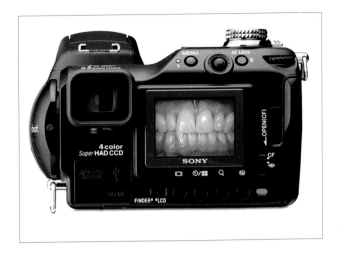

Fig. 17.130b   Result: natural-looking inserted picture.

17.6.10   Sepia effect

A very traditional effect in photography was the sepia effect. It was a simple photographic effect, which gave a black and white photograph the impression of color.

Step 1: The photograph is opened (Ctrl. + O). The plan is to create a black and
         white photo first using the gradient effect to get more contrast. Select
         black as foreground color (press "D"), then activate the icon "Create new
         fill or adjustment layer" (third from right, bottom of the layers box) and
         select "Gradient map". As soon the dialog box opens, the photograph
         turns black and white (Fig. 17.131). Press OK.

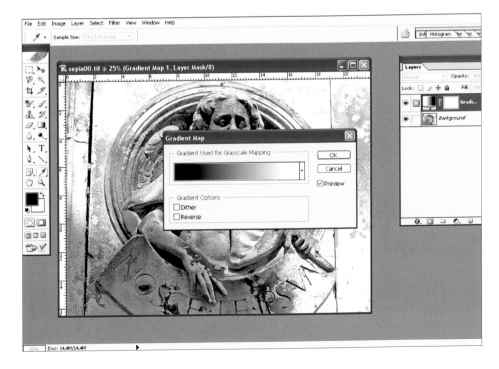

Fig. 17.131   To add a sepia ef-fect, the image is converted into a black and white image first.

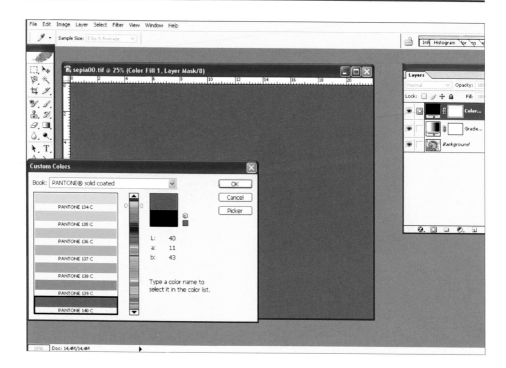

Fig. 17.132
A brown color is selected.

Step 2:   Again activate the icon "Create new fill or adjustment layer" (third from right, bottom of the layers box) and select "solid color". The color picker box opens. Select CUSTOM. The Custom Colors Box opens. Under Book, "Pantone® solid coated" is selected. A color is selected (Fig. 17.132), then click OK. The whole image gets the selected color and turns brown.

Step 3:   Go into the Layers Palette and change the layer blending mode from "Normal" to "Color". The image appears with the sepia effect (Fig. 17.133).

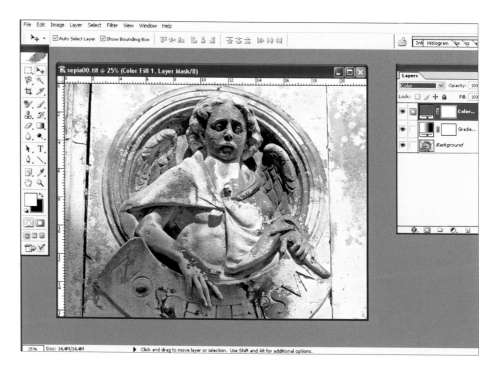

Fig. 17.133
Image with sepia effect.

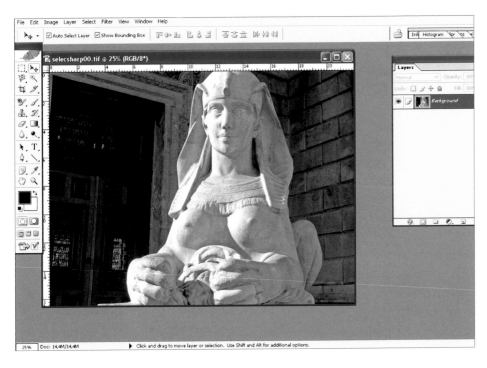

Fig. 17.134   Image is opened.

17.6.11   Selective sharpness

Sometimes overall sharpness is not the best for a picture. A selective sharpness may enhance a picture by adding a certain three-dimensionality.

Step 1: Picture is opened (Fig. 17.134).

Step 2: With the magic wand, the object is selected (Fig. 17.135).

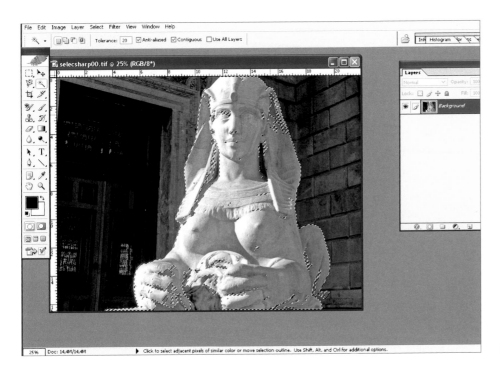

Fig. 17.135   Object is selected.

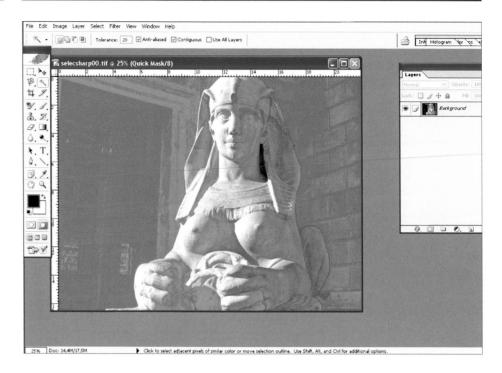

Fig. 17.136   The Quick Mask
Mode facilitates selection of an
object.

Step 3: Change to the quick mask mode ("Q") (Fig. 17.136).

Step 4: Eraser is activated ("E"). Remove all red parts within the object. To work
more precisely, the image can be zoomed in. If necessary, add red color
outside the object by using the brush.

Step 5: Change from the Quick Mask Mode to the normal mode again ("Q").
Selection must be expanded by SELECT>Modify>Expand 3 pixels (Fig.
17.137). Then selection is inversed: SELECT>Inverse (or Shift + Ctrl. + I).

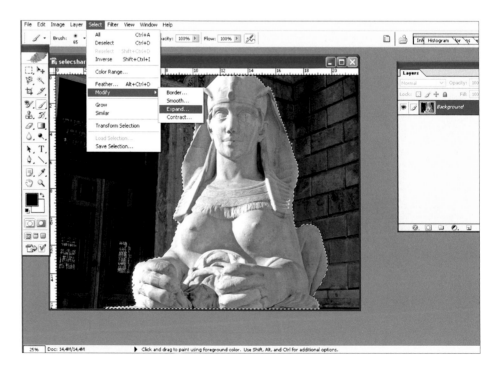

Fig. 17.137   Selection is
expanded to avoid a margin
around the selection.

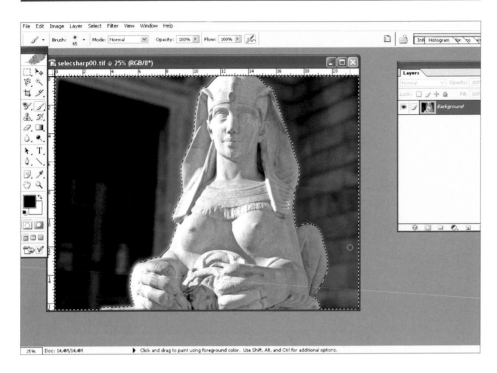

Fig. 17.138
Inverted selection is blurred.

Step 6: Blur the selection: FILTER > Blur > Gaussian Blur (radius 4 to 8). Blurring can be repeated by Ctrl. + F (Fig. 17.138) until the desired effect is created. Then deselect Ctrl.+D.

Slide presentations with PowerPoint® 18

Screen presentations can be used in the context of dental photography for patient information, displaying information about the practice, web presentations, and scientific lectures. Within only a couple of years, conventional slide presentations have disappeared almost entirely, having been replaced by screen presentations.

The most common program used for this purpose is Microsoft PowerPoint®. Other programs are:
- Keynote (Apple Corp.)
- Impress (www.openOffice.org)
- ActiveSlide (www.activeSlide.com)
- Corel Draw
- …

Because the most commonly used program is Microsoft PowerPoint®, this chapter refers mainly to this program.

There are hundreds of books dealing with the PowerPoint® program and its possibilities. Additional information is available in the Internet, where tutorials and examples (both bad and good) can be found. In the context of dental photography, this chapter will not add another book. The information compiled in this book aims at the beginner to facilitate his or her first steps with PowerPoint® or similar programs. It gives some general information about how to plan a presentation and create effective slides.

Some advantages of screen presentations are:
- Image elements can be animated, not only drawing attention to the presentation in general, effectively making important points and thus improving the didactics of a presentation. These allow dynamic developments and relationships to be presented with a great deal of finesse, bordering on the possibilities of animated films.

- Sound and video can be added.
- The layout of entire series can be easily changed.
- Individual "transparencies" can be added from existing presentations at the touch of a button.
- Storing and archiving presentations is much easier. No need to "re-archive" slides after a lecture, with the associated problems.
- The lecturer's logistical problems are greatly reduced, as it is no longer necessary to carry around bulky slide trays; he or she now brings the presentation along on a CD, if the presentation means are available at the lecture hall.

Disadvantages of screen presentations
- Image quality is still inferior to that of a slide presentation. The beamer resolution is still the limiting factor.
- Dependence on complex technology, with compatibility problems still prevalent.
- Presentation equipment still not available in adequate quality at all higher learning facilities.

A computer program for presentations is not an end in itself. It is only a tool, probably a powerful one, to transfer ideas and information to the audience. One of the main problems of "slideware" (programs for presentations) is that these programs elevate format over content. This must be avoided.

Nevertheless, the visual expectations of the audience must be taken into account. It can be assumed that people of the "videoclip generation", who are constantly being bombarded by overpowering visual images, will need to have their attention held by different visual means than their parents did. Consumer surveys of US television audiences have shown that 35% of viewers are "flippers," that is, they keep changing from one channel to another. Even short periods of boredom are not tolerated, but are relieved by a quick click of the TV control. This, of course, also has an effect on an audience's expectations of the visual content of a scientific presentation.

18.1   Preparing the presentation

Mark Twain quipped: "It usually takes me more than three weeks to prepare a good impromptu speech." To prepare a presentation, the SPAM model can be used:
- **S**ituation
- **P**urpose
- **A**udience
- **M**ethod

18.1.1   SPAM model

Situation

Take the time and the place of the presentation into account. Is it a seminar presentation? Or is it a scientific lecture? How many people will be in attendance?

Purpose

A presentation may have more than one purpose, but it should have at least one. Before starting the preparation, the following questions should be answered:

Why I am speaking? What are my objectives? What is the "take-home message"? What do I want to achieve?
- Dissemination of information
- Motivation
- Persuasion

In many cases, the purposes of a presentation are a mix of conveying a message, giving some information, motivating the audience, and helping them finding additional learning resources.

Audience

Consider your audience. Put yourself in their place. Why are people there? Are they there for coursework, practical improvement, entertainment? Is it a mandatory educational lecture? Are they attending the presentation voluntarily or are they obligated to attend?

What do the people expect, to whom the speech is directed? Participants of a scientific congress may expect results of solid research. Workshop participants may expect practical instructions. Laypeople may expect some general information.

How much does the audience already know about your topic? What is their knowledge level? Are they students, practitioners, nurses, laypeople? How much does the audience need to know? And how much do people want to know?

In most cases there is a mix of people, some with and some without a certain level of knowledge. In this case, the interest of the majority should be maintained. The presentation should not be reduced to the lowest common denominator. Then you lose the attention of the majority. Parts of the presentation can be above the heads of part of the audience, as long as continuity is not interrupted. Nevertheless, a good presentation should try to reach everyone in the audience.

Method

Which presentation format will best accomplish the purpose of my presentation?

- Public address?
- Lecture with blackboard?
- PowerPoint® slides?
- Movie/Audio?
- Demonstration?

As the Oriental proverb goes, "I listen and forget, I see and remember, I do and comprehend." It is frequently cited that we remember approximately 25 percent of what we hear, 40 percent of what we see and hear, and 75 percent of what we hear, see, and do. Apart from "hands-on-seminars", we do not have the opportunity for practical exercises during most lectures. This is the advantage of lectures where images are used. We can use images to anchor our information in the brains of our audience, using impressive and readable illustrations and charts. And we can use animated illustrations to develop ideas.

The very ambitious goal of presenting a lecture is that the audience should retain as much as possible of that which we relate and show. That which we perceive and have understood should remain as much as possible in our memory.

Images and graphics are an aid to presenting complex concepts in a simpler manner. They improve understanding and reduce the amount of explanation needed: "One picture is worth a thousand words." Presenting information in a visual form aids in remembering the spoken word, since a second "information channel" is being used. We remember more of what we have seen than what we have heard or read. The old boxer's maxim holds true here: "A punch on the eye is worth three on the ear." Combining oral and visual information increases the amount of information recalled. This is aided by images, which are the anchor for memory.

Real images intensify the impact of the information, since they appear authentic. Images are also able to sway an audience's emotions and intensify the message. Text and graphic slides in particular are helpful in structuring the lecture. This not only helps the listener to better understand the ideas in context, but also forces the lecturer to better structure his or her presentation, with the slides being the main thread.

18.1.2   Structuring the content

The number of key points the audience will remember is limited. Most sources speak of five key points the audience will take home. The problem is you do not know if your key messages and the points remembered by the audience are the same. Therefore, you have to put them down and show them to the audience.

Outlining your presentation can be done using PowerPoint® or Word® or other computer programs. A piece of paper and a pencil will do as well.

Introduction

There is an old but successful rule of structuring a presentation, the "rule of tell 'em": "Tell them what you are going to tell them, tell it to them, and then tell them what you told them." That means: Start with a big picture, with a presentation of an overview of your lecture. Tell the people what they will learn. Then provide the information and finally summarize the results.

Experienced speakers recommend starting with the last slide when preparing the lecture. The conclusion or summary slide is put down without considering all the details and the presentation's organization. Then it is relatively easy to build the whole presentation around these main points, facts, concepts etc.

The main part (body)

The most important point for structuring the lecture is to have done the research completely and to have understood the main problems involved. A second important point is to start early with the preparation of a presentation.

Structure of content

Research presentations should be organized according to a fixed scheme.

1. Title
2. Introduction of scientific problem
    a.   Statement of problem and purpose
    b.   Identification of framework
3. Methodology
    a.   Design
    b.   Sample size
    c.   Identification of data analysis methods
4. Results
    a.   Major findings
    b.   Conclusions
    c.   Implications for the audience addressed
    d.   Recommendations for further research

If the context of the presentation allows more freedom, it is important that at least the following topics are covered:

- What is the problem and why is it a problem?
- How was this problem approached/solved before?
- Which approach is preferred by the lecturer?
- What are the advantages of this new approach?
- What are future possibilities and aspects?

The body of your presentation has to be divided into subtopics with introduction, conclusion and proper transition into the next subtopic. There are different ways to give your key points and subtopics a structure.

- Topical: e.g., presentation of four different filling materials.
- Chronological/sequential: e.g., history of dentin adhesion materials.
- Cause/effect: e.g., vitamin deficiencies and the related diseases.
- Structural/graphical: e.g., showing organs which produce hormones and their relationships.
- Problem-solving: e.g., showing most common faults in making radiographs and how to improve the technique.
- Spatial: e.g., showing the most common skin lesions and their chief locations

Breaking down the main topics in such a structure will help the audience to follow along, even if attention has been distracted by other things for a short time.

During the main part of the lecture, methods to achieve the objectives are presented. When introducing novel concepts, the background must be explained and the listeners provided with clear information. Explaining the methodology is normally followed by showing typical results together with statistical analyses. Finally, the results are discussed, not only the successes, but also the mixed outcomes and failures. At the end of the presentation, proper acknowledgments must be given.

Maintaining attention

The attention span of an adult listener is 15 to 20 minutes. Therefore a (sub-)topic should not be discussed longer than 15 to 20 minutes. Varying the pace of a presentation by inserting a question period, some interactive activities or by showing a short movie helps to maintain attention. Explaining how each subtopic fits into the whole context allows the listener to follow more easily.

Rather than say more, the presenter should say less, concentrating on 3 to 5 major points. A presentation is not the place to say everything you know about a problem. Leave some details for the discussion at the end. Instead of listing details endlessly, tell stories. The human mind is receptive to information through storytelling, as myths, verbally transmitted experience, and epic poetry did thousands of years before. A story is capable of anchoring the message in the mind of the listener better than the mere description of facts.

Always keep your presentation focused on the message. Before inserting a new slide ask: Is this slide essential for my lecture? Or does it carry away the audience?

Repetition is the mother of learning and remembering. Nobody in the audience is able to pay attention constantly. Therefore, repetition of the key-points is essential.

Never read a speech, as reading is monotonous and lacks dynamics. If a manuscript is prepared, it has to be prepared in a spoken, conversational language. An exception to this recommendation is the international congress, where translators need a manuscript in advance. After preparing themselves, good translators should be able to translate a conversationally spoken presentation.

Keep it simple

An ancient, but still valuable adage is KISS – Keep it simple, stupid. The more sophisticated the technology is, the more problems are to be expected. Using links within a presentation can be very helpful to be prepared for different situations, but if the links are too complex, there is always the danger of getting lost in your own presentation. The more complex the technical setup, the more likely is a technical breakdown. Using two beamers at a time, starting short movies out of a program or running different programs can attract the attention, but—if exaggerated—these visual special effects can distract the attention as well. In addition, it can end in a technical disaster in the worst case. Never use rented equipment without having checked (and rechecked) it.

Check the time

The content of the main part of the presentation has to be checked to keep within the allotted time. By eliminating all slides not properly focused on the main topics, the lecture can be boiled down. Speaking faster is not the solution for a presentation with too much material. The shorter the speech, the more difficult is the preparation. Goethe once wrote: "I intended to write a shorter letter, but I had no time for it."

Finishing the presentation in time or some minutes before allows more time for the discussion. No audience has ever become angry with a speaker for coming to an end too soon. But everybody has experienced speakers spoiling their own presentation by talking hastily at the end of their lecture or—even worse—by not being allowed to say their concluding remarks, as the chairmen has switched off the microphone.

Summary/conclusion

The summary at the end of a lecture is the most important part. It is the last chance to transfer the relevant messages to the audience. The worst thing you can do is to finish your lecture with a feeble "Well, that's it."

The summary slide should emphasize the key points again. The concluding statement can be a little bit emotional. You want your audience leave the room and discuss your ideas. Finally thank the audience, make materials (hand-outs) available, if you have prepared them, and be ready for a discussion.

As time is always limited during a congress, provide the listeners with your e-mail address, internet homepage, or another way to get in touch with you. Try to get feedback; it is the best way to improve your presentations in the future.

18.2 PowerPoint® basics

18.2.1 Creating a PowerPoint® slide

In this context, it is not possible to provide the step-by-step procedure of every detail. There are numerous books providing the user with valuable information. In addition, there is a lot of information accessible via the Internet. Here, only some important details are mentioned.

To create a new presentation there are four choices offered after opening the program:

- Autocontent wizard
- Design template
- Blank presentation
- Open an existing presentation (Fig. 18.01)

You can use design templates with color schemes or you can construct your own slides using master slides (title master and slide master) in order to maintain unity in design from slide to slide. For backgrounds and text, different styles and colors can be used.

A new slide can be added by selecting the INSERT menu and selecting NEW SLIDE or clicking on the New Slide button on the toolbar. The new slide appears as a slide with a title box and a text box. Beside this, the task pane will display the slide layout options. Here, a variety of slide layouts (text, content, combinations) is offered. To

Fig. 18.01 There are different options to begin a new presentation.

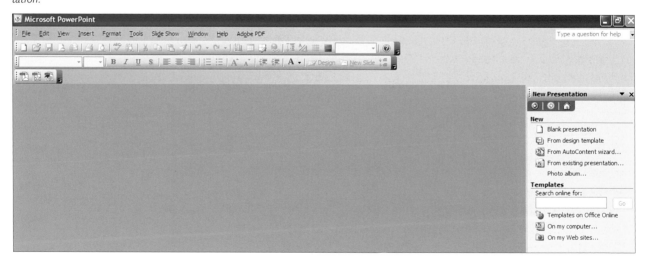

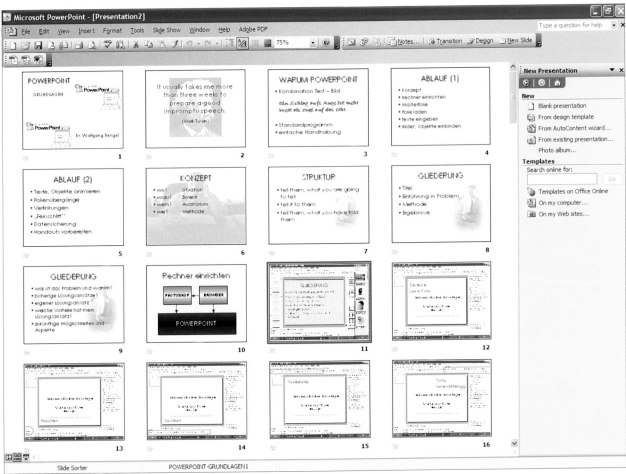

Fig. 18.02   The Slide Sorter View offers a fast possibility to add new slides.

select any layout, its thumbnail image is selected. By this means, the slide will change automatically.

A very fast and elegant way to add new slides is by copying single slides in the Slide Sorter View (Fig. 18.2). For example, you have just finished a text slide. Now you need another slide with the same formatting. The text slide is selected and copied by Ctrl.+ D. Double-clicking the copied slide opens it. Then you double-click the items to be replaced by new text, and just start typing the new text. The same works with all types of slides. If you need a type of slide generated before, select it, duplicate it, and move it with the mouse to the place where you need it.

18.2.2 Background

The main function of a background is to provide sufficient contrast for text or graphic elements. An object is only visible if there is a contrast between the object and the background. A second important point is that the background should visually remain in the background. Red is not a background color (see below). One of the reasons is that red is perceived on a different plane than, for example, blue.

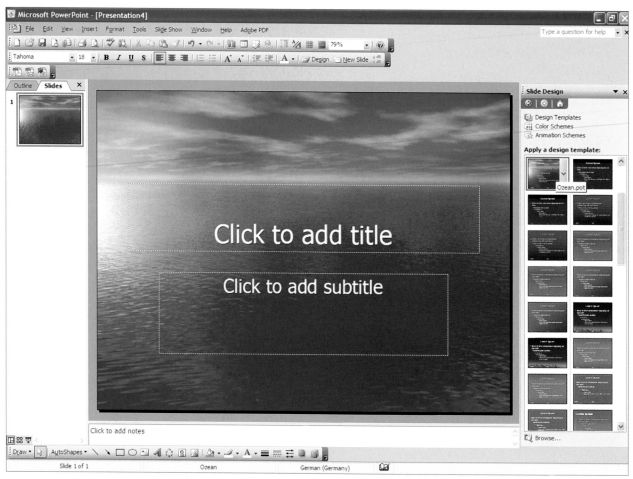

Fig. 18.03
Design Templates can be used.

Tips for color selection

One of the most common mistakes made by beginners is to use a huge variety of colors. They should be used sparingly. The intention is to use the visual attractiveness of colors without overwhelming the audience. To be on the safe side, use the predefined color schemes of PowerPoint®. In these schemes, different colors are combined successfully.

To open the color schemes, NEW PRESENTATION is opened and the DESIGN TEMPLATES are selected (Fig. 18.3). To access color schemes, we select COLOR SCHEMES from the SLIDE DESIGN menu. Here PowerPoint's standard color schemes are stored (Fig. 18.4). These schemes can be edited individually: select EDIT COLOR SCHEME and then select CUSTOM. Now every color element in the display can be modified. After editing, the CHANGE COLOR button is clicked. The color of the background can be changed in the same way. Individual mixing of the color is also possible. After that, the APPLY button has to be clicked and the newly developed scheme is displayed in the color scheme menu.

As colors look different when projected by different beamers, it is advisable to test the color combinations before starting the presentation. If there are problems, colors can be rearranged. Using colors is a means of conveying an additional message, because colors have a subjective message themselves which varies according to bi-

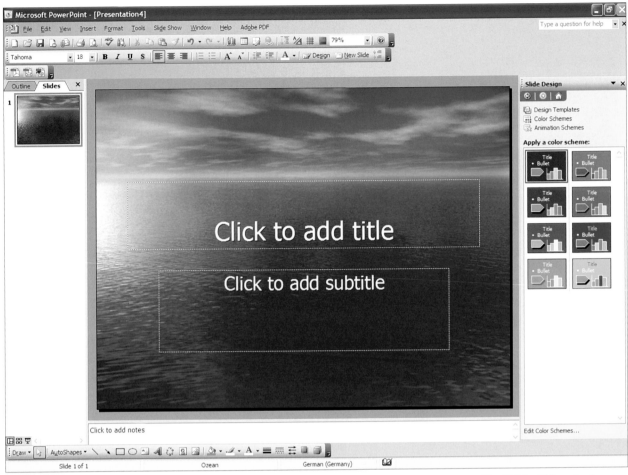

Fig. 18.04   Different color
schemes can be selected.

ological, cultural and individual factors. Our retinas contain more color receptors for red (about 64%) than for green (about 34%) and blue (only 2%). In our culture, black is associated with death and evil. In Egypt, black stands for reincarnation and resurrection, and in the Hebrew culture, black means understanding and sympathy. In addition, everybody has certain color preferences and aversions which can change over time, influenced by personal experiences and fashion.

Some examples for the meaning of colors (Western world):

Red:	hot, stop, fire, aggression
Pink:	cute, female, cotton-candy
Orange:	autumn, Halloween, warm
Yellow:	happy, sunny, cheerful, slow down
Brown:	warm, autumn, dirty
Green:	envy, jealousy, pastoral
Blue:	water, peaceful, sad, male, cold
Purple:	royal
Black:	night, evil, death, fear, mourning
Gray:	overcast, gloom, old age
White:	clean, innocent, cold

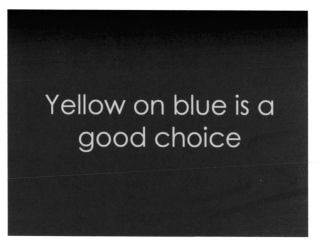

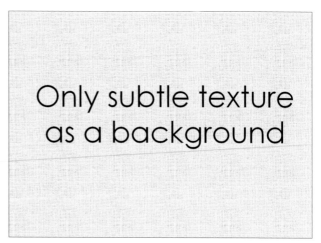

Fig. 18.05   Classical choice for text slides: yellow on blue.   *Fig. 18.06   Textures as background should be subtle.*

For background/text combinations, not more than three additional colors should be used. For ease of reading, high-contrast colors should be selected. Good combinations are white on black, blue-violet on yellow, black on yellow, yellow on blue, white on blue (Fig. 18.5). In general, cool colors (blue) are most suitable for backgrounds. One of the reasons is that the human eye is not very sensitive to blue.

When graphics are used in combination with text, colors of the graphic should be used as text colors in order to avoid a confusing and disturbing color variety and to achieve a more uniform appearance.

Sometimes a textured background with a neutral color is a good choice, but only if the pattern is subtle, related to the topic, and conveys additional meaning (Fig. 18.6). If different colors are combined for the background, analogous colors (neighboring colors in the color wheel) work well. Up to 10% of males have some kind of color-perception deficiency. The most common is a red-green deficiency. To avoid problems, red-green combinations should not be used.

Some tips may help select a background:
- Select a medium or bright tone: slides with white background allow a brighter room illumination. If the projection is very bright, this can literally dazzle the audience. If the background is too dark, people soon feel sleepy, since the ambient light is reduced too much. Changing brightness in a series is to be avoided if possible.
- Create good contrast with the text: light text on a dark background is more legible than vice versa. If the room illumination is not reduced too much, dark text (black or blue) on a white background also works well.
- Background color should remain in the background in visual terms; that is, do not use red, since this color is focused on a different plane than those of other colors. Red is perceived in the foreground.
- Reduce the number of background colors to allow images from other series to be used.

- Use uniform color for a series.
- In case of doubt, blue should be selected as a background color. Since the human eye is relatively insensitive to blue, it provides good contrast and does not tire the audience if they have to look at a blue background for a long time.
- Backgrounds with real images should be avoided or used only if the image stays in the background visually ("softened" pictures with reduced contrast and increased brightness).

The general rule of thumb: keep it simple. The listener/observer has attended the lecture to learn new information in his or her field and not what the latest computer graphics program can do.

18.2.3 Text

Most slides contain text elements. Frequently, the only content of a slide is text. To add text to the slide, click in the box labelled "Click to add text" and type the text (Fig. 18.7). If it is too long for the line, PowerPoint® automatically wraps the text to the next line. If text has to be added to a different part of the slide, a new text box

Fig. 18.07
Adding text is simple.

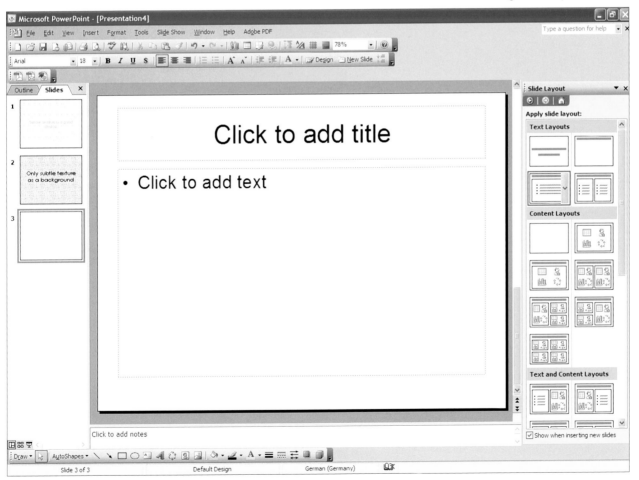

has to be inserted: INSERT menu > TEXT BOX. The new text box can be drawn with the mouse and moved to the proper position.

Text is the most essential part of a PowerPoint® slide. Therefore, selecting the right font is of utmost importance.

BACKGROUND

Serif or Sans serif

An important distinction can be made between fonts with and without serifs. Serifs are small decorative strokes (they look like little feet) that are added to the end of a letter's main strokes. An example is Times New Roman (Fig. 18.8).

We read words as a whole, not letter by letter. Serifs help us recognize the words grasped as a whole by comparing them with acquired samples in our brain. They improve readability by leading the eye along the line of type linking the words together. Therefore, serifs are best suited for long blocks of text. Serif fonts are more difficult to read in small scale (smaller than 8 pt) and in very large sizes. It is often said that serifs are not suitable for screen display. If the serifs are not too thin, they can be used for presentations without problems, as modern monitors have a higher resolution than the monitors used a few years ago.

Sans serif fonts don't have the little feet on each character. The appearance of the letters is reduced to the essential figures. An example of a sans serif font is Arial. Readability is not as good as with serif fonts, as the text has to be read letter by letter. It is recommended that you use sans serif faces for small (smaller than 8 pt) and very large sizes. Sans serif fonts are more informal and work better in smaller pieces of text. Serif fonts look more formal.

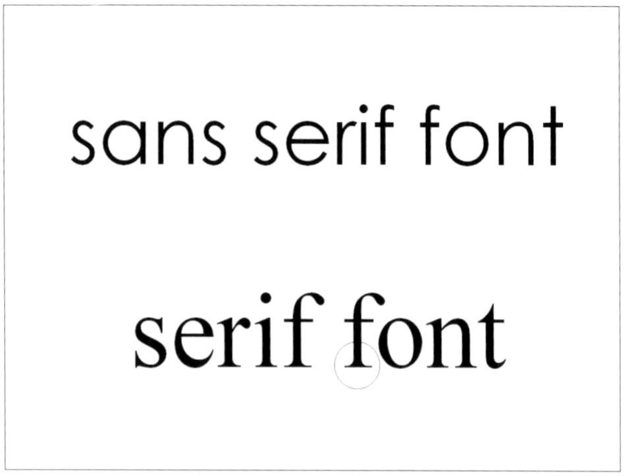

sans serif font

serif font

Fig. 18.08   Serifs are the small "legs" at the end of the characters.

Selection of a font

Selection of a suitable font for a presentation depends on many considerations. Is it a formal presentation or an informal one? Formal presentations need formal fonts. Children, for example, like fancier fonts more.

Content fonts

Fonts for the body text should be easy to read and clear, independent of their size. Simple sans serif and serif fonts fall into this category. A good choice are fonts out of the Bookman family, Garamond or Century Schoolbook. These fonts are easy to read and not as over-used as Times New Roman (Fig. 18.9). It is advisable to find a small selection of content fonts and to stick with them, depending on the content to be com-

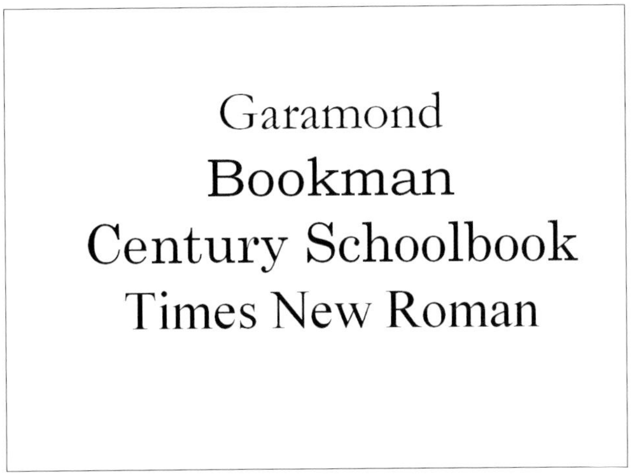

Garamond
Bookman
Century Schoolbook
Times New Roman

Fig. 18.09   Examples of easy-to-read fonts with serifs.

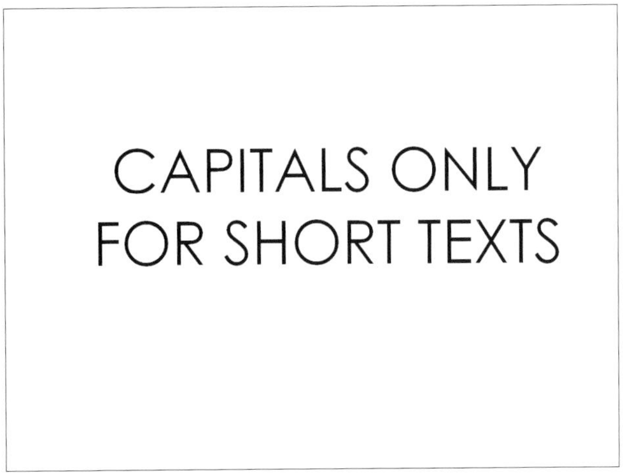

CAPITALS ONLY
FOR SHORT TEXTS

Fig. 18.10   Capitals should be used only for short texts.

municated. Do not use italic fonts and do not use text written only in capitals (Fig. 18.10). Use attributes (bold, italic, underline) only sparingly. Do not use condensed or narrow fonts. They are difficult to read under bad conditions. Care must be taken that font type and content of text suit each other.

Fonts for titles and labels

Title fonts can be a little bit less formal than content fonts. Often fonts like Arial are used. A nicer font is Tahoma. Comic sans is slightly over-used and appears overly informal (18.11).

Display fonts

Display fonts try to grab the audience's attention. Script fonts, block fonts and many others belong to this category. It should stand out from the other fonts selected, but match the content font for the body text. Display fonts should be used for short text elements only.

Font size

Selecting a font which is too small is one of the most common mistakes seen in presentations. Characters should always be big enough to be readable by the whole audience, even from the back of room. That means at least 28 points for body text and 48 points for titles (Fig. 18.12).

If you are not sure about the readability, make the following test ("floor test"). Print out the slide (one slide per page filling the format), put it on the floor and try

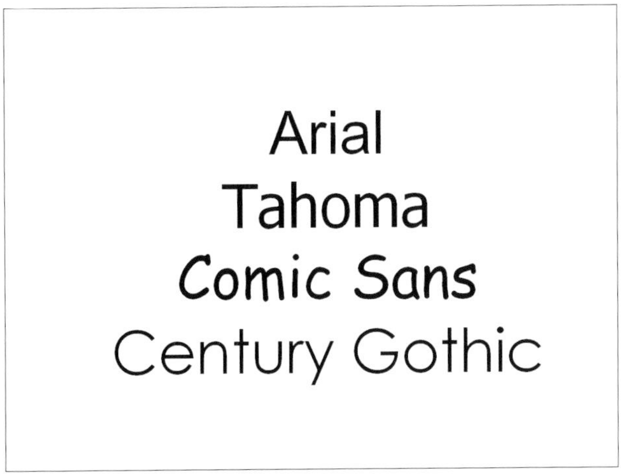

Arial
Tahoma
Comic Sans
Century Gothic

Fig. 18.11   Examples of good sans serifs fonts.

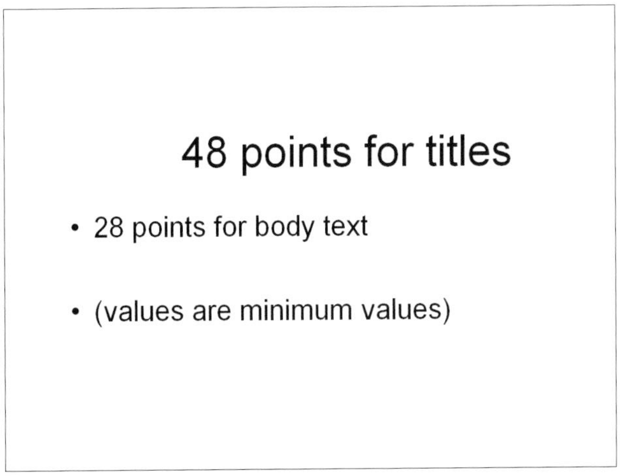

48 points for titles

• 28 points for body text

• (values are minimum values)

Fig. 18.12   Font size for titles and body text.

A good text slide should have

- not more than 25 characters per line
- not more than six words per line
- not more than 15 – 25 words
- not more than 6 – 7 lines
- no abbreviations or acronyms

Fig. 18.13   What a good text slide should have.

to read standing in an upright position. If you can, everybody in the audience will also be able to read the text. In other words: If the text on the original can still be read when viewed from a distance equal to six times the width of the original, the text on the slide will also be legible.

Arranging the text

Do not use the text slides as a teleprompter and do not read the text. The audience can read, too. Avoid more than 6 words a line and more than 6 or 7 lines per slide. Use no more than 15 to 25 words and no more than 25 characters (including spaces) per line. Avoid long sentences. Avoid abbreviations and acronyms (Fig. 18.13).

Do not arrange the text or other elements too close to the slide margins. Beamers frequently cut off the slides a little bit. All peripheral items are in danger of not making it onto the screen, if there is no safety margin.

Text can also be structured by varying the space between lines and by using indented text. The amount of text should be reduced by conscious use of meaningful concepts and phrases. If this is not sufficient, then the text should be divided into several slides.

Lists and longer text passages should be flush left; setting these flush right makes it more difficult to read text passages. Bibliographical data, however, can be set flush right. Centering is advantageous only for short bits of text or titles.

The point order is also important. The first point will get the most attention, followed by the last point. The points "in between" will receive less attention.

*Fig. 18.14
Red on blue should be avoided.*

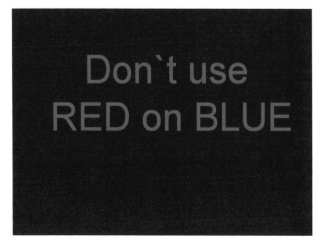

Colored text

Above all, the color of the type should contrast with that of the background, both in terms of the color itself and also for its brightness. It must also be kept in mind that different colors are focused at different planes. Thus, red type on a blue background is not good, especially when they are equally bright (Fig. 18.14). A large mixture of colors, especially against a black background, should be avoided, because the viewer is quickly tired by having to focus on the various colors (Fig. 18.15). Suitable colors for text are white, yellow and bright blue, for example.

Blue text should never be used on a black background, or—even worse—black text on a blue background, since the eye is not sensitive to blue, resulting in too little contrast (Fig. 18.16). The complementary

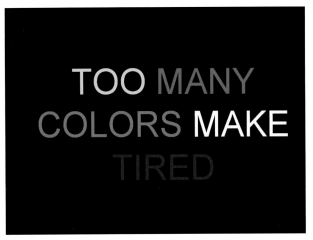

Fig. 18.15   *Too many different colors should be avoided.*

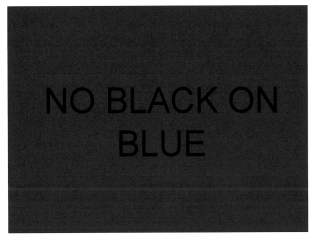

Fig. 18.16   *Black on blue should also be avoided.*

pairs of red-cyan and green-magenta should be avoided; on the other hand, the combination of blue-yellow is tolerable (Fig. 18.17).

The use of colored text can give some additional information to the audience by indicating relationships between information items. Some colors have common associations in our society. Red and green are used for "Stop" and "Go". But be aware that these associations may differ from country to country.

The same word written in different colors can convey different meanings. For example, the word hot written in red or orange colors appears completely different from hot written in blue (Fig. 18.18).

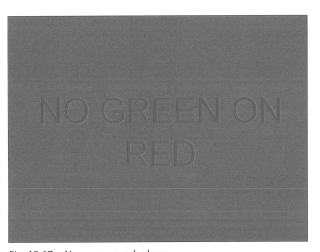

Fig. 18.17   *No green on red, please.*

18.2.4   Including graphics

Drawings should be simplified to the point that they can be perceived in the short time during which the slide is on the screen. Drawings should only be included if they are high quality. Beware of gimmicks like primitive cliparts, poorly animated gifs etc., as they only obscure your message. Cliparts are very often overworked and have lost their value.

To add shapes to the slides, simple drawing tools are offered by PowerPoint®. The drawing toolbar is located on the left-hand side at the bottom of the window (Normal View). The shape icon is clicked and the mouse cursor is moved to where the drawing is to be placed.

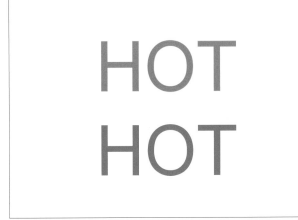

Fig. 18.18   *Different colors convey different messages.*

Then the mouse is dragged with the left mouse button held down. In addition, several AutoShapes are available.

18.2.5 Including charts

There is a vast variety of different charts available. In this context, only some general recommendations are given (Fig. 18.19).

Despite the fact that modern chart programs allow us to quickly produce a wide range of diagrams, we should keep in mind that they should be as simple and uniform as possible. Anyone looking at charts must first learn to perceive even the simplest graphic. If the content of a lecture is presented using many types of graphics, the viewer is compelled to exert an effort to comprehend each new one that is introduced.

The x-axis (lower, horizontal axis) is the base of many graphics, for example, elapsed time can be represented, in accordance with the Central European convention of reading from left to right. Values are generally placed on the y-axis (vertical

Fig. 18.19   Adding charts into PowerPoint® is rather simple.

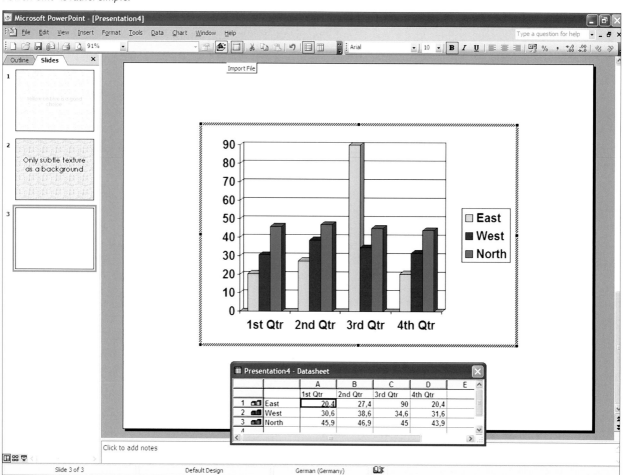

axis). These include not only the title of the axis (for example, units of measurement) but the corresponding scale with a minimum and maximum. The x-axis usually represents the value of 0. With percentage, the maximum is 100. The scale should be kept uniform to allow graphics to be compared. Gridmarks can improve the legibility of diagrams, especially if values are close together.

As in the case with a text chart, the title should be short and pithy; subtitles can underpin the message.

Values such as percentages, years, etc. should be written directly on the diagram if possible. Keys to parts are difficult to read and cause the viewers eye to flick back and forth between the list and the point in the graphic.

It is tempting to let colors get out of hand in a graphic, but these should be confined to a few easily distinguished ones. Shading and patterns can be used effectively in graphics in black and white.

Many types of graphics can be presented so that they appear three dimensional, such as a circle cut up into a pie chart. In principle, three dimensional presentation is more optically pleasing, but more difficult to read. In case of doubt, they should be left out.

18.2.6   Including photographic images

Photographs are very important for slide presentations in dentistry. They can be part of the slide content or can be the only content. To insert a picture, it must be saved in a graphic format PowerPoint® understands. Such formats include GIF, TIFF and JPEG.

Requirements

Photographic images are produced for different reasons. Their later use imposes various requirements on the images. Since the ultimate use of an image is not always known at the time it is created, it is generally advisable to take the images so that they can be viewed under difficult conditions.

Documentary images should be made under reproducible conditions. Images for print can be made with more content than images for lectures, since the reader has better conditions under which to take in these images than a person looking at slides at a lecture. In the latter case, the length of time the slide is on the screen determines the time in which she or he can comprehend the content. With book illustrations, the reader alone determines how long he or she wishes to examine an image. The viewer of a presentation does not have the ability to turn back the page, nor can she or he get closer to the image to see the details more closely as in looking at a book illustration. Real images are frequently used to implant the information in the listener's memory, in keeping with the motto: "Memory cannot be forced, but it can be cajoled".

Requirements for a real image used in a lecture are thus:
- High technical quality.
- Fill the frame; if possible, uniform horizontal format.
- Reduced content.
- Optimum perceptibility.

Content can be reduced by:
- Using the whole format ("Get close to the subject!").
- Selective depth of field.
- Selective illumination.
- Isolating the subject.
- Dividing complex content into several slides.

Aside from its technical details, the perceptibility of an image is influenced by:
- Correct orientation.
- Angle from which photo is taken permits three-dimensional perception of image content.

Fig. 18.20   Menu structure for inserting pictures.

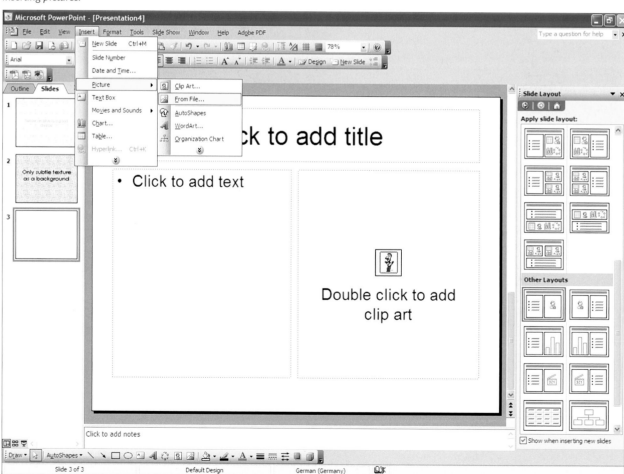

- Geared toward observer's experience (observer not overwhelmed; has been introduced to the subject).
- Sufficient contrast with background.
- Correct illumination, main light from above.
- Correct arrangement of center points of perception; with text slides, observing the direction the way in which the observer would read..

Adding images

To speed up the production of a PowerPoint® presentation, adding an image should be as fast as possible.

1. The normal procedure is (Fig. 18.20):
- In the desired slide, from the INSERT menu, select Picture → From File...
  The Insert Picture dialog box appears.
- Using the Look in pull-down list, locate and select the image to be added.
- Click INSERT.
  The image appears in your slide and the Picture toolbar appears.

Fig. 18.21   Images can be imported using the drag and drop function.

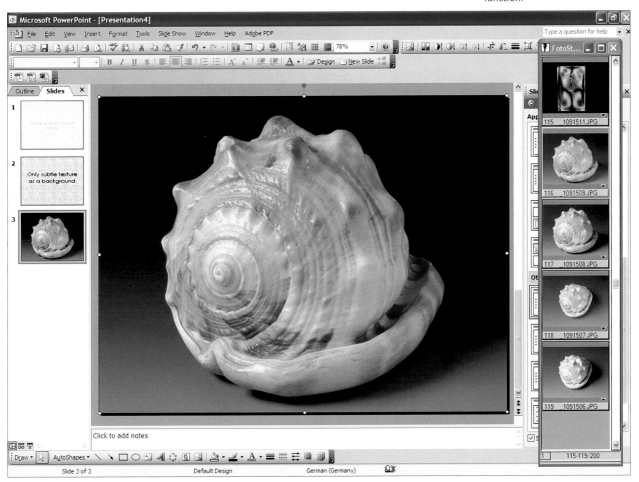

2. Drag and drop

Another very fast way to add images is to use the drag and drop function of archiving/browsing programs. PowerPoint® and the image browser (e.g., Fotostation®) are open. The screen window of Fotostation can be reduced to a small band, where pictures are arranged vertically as thumbnails. The desired PowerPoint® slide is selected. By selecting the Fotostation® thumbnail and dragging it into the PowerPoint® slide, it is added to the slide in a second (Fig. 18.21).

3. Clipboard

To paste an object from another application, go to the host application and copy the object to the Clipboard (Ctrl + C). Then go to the slide in PowerPoint® where you want the object pasted and select the EDIT menu>PASTE (Ctrl. + V). The object will now be pasted onto the slide, if the file volume is not too big.

Sometimes it is necessary to update the object automatically in PowerPoint® whenever changes are made to the object in the original application. In this case, choose the Edit menu>PASTE SPECIAL and click on the PASTE LINK option. This forms a link between the object in PowerPoint® and the object in the original application. Be aware of the fact that these objects are not embedded, but linked only. Storing the presentation does not store the linked object. This has to be done individually, e.g., when taking the presentation away on a CD.

Resolution

Quality of digital photographic images depends very much on their resolution. Making high quality images with modern DSLR cameras is not a problem. The problem is that high quality images increase the file size of PowerPoint® presentations dramatically. This may have an influence on the performance of the presentation. Which resolution is necessary? The limiting factor in image quality projected by a beamer is the resolution of the monitor (96 dpi at best) and of the beamer itself. Most projectors have a resolution of only 1024 x 768 pixels. Only a few beamers offer higher resolutions. Therefore, it does not make sense to include 18 MB images in the PowerPoint® presentation. The quality will not be better than with a 1024 x 768 pixel image.

It is recommended to downsize the image before including it in the presentation. If the image fills the whole frame, a size of 1024 x 768 pixels is appropriate. If it fills only half of the image, a size of 512 x 384 is enough. Downsizing an image can be done using image editing software. Some programs offer prefabricated actions to downsize an image by a mouse click. Reducing the image size can be performed by archiving or browsing programs as well, for example, by FotoStation® Pro.

Removing the extra resolution data makes your file smaller and more manageable without compromising the quality of the image.

Compressing a picture

In addition to the possibility of downsizing a picture before adding it to the Power-Point® presentation, there is another way: first add the picture and then compress it.

The following steps are necessary:
- Select the image in your presentation that you want to compress.
- In the Picture toolbar (View menu > Toolbars > Picture), select the "Compress button" (Fig. 18.22). The "Compress Pictures window" will appear.
- In the Apply to section, choose whether to apply the compression to all the pictures in the presentation or just the selected one.
- In the Change resolution section, select the Web/Screen option if you will primarily be displaying your presentation on a screen or on the web. This will change the resolution of your image to 96 dpi.
- In the Options section, check the Compress pictures box. If you have cropped the image using the Crop tool in the Picture toolbar, you can also select the option to delete any information that has been cropped from your picture by checking the appropriate box (Fig. 18.23).

Fig. 18.22
Compress button is selected.

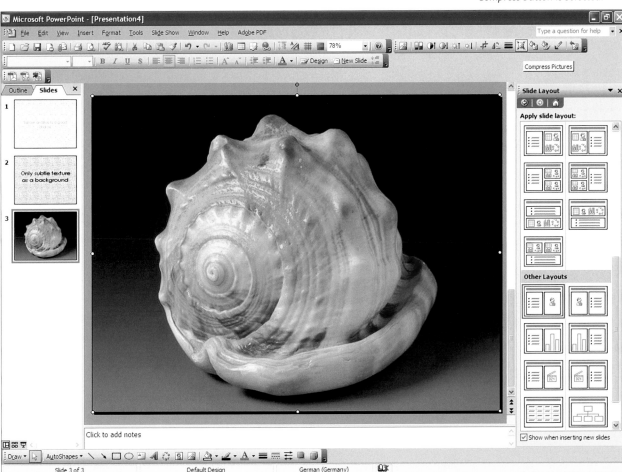

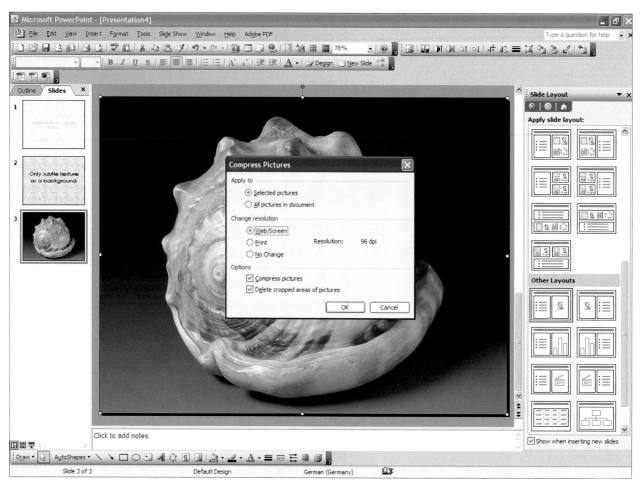

Fig. 18.23   *Compression can be applied to one single or to all pictures.*

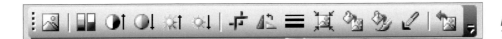

Fig. 18.24
Toolbar for image editing.

Editing images

When the photograph is added to the PowerPoint® slide, the Picture toolbar appears (Fig. 18.24). Numerous buttons offer different options for formatting the image.

Button	Action
Insert Picture	Opens the Insert Picture dialog box so you can insert a saved image
Color	*Image Control* options include the following: **Automatic, Grayscale, Black & White,** and **Washout**
More Contrast	Increases image contrast
Less Contrast	Decreases image contrast
More Brightness	Brightens image colors
Less Brightness	Dims image colors
Crop	Cuts or crops unnecessary elements
Rotate Left 90°	Rotates the image 90° to the left
Line Style	Creates an image border
Compress Pictures	Compresses your pictures to reduce file size **NOTE:** If pictures are compressed, image quality may be diminished.
Recolor Picture	Opens the *Recolor Picture* dialog box so you can change image colors
Format Picture/AutoShape	Opens the Format Picture or Format AutoShape dialog box so you can edit and format your image
Set Transparent Color	Changes the image background color to the background color of the document
Reset Picture	Resets the image back to its original size

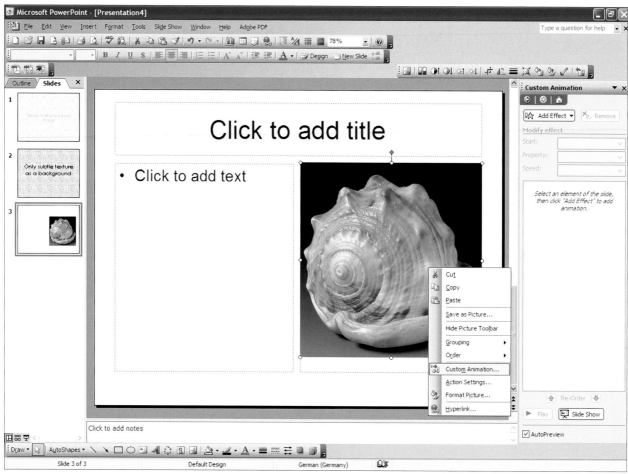

Fig. 18.25   Shortcut menu to
add an animation.

18.3   Animating objects

Text and objects can be animated. For example, you can have your text fly in from the left, one word at a time, or hear the sound of applause when a picture is uncovered.

An animation makes it possible to control the flow of information, and it may help to focus interest on important points. However, every animation that is added to the presentation contributes to an overall restless impression of the whole show, and it may distract the audience from the main points you are making.

Therefore, animations should be used sparingly, and only in cases where the animation adds information itself, e.g., showing a progression of events. If you need ten or more mouseclicks to bring the whole content on the screen, the audience is forced to be in sync with you and it forces you to concentrate on the mouseclicks more than on getting your point across.

Avoid sounds if possible. Include sounds only in specific context, where sound is required.

Custom animations can be applied to items or placeholders of a single slide, the master slide, or a group of slides.

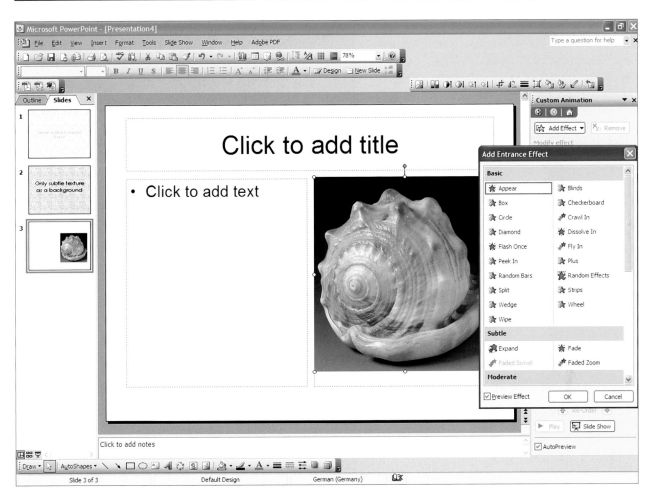

Click to add title

• Click to add text

Fig. 18.26   Different entrance effects are displayed.

An animation can be added by the following steps:

- Right click on the object (image, clipart, text etc.) you want to animate.
- From the shortcut menu click CUSTOM ANIMATION (Fig. 18.25). The task pane will appear at the right.
- Click on the ADD EFFECT down arrow. A drop-down menu appears.
- Click on an effect from the list (Fig. 18.26).
- Click PLAY to preview.

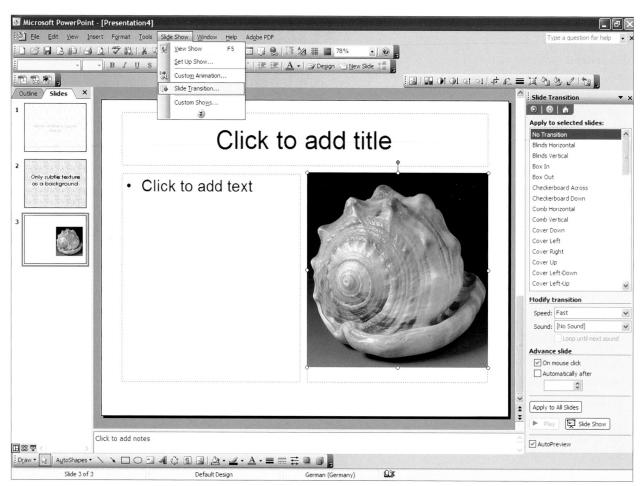

Fig. 18.27
Transition options are displayed.

18.4   Slide transitions

The way in which slides change from one to the next can be defined by the Slide Transitions. Including transition effects helps break the monotony of changing slides, but carries the risk of making the audience nervous, as there are more than 50 possibilities.

The following steps are necessary:
- Move to the slide to which you want to apply the transition (slide sorter view recommended).
- Select SLIDE SHOW and SLIDE TRANSITION. The Slide Transition task pane appears (Fig. 18.27).
- Click the slide transition you want.
- Adjust the transition speed if necessary.

If you want the slide to advance automatically, the "Automatically after" check box is marked and the number of seconds is set. Choosing the Apply to All Slides option applies the selected transition to all slides.

The same recommendations are given for slide transitions as for the other animations: do not use too many different transitions. Use a calm transition, e.g., "fade smoothly" or "fade through black". It is good practice to arrange the items of your slides in a way that only parts of the slide change during transition from one slide to the other. For instance, the title and image remain the same while the text changes. This technique lets the presentation flow, unlike conventional slide presentations of the past.

18.5   Videos and sounds

Inserting movies can add valuable information to the presentation. But it also can add some trouble during the presentation. Moreover, adding a movie changes the pace of a presentation and gives the audience the opportunity to relax a little bit while the concentration level drops. It is important to save the movie files with the Power-Point® presentation or else it will not work. It is recommended that a folder be created to save the presentation and media clips together.

With the use of Media Player you can insert a movie object on the slide. The computer must have these applications installed to use the multimedia capabilities of PowerPoint®. It is absolutely necessary to test the presentation on the computer to be used to make sure the necessary applications are installed on the computer. Some media formats are not fully compatible on Macintosh computers in PowerPoint®. More and more congress organizations do not allow lecturers to use their own notebook. A network server is used instead. Especially in this case, a test is absolutely necessary.

To insert a movie following steps are necessary:
- Select the Insert menu > Movies and Sounds menu > Movie from File. The movie dialog box will appear (Fig. 18.28). Navigate to the folder containing the movie file.
- Select the movie file and click Open.
- The initial frame of the movie appears in the center of the slide. A dialog box will ask if you would like the movie to play immediately, when you navigate to the slide or when you click on it. Select the option that works best for your presentation.
- To see the movie play during a slide show, click the Slide Show button.
- Click anywhere on the movie frame to play the movie if you set it to "play when clicked".

PowerPoint® 2003 enables playing movies in full screen format while the slide show is in progress.

To view a movie clip full screen:
- Right-click on the movie after you have inserted it into PowerPoint®.
- Select Edit Movie Object on the shortcut menu.
- Check Zoom to Full Screen.

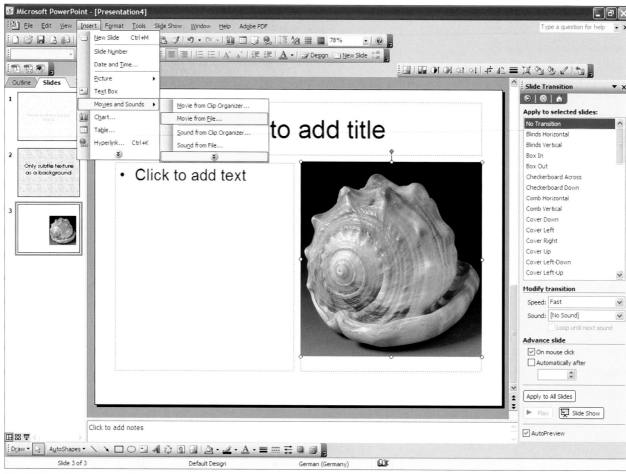

Fig. 18.28   Menu structure to
insert a movie.

The same remarks made above for movies are true for sound clips. Only add a sound
clip if it conveys additional information to the presentation. This is not often the case.

To insert a sound clip following steps are necessary:

- Select the Insert menu > Movies and Sounds > Sound from File. The sound dialog box will appear. Navigate to the folder containing the sound file to be used.
- Select the sound file and click Open. The sound clip icon will appear in the middle of the slide. A dialog box will ask you if you would like the sound to play
  immediately when you navigate to the slide or when you click it. Select the option that works best for your presentation.
- To hear the sound clip play during the slide show, click the Slide Show button.
- Click on the sound clip icon to hear the clip play if you set it to "play when
  clicked".

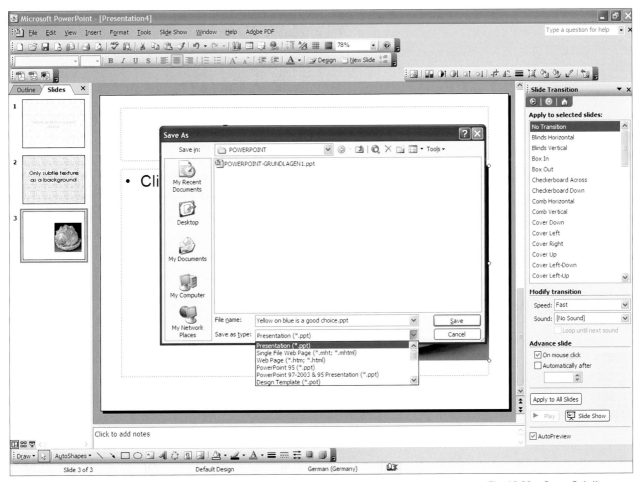

Fig. 18.29   PowerPoint® presentations can be saved using different options.

18.6   Storing the presentation

Storing the presentation can be done according the usual options. Selecting the File menu > Save will save the current presentation. To save a presentation under a different name or in a different folder, select the File menu > Save As... from the menu as usual (Fig. 18.29). There is also an option to save the presentation in different formats, such as Windows Metafile, JPEG, etc. The html-option makes it possible to put the presentation on the Internet.

Not all features are available after transforming to the webpage.

Converting PowerPoint® presentations into a PDF File
Sometimes it is necessary to convert PPT files into PDF files. This cannot be done directly from PowerPoint®. If you have the full version of Adobe Acrobat (not only the reader) there are some icons for PDF conversion on top of the PowerPoint® window (Fig. 18.30). Special tools and programs allow a conversion as well, e.g., Prep4PDF, FlashPaper® (Macromedia). Not all conversion programs preserve all interactive features. Therefore, before buying such a converter, try the functionality with a try-out version of the program.

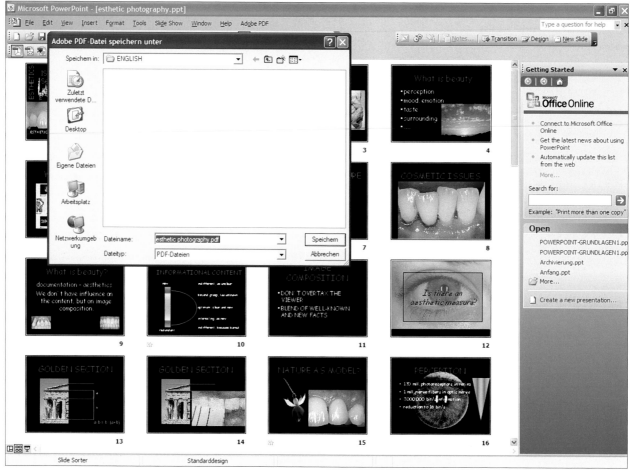

Fig. 18.30   A PPT presentation can be saved as a PDF file.

Package for CD

A powerful feature in the 2003 version of PowerPoint® is "Package for CD". Guided by a menu, all files necessary to play the presentation on another computer without PowerPoint® are collected. The feature can be found under FILE > Package for CD.

A dialog appears with different options. First the CD is given a name. Package for CD reads the presentation, identifies all links, locates the linked files, and ensures that the link addresses are pathless.

Normally you don't have to specify any files that need to be included on the CD.

In case you want to add some material to the CD (e.g., research papers, background information) you have to click ADD FILES and select the files in the following dialog. By clicking OPTIONS, you can check whether all necessary files are included. By default, the PowerPoint® Viewer and all linked files will be included. True type fonts are embedded if you want and if there are no copyright restrictions. Passwords can secure the presentation. Finally, two buttons can be clicked to write the CD: Copy to CD (Windows XP) or Copy to Folder (Windows 2000).

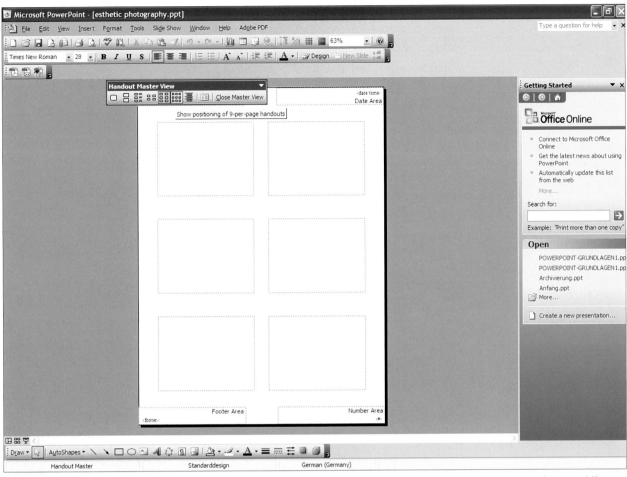

Fig. 18.31   There are different handout styles.

18.7   Printing handouts

PowerPoint® offer four options for printing:

- Outline
- Audience handout
- Notes page
- Slides

If you want to give the audience a handout for making comments on each slide, use the option "handout". PowerPoint® places three slides on the left side of the page, leaving writing room to the right of each slide. All printing is started from the Print dialog box, which is displayed when you choose the File menu > Print. You can select the slides to be printed or print all slides. A handout can have 1, 2, 3, 4, 6, or 9 slides. You can print in color, gray tones, or black and white.

Handouts can be formatted by adding headers, the date, page number, etc. To format the handout, select the View menu > Master > Handout Master (Fig. 18.31). Then choose the icon representing the number of slides you want to be displayed on each handout page. Choose View > Header and Footer command to add text that you want to be printed on each page. You can also add background graphics. When you are satisfied, click Close on the Master Toolbar.

Headers or footers added on the Handout Master are not displayed. They only appear on the printed handout page.

Conversion to PDF Handouts

To convert the PowerPoint® handouts into the popular pdf format, the following steps are necessary:

- Select File > Print Preview.
- Select Print What > handouts from the pull-down menu.
- Close print preview.
- Using the Adobe buttons at the top of the PowerPoint® screen click on "Convert to Adobe PDF.

Alternatively, Adobe PDF can be selected as a printer: File > Print >… (older computers may use the "Adobe Distiller" function).

18.8   Helpful tricks and special effects

There are thousands of possibilities which can be used with Microsoft PowerPoint®. Many of them can be found in the literature and in the Internet. Some of them are compiled here.

18.8.1   Link different parts of the presentation

Linking different parts of a presentation increases the flexibility. This is an elegant technique used for longer presentations. An example: the topic of a presentation is the diagnostic procedures for oral lesions. You are talking about clinical inspection, palpation, biopsy, brush biopsy, photography etc. The brush biopsy slide contains an element which can be used as a trigger to start another PowerPoint® file, dealing with more details about brush biopsy. If you see during your seminar that you have enough time, or if there are some questions referring to the brush biopsy, you move the mouse on the trigger element and by clicking start the secondary PowerPoint® file, deviating from your main topic. Nobody will be aware that this deviation is only an option, as the last slide will automatically lead back to the main lecture (Fig. 18.32).

The same technique can be used to prepare some slides for expected questions. Clicking on certain items of your slides let you jump to the answer of the question – very impressive for the audience. There are many implementations for this linking tool, but if the structure of a presentation becomes too complex, there is also the risk of getting lost in one's own presentation.

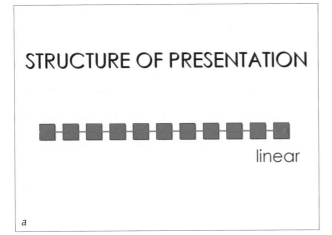

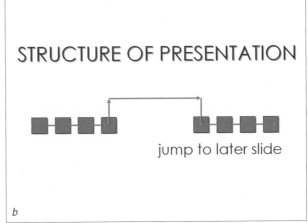

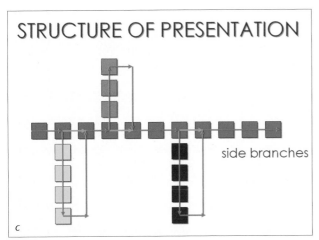

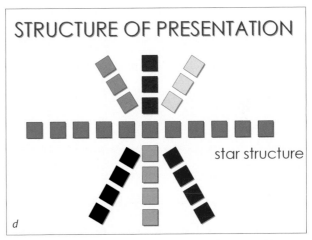

Fig. 18.32   Linking together different parts of a presentation offers very useful options. Normally the presentation is a linear one (a). Jumping from one slide to a later slide can save time (b), side branches of a presentation can be an option to go more into detail, if necessary (c). Detouring from one slide to different directions (d) is possible if the presentation has a star structure.

It is very easy to add a trigger function to an object:

- Select the object.
- Rightclick the object.
- Select "Action settings" in the pop up menu (Fig. 18.33).
- Check "Hyperlink to" – box.
- Select "Other PowerPoint® presentations", if you want to start a second presentation (Fig. 18.34).
- Select other options according to the situation.

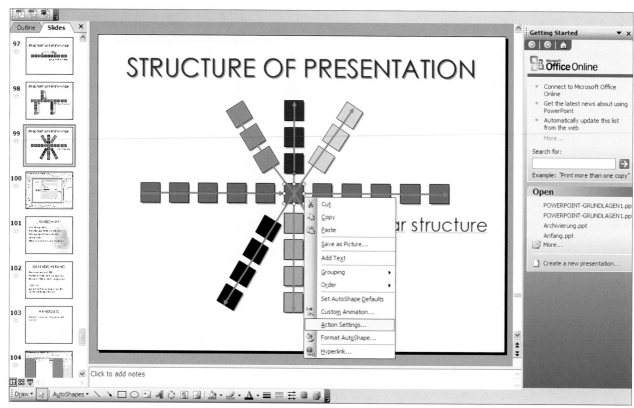

Fig. 18.33   *An action can be added to a selected object using the pop-up menu after right-clicking the object.*

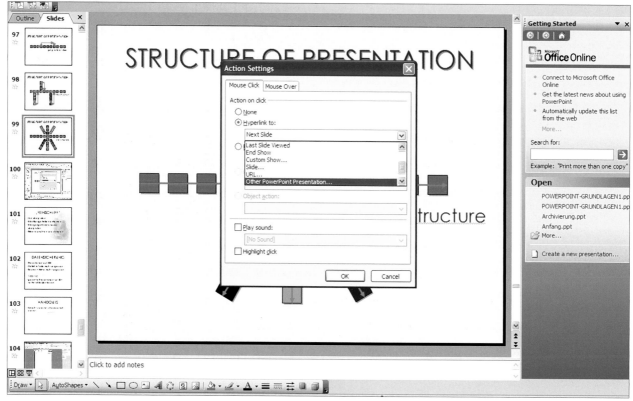

Fig. 18.34   *Linking to another PowerPoint® presentation.*

18.8.2 Write on your slides

Sometimes it can be necessary to write down text or emphasize some details of the slides. For this, the new pen feature can be used when presenting in Slide Show View. Different pens in different colors and a highlighter are offered. The menu is located at the bottom left. In addition the ink can be removed using an eraser tool (Fig. 18.35).

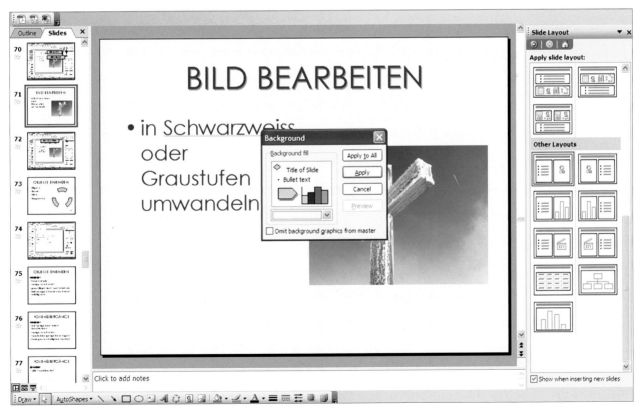

18.8.3 Change the background color of a single slide

If color schemes or slide masters are used, all slides have the same background. To emphasize a message it can be necessary to change the background color of a single slide. Select Format > Background. In the pop up menu a background can be chosen. By checking the "omit background items" box, you ignore the Slide Master design (Fig. 18.36). These changes can be applied to a single slide or many slides selected in the Slide Sorter View. One problem has to be taken into account: If you place a photographic background on many of your slides instead of doing it once on the Master, the file size may increase dramatically. Newer versions allow different master slides.

Fig. 18.35 A presentation may become more vivid, if the pencil tool is used.

Fig. 18.36 Single slides can be given backgrounds differing from the Master Slide background.

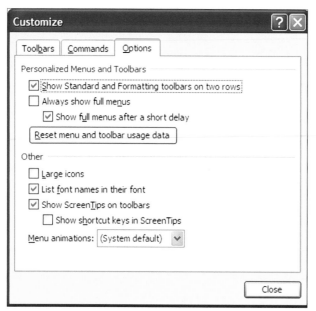

*Fig. 18.37   The check box
"Show shortcut keys in screen
tips" has to be marked.*

18.8.4 Displaying keyboard shortcuts in Tool Tips

To speed up the work, the use of keyboard shortcuts is recommended. In order to become familiar with these shortcuts, you can make them appear on the screen. Go to Tools>Customize, click on the Options tab, and click on "Show shortcut keys in screen tips" (Fig. 18.37). Every time you select a tool, its shortcut is displayed when moving the mouse over it.

Some of the most important short keys are listed below:

- Ctrl + A   Select All   all objects on a slide are selected.
- Ctrl + D   Duplicate   duplicates the selected objects.
- Ctrl + C   Copy   copies the selected object to the Clipboard.
- Ctrl + V   Paste   pastes the contents of the Clipboard to the current slide.
- Ctrl + X   Cut   removes the selected object and places it on the clipboard.
- Ctrl + Z   Undo   this will "undo" the last operation.
- Delete   deletes the selected object(s). If no objects are selected it will delete the current slide.
- F4   repeats the last action.

A complete list of keyboard shortcuts can be found under:
www.bitbetter.com/poerkeys.htm

18.8.5   Copying objects

Very often it is necessary to copy an object of a slide. There are two quick ways to do this.
a. Select an object>press Ctrl. and "drag it off" using the mouse.
b. Select an object>and duplicate it by Ctrl. + D.

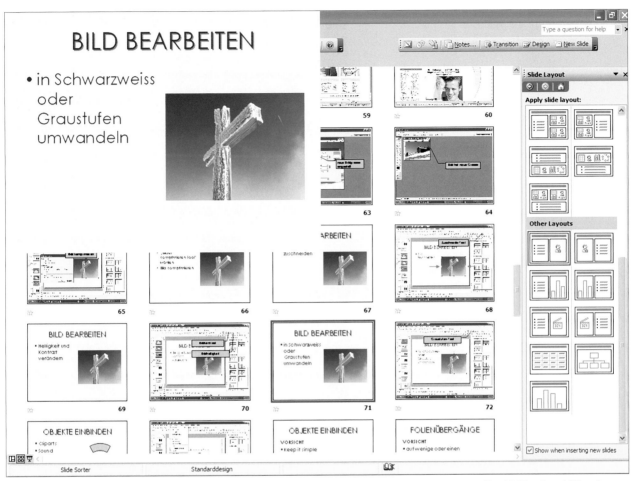

Fig. 18.38   An additional preview window can be useful when editing a slide show.

18.8.6   Preview slide show effects

While editing a presentation, press the Ctrl. key while clicking the Slide Show View button. A small preview window opens showing that slide in Slide Show mode (Fig. 18.38).

18.8.7   Changing from caps to lower case

If there is text in the wrong case, select this text and then press Shift + F3 repeatedly. By this you can switch between ALL CAPS, lower case, and Initial Capital style (ABCDE, abcde, Abcde).

18.8.8 Moving objects

Moving objects with the mouse is sometimes very difficult (especially for notebook users with a touchscreen). You can move the object with the arrow keys. Select the object, and every time you press an arrow key, it will move the object one "grid unit" (1/12th of an inch). If the grid is turned off, or if you hold down the ALT key, the objects are moved one pixel at a time.

18.8.9 Selecting small or hidden objects

Selecting small objects or objects hidden by larger ones is often difficult. Press the ESCAPE key to deselect the current selected object. Then repeatedly press the TAB key until the object you want is selected.

18.8.10 Enlarge slides within the slide sorter view

Sometimes there are slides which cannot be distinguished very well in the sorter view. They can be enlarged by pressing Ctrl. and scrolling the mouse wheel simultaneously.

18.8.11 Locating and storing templates

Design templates can be purchased or downloaded, or they can be created individually and stored in a folder. To find out where this folder is, you can procede as follows:

- Open PowerPoint® and go to View>Master>Slide Master.
- Select File>Save As and click on "Design Template .PPT" in the "Save as file type" box (Fig. 18.39). The "Save In" box will show the folder where PPT plans to save the file. When clicking the arrow on the side of this box, a drop down menu will show the full path to the folder where your templates are expected to be.
- Exit PowerPoint® and place new templates in the correct folder, or create a new folder at the same level and save them there. I like that method because I can have a folder called "\My Templates", for example.
- Open PowerPoint® and go to Format>Slide Design and you will see all of the available templates in the Task Pane.

Design Templates embedded in PowerPoint® when just purchased and installed will be stored in the following locations:

C:\Programs\Microsoft Office\Templates\Presentation Designs

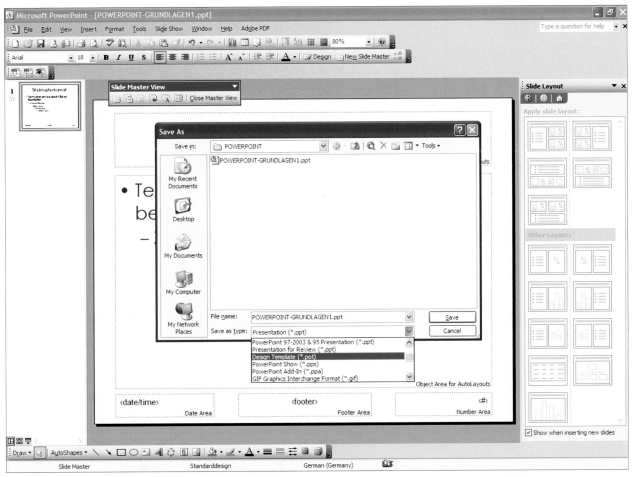

Fig. 18.39
Here templates are stored.

The paths on your system may vary, depending on where you have installed Power-
Point®. On the same level, a new folder named "My templates" can be placed beside the "Presentation design folder" to store the individually created new templates.

18.8.12 Guides

Guides are very useful for checking the layout and aligning objects. After selecting
VIEW>Guides, there is only one vertical and one horizontal guide visible (Fig. 18.40).
These guides can be cloned: hold down the Ctrl key, select a guide and clone the
guide by dragging the new guide (left mouse button pressed down) into the new
position.

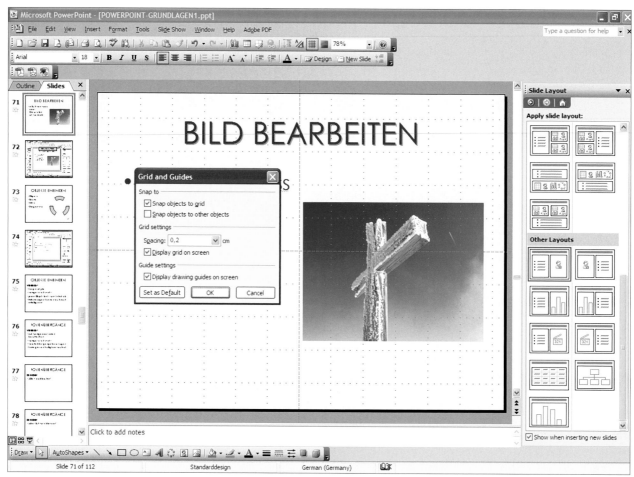

Fig. 18.40   Grid and guides help arrange the objects.

18.8.13 Repeat the last action – use F4

F4 is a handy key which repeats the last action. If multiple text elements have to be treated in the same way, use F4. If an object has to be duplicated several times, duplicate it and then use F4.

18.8.14 Select multiple objects

If you want to select multiple objects in one stroke, draw a box with the mouse around them: press the left mouse button, keep it pressed and drag to create a rectangle around the objects. After the mouse button is released, all objects are selected and can be treated (moved, deleted etc.) as a group.

18.8.15 Format painter for objects

The format painter is a handy tool to transfer format settings from one object to the other. Select the source object, click on the format painter in the toolbar, and click on the destination objects. The whole formatting (color of objects, fonts used for text) can be transferred easily by this small tool.

18.8.16 Beamer resolution

Check if beamer resolution is the same as laptop resolution. If not, images may be cropped.

18.8.17 Switch off standby Power Management

Check the Power Management of your laptop: Control Panel>Power. If you are inactive for a while during the presentation (e.g., answering questions, discussing a detail) the Power Management tool may switch off your computer. Sometimes waking up your computer takes a while, or it may be necessary to reboot the PC.

18.8.18 Remove the screen saver

You are running into trouble if the screen saver turns on during inactive parts of your presentation. Turn it off or remove the screen saver.

18.8.19 Presentation on other computers

Don't think your presentation will work on another person's PC. There are a lot of possible mismatches: program versions, hard drive space, memory size, missing programs, missing drivers, screen savers not deselected etc. The only way to be sure it works is to try it. Do not try only two or three slides and assume that the rest will work as well, but try the whole presentation.

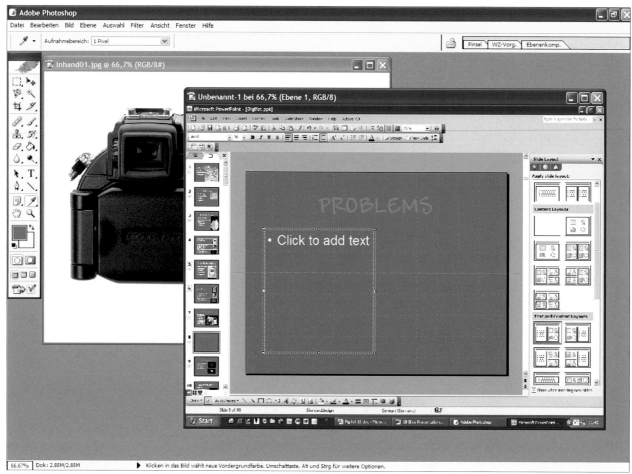

Fig. 18.41a   The foreground
color in Photoshop taken from a
PowerPoint® screenshot.

18.8.20 Import images with identical background color

Bitmap images are rectangular, even when objects show on a white background. When such an image is imported into PowerPoint® with a colored background, the disturbing white rectangle of the whole image appears on the screen. Recoloring the background of the image with the same color used as background in PowerPoint® will improve the result: the object appears without the white rectangle.

The problem is to match the background of the image with the background color in PowerPoint®. Open PowerPoint® showing an empty slide with the background color. Make a screenshot by pressing the PrtSc key. The content of the whole screen is copied into the clipboard.

Open Photoshop (or another image editing software) and generate a new empty image by FILE>New (or Ctrl. + N). The NEW dialogue opens. Normally "Clipboard" is preset; if it is not, you have to select "Clipboard" and press OK. An empty white image with the same dimensions as the screenshot opens. The content of the clipboard is copied into the new image by Ctrl. + V. Now you select the foreground color with the pipette.

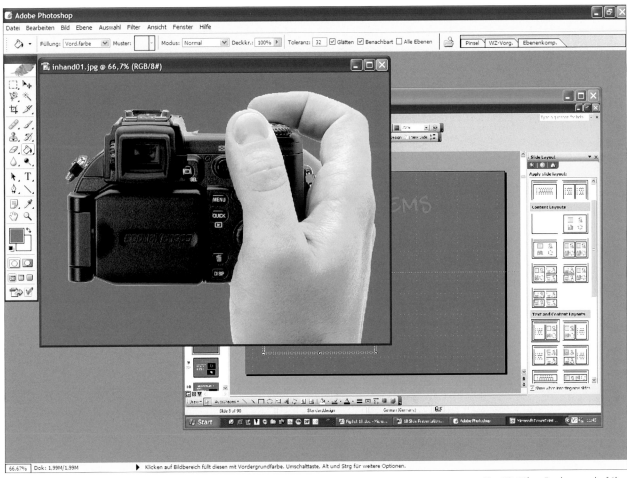

Fig. 18.41b Background of the image with same color as PowerPoint® background.

Move it just over the background of the PowerPoint® slide on the screenshot and click. The foreground color in Photoshop is now the same as the background color in PowerPoint® (Fig. 18.41a).

Open the image which has to be recolored and imported into PowerPoint®. Select the white background with the magic wand tool and fill the selected area with the new foreground color using the paint bucket tool (press G, move the cursor over the white selected background and click left). The background color of the image changes (Fig. 18.41b). Save the image and import it into PowerPoint®. Now the two background colors match perfectly. The object appears as if cut out along its contours (Fig. 18.41c).

If the background of the image to be imported is perfectly uniform the tool "Set Transparent Color" from the image tool box can be used as well.

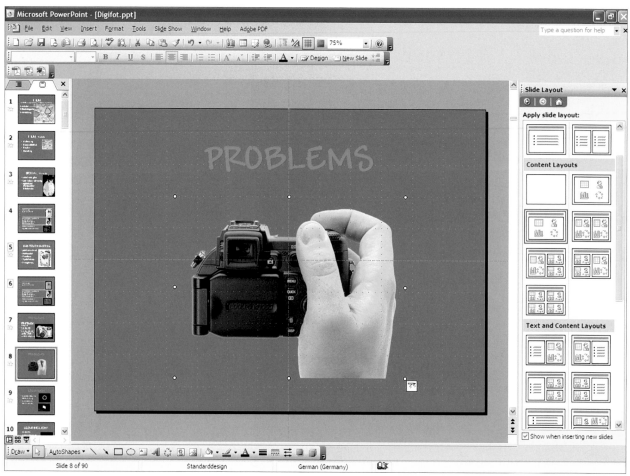

Fig. 18.41c   Result: Perfect
match of the two background
colors.

18.8.21 Using an alpha channel to import "cut out images"

The method described above works very well for uniform backgrounds, but for grad-ed backgrounds there is no perfect color match. A Photoshop® alpha channel will help. The image containing the object to be imported into PowerPoint® is opened (Fig. 18.42a). For an easy selection, it is recommended that an image with only one background color be used. But this is not absolutely necessary.

Open the Layers palette, doubleclick on the background layer and press OK. In this way, the background layer is converted into a normal layer (called layer 0) to which an alpha channel can be added. Select the background or the part of the im-age which should later appear transparent by using the Magic Wand Tool (press W). Then invert the selection by SELECT>Inverse (or Shift+Ctrl.+I) (Fig. 18.42b). Now the object is selected which will not appear transparent.

Open the Channels palette and click on the icon "Save selection as Channel". The new Alpha Channel (Alpha 1) appears on the palette (Fig. 18.42c). Areas to be trans-parent in the PowerPoint® slide appear black in the alpha channel, areas with no transparency appear as white. To be sure that the mask has a 100% opacity, open

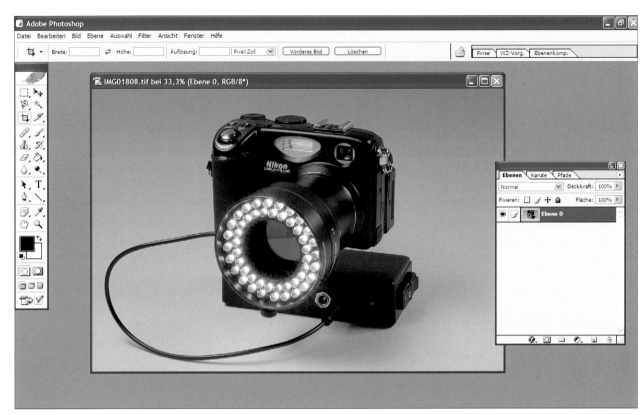

Fig. 18.42a   *Image containing the object is opened.*

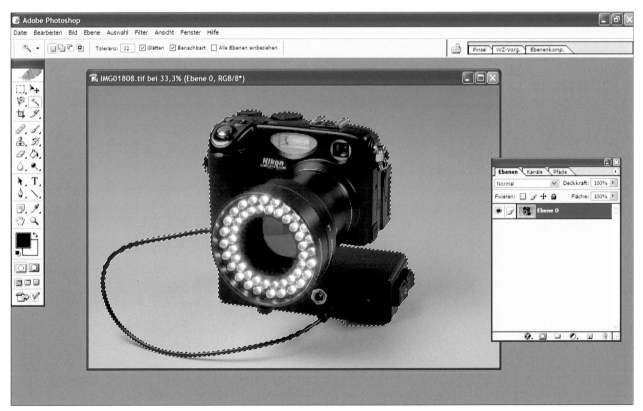

Fig. 18.42b   *Object is selected.*

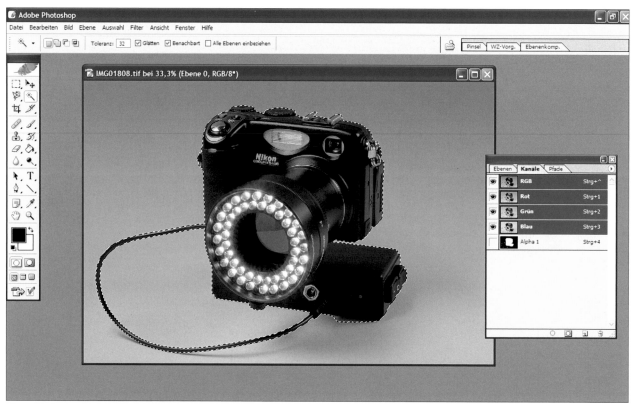

Fig. 18.42c   Channels palette is opened and selection is saved as a channel.

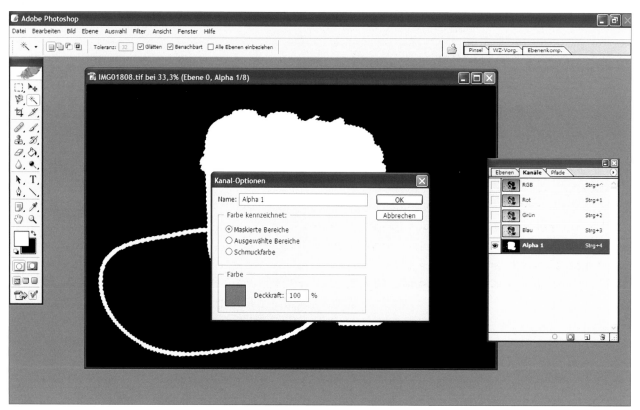

Fig. 18.42d   Opacity of masked areas is set to 100%.

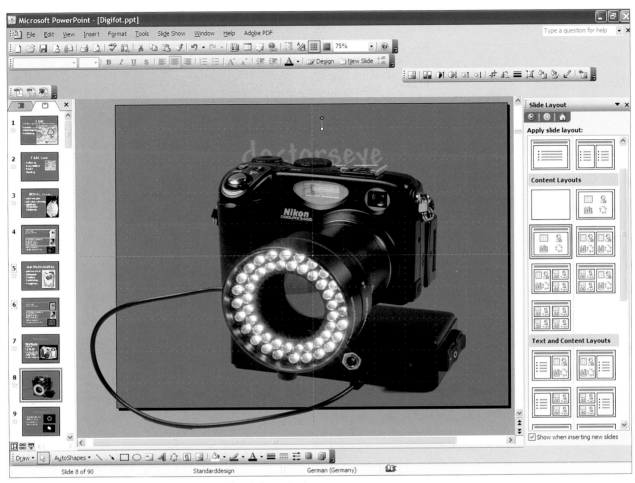

Fig. 18.42e   Image inserted into PowerPoint®. It has to be resized.

the Channel options by double-clicking into Alpha 1 channel of the channel palette. Then set "masked areas" to 100% opacity, press OK (Fig. 18.42d).

After this, save the image together with the new Alpha channel in Photoshop as a TIF file. Now this image can be imported into PowerPoint® with the object selected and the disturbing background transparent, which means it is not visible (Fig. 18.42e).

Finally, the image has to be resized (Fig. 18.42f).

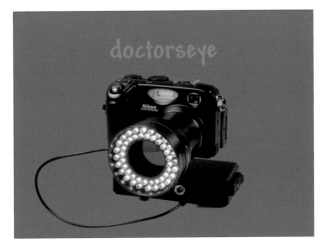

Fig. 18.42f   Result after resizing.

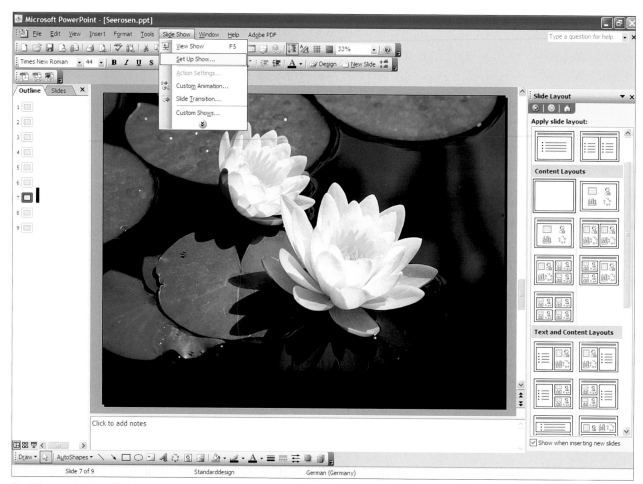

Fig. 18.43a   "Set up show" option is selected from the Slide Show menu.

18.8.21 Creating a self-repeating opener

Sometimes an opener can be used to fill the time before the main presentation starts. This attracts the attention of the audience to the screen while people are taking their seats. Such an opener is a short PowerPoint® presentation, which is linked to the main presentation.

The first step is to generate the opener presentation as a PPT file. Then select "Slide Show > Set up show (Fig. 18.43a) and select the option "Loop continuously until Esc" (Fig. 18.43b). Then the slide transition with an automatic function is selected and the transition time is adjusted (Fig. 18.43c).

Now this short opener is linked to the main presentation. In the main presentation, the first slide is opened. An object on this slide is selected and then—by clicking right —"Action Settings" is selected. Then a hyperlink is generated: hyperlink to > other PowerPoint® presentation. The hyperlink is linked to slide Number 1 of the opener presentation. After that the main presentation including the hyperlink is saved.

To begin the opener presentation, the main presentation is started and the linked object is clicked. Now the opener starts and repeats itself until it is finished by "Esc". When "Esc" is pressed the main presentation starts. Check that the cursor is not on

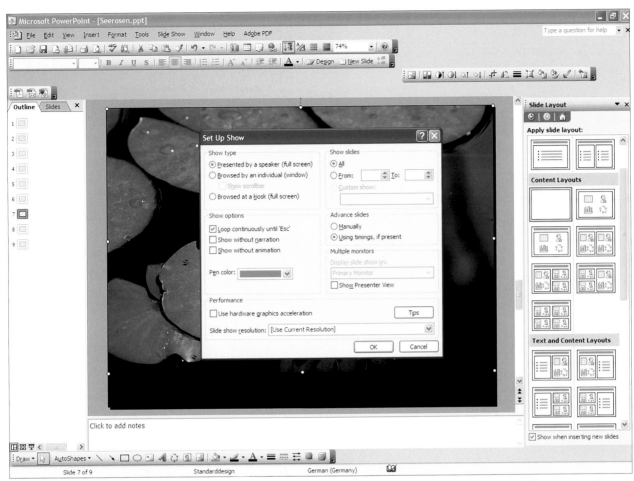

Fig. 18.43b   "Loop continuously until Esc" is checked.

the linked object. If it is, move it away, otherwise you start the opener again. Do not
press the Esc key twice. If you do, you will leave the presentation mode completely.
Be aware that only the main presentation file is opened, not the opener file as well.

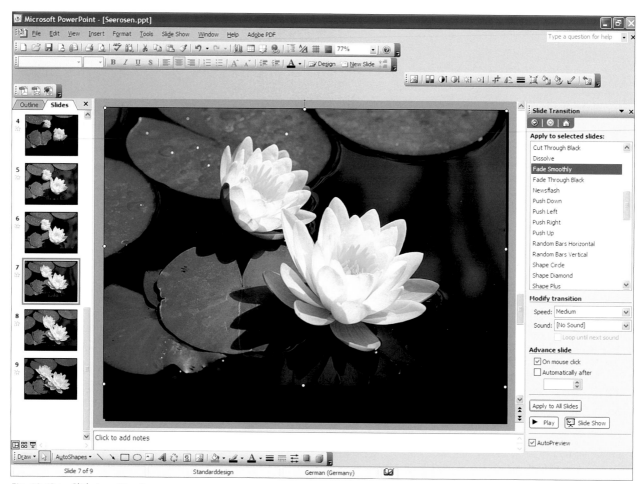

Fig. 18.43c   Slide transition is
selected. "Automatically after"
has to be checked.

Internet addresses

This list is not exhaustive, and the presence or absence of a company does not indicate any judgement.

Industry

www.canon.com
www.casio.com
www.epson.com
www.fujifilm.com
www.fotowand.com
www.jvc.com
www.kaiser-fototechnik.de/en/index.htm
www.kodak.com
www.leica-camera.com
www.minolta.com
www.nikonusa.com
www.olympus.com
www.ricoh-europe.com
www.sony.com
www.toshiba.com
www.yashica.com

Scanners

www.avision.com
www.epson.com
www.microtek.com
www.mustek.com
www.plustek.com
www.umax.com

Storage media

www.crucial.com
www.ibm.com
www.iomega.com
www.lexarmedia.com
www.sandisk.com
www.simpletech.com

Software

www.adobe.com
www.corel.com
www.download.com
www.gimp.org
www.grafik-software.de
www.lemkesoft.com
www.micrografx.com
www.microsoft.com
www.photoshopuser.com/
www.ulead.com

Companies

www.bitsinstyle.de
www.chriscamera.com/dental.htm
www.digident.com/camerachoices.htm
www.digitale-fototechnik.de
www.dinecorp.com
www.discdirekt.com
www.d-store.com/d-store/
    Digi-Slave/rf50.html
www.foto24.de
www.kodak.com/US/en/health/dental/
    products/digPho/digiPhoKit.jhtml
www.ny-camera.net
www.photomed.net
www.tiffen.com

Magazines/Communities/Information

www.digit.de
www.dpreview.com
www.fotoline.ch
www.megapixel.net/
www.pcphotoreview.com/
www.peimag.com
www.photolink.de
www.photoweb.de
www.robgalbraith.com/
www.shortcourses.com/
www.tambcd.edu/res/photo.html

Organizations

www.photosuisse.ch
www.psa-photo.org

Bibliography

Adams CP. Dental Photography. Bristol:
John Wright & Sons 1968.

Adobe. Adobe Photoshop CS -User Guide.
Adobe Systems Inc. San Jose CA 2003.

Ahmad I. Dental Photography. Chicago:
Quintessence 2004.

Altmann R. Digitale Fotografie und
Bildbearbeitung. Zürich: Midas 2001.

Baker CM. Introducing dentistry to
the 21st century via the intraoral camera.
Dent Today 1996;15:94–95.

Baumann D, Künne C. Digitales Atelier.
Hamburg: Rowohlt 2004.

Baumann H.D. Digitale Mal- und
Grafiktechniken. Köln: DuMont 1993.

Bengel W. Die Photographie in Zahnmedizin und
Zahntechnik. Berlin: Quintessenz 1984.

Bengel W. Sailwind MacroMate:
Für Objektbeleuchtung im Nahbereich.
Photomed 1992;5:90–93.

Bengel W. Einfache Fotografie kleiner Objekte
unter Verwendung einer neuen Faser-
lichtquelle. Quintessenz 1992;43:293–309.

Bengel W. Zahnärztliche Sach- und
Reprofotografie. Zahnarztl Mitt
1997;17:2044–2050.

Bengel W. Möglichkeiten der digitalen Fotografie
in der Zahnheilkunde. Quintessenz
1997;4:517–536 und 5:671–683.

Bengel W. Bildschirmfotografie. Quintessenz
1997;10:1381–1387.

Bengel W. Dentale Fotografie – konventionell
und digital. Berlin: Quintessenz 2000.

Bengel W. Mastering Dental Photography. Berlin,
Chicago: Quintessence 2002.

Bengel W. Digital Photography and the Assess-
ment of Therapeutic Results after Bleaching
Procedures. JERD 2003; Vol. 15,
Supplement 1.

Besser H. In: Sitts M (ed.). Handbook for Digital
Projects: A Management Tool for
Preservation and Access. Andover MA:
Northeast Document Conservation Center
2000:155–166.

Blaker AA. Handbook for Scientific Photography.
2nd ed. Boston: Focal Press 1989.

Brown EM. Medical Photography of Patients.
London: Lewis & Co 1968.

Claman LJ, Rashid R. Techniques for Dental
Photography.In: Vetter JP (ed.):
Biomedical Photography.
Boston: Butterworth-Heinemann 1992.

Deininger HK. Die Reproduktion
von Röntgenaufnahmen.
Photomed 1993;6:19–24.

DiSaia JP. Digital photography for the plastic
surgeon. Plast Reconstr Surg
1998;102:569–573.

Enk D, Filler T. Optimierte Bildschirmfotografie.
Photomed 1992;5:42–49.

Fan PP. Choosing the Right Clinical Camera.
Part I-III. Oral Health 1998;4–6.

Farr C. Video Imaging. Dent Today 1993;11,12.

Fleischer G. Dia-Vorträge. Stuttgart: Thieme 1986.

Freehe CL. Symposion on Dental Photography.
Dent Clin North Am 1968;Part II.

Freeman M. The Photographer's Studio Manual.
London: Collins 1984.

Freund U. Picture Publisher 4.0 – das offizielle
Handbuch.München: te-wi-Verlag 1994.

Frey S. Die Macht des Bildes. Bern: Huber 1999.

Garber DA. The Changing Face of Dentistry. Vor-
trag gehalten am 16.02.1992. Chicago:
Midwinter Meeting.

Gehrman RE. Dental Photography. Tulsa:
PennWell 1982.

Goldstein CE, Goldstein RE, Garber DA:
Imaging in Esthetic Dentistry.
Chicago: Quintessence 1998.

Gradias M. Computergrafik in der Praxis. Reihe: Medien in der Wissenschaft, Bd 3. Gesellschaft für Medien in der Wissenschaft e. V. (Hrsg.). Göttingen 1994.

Grey T. Color Confidence. Sybex, Alameda CA 2004.

Händel K. Rechtsfragen der medizinischen Photographie. Photomed 1990;3:281–286.

Hansell P (ed.). A Guide to Medical Photography. Lancaster: MTP Press 1979.

Kelby S. The photoshop CS book for digital photographers. New Riders Publishing, 2003.

Kelby S. Photoshop Classic Effects. München: Addison-Wesley 2005.

Kommer I, Held B. Microsoft PowerPoint – Das Profibuch. Unterschleißheim: Microsoft Press 2004.

Koren G, Buchinger F. Adobe Photoshop CS professionell. Bonn: Galileo Press 2004.

LeBeau LJ. Photography of Small Laboratory Objects. In: Vetter JP (Hrsg.): Biomedical Photography. Boston: Butterworth-Heinemann 1992.

LeBeau L. Fotografie kleiner biomedizinischer Objekte. Photomed 1993;6:159–167.

Maro F. Sicher Präsentieren. Düsseldorf: Econ 1994.

Maschke T. Digitale Aufnahmetechnik. Berlin: Springer 2004.

Maschke T. Digitale Bildbearbeitung. Berlin: Springer 2004.

Maschke T. Digitale Kameratechnik. Berlin: Springer 2004.

McLaren, EA, Terry DA. Photography in dentistry. J Calif Dent Assoc 2001;29:735–742.

Meyer T. Die Inszenierung des Scheins. Frankfurt: Suhrkamp 1992.

Nathanson O. Dental imaging by a computer: a look at the future. JADA 1991;122:45–46.

Rashid R, Claman LJ. Equipment for Dental Photography. In: Vetter JP (ed.): Biomedical Photography. Boston: Butterworth-Heinemann 1992.

Ratcliff S. Digital Dental Photography. Pankey Dental Foundation 2004.

Riedel H. Fotorecht für die Praxis. München: Verlag Photo Technik International 1988.

Schirra C, Haak R. Bitte lächeln! Die zahnärztliche Fotografie als Hilfsmittel bei der Patienten-dokumentation und -kommunikation. Quintessenz 1999;4:377–384.

Schlicht H-J. Digitale Bildverarbeitung mit dem PC. Bonn: Addison-Wesley 1993.

Schlicht H-J. Anwendung und professionelle Nutzung der Kodak Photo CD. Bonn: Addison-Wesley 1995.

Schröder G. Technische Fotografie. Würzburg: Vogel 1981.

Schuler G. Adobe Photoshop CS – Retusche, Montage & Farbkorrektur. Bonn: Galileo Press 2004.

Seino H et al. Dental Imagination – A Record of Techniques and Feelings. Tokyo: Quintessence 1988.

Snow SR. Dental Photography Systems: Required Features for Equipment Selection. Compendium May 2005; Vol. 26.

Spanik C. Elektronische Bildverarbeitung mit dem PC. Würzburg: Vogel, 1994.

Thissen, F. Kompendium Screen-Design, 3. Aufl. Berlin: Springer 2003.

Thomas JR et al. Analysis of patient response to preoperative computerized video imaging. Arch Otolaryngol Head Neck Surg 1989;115:793–796.

Van der Veen G. Die Archivierung von Dias und Videobändern: Ein Minimalansatz. Photomed 1988;1:285–288.

Vetter JP (Hrsg.). Biomedical Photography. Boston: Butterworth-Heinemann 1992.

Vonow P. Zahnärztliche Fotografie: Das Contax-Dental-System. Schweiz Mschr Zahnheilk 1983;4:252–257.

Walz P. Photo-CD mit dem PC. Würzburg: Vogel 1994.

Wander P, Gordon, P. Dental Photography. London: BDJ 1987.

Wesche H. Photoaufnahmen abseits der Routine – ein Praxisbericht. Photomed 1989;2:191–194.

Wesche H. Diakopie mit dem Farbmischkopf. Photomed 1990;3:49–54.

Williams AR. Medical Photography Study Guide. Lancaster: MTP Press 1984.

Williams AR. Positionierung und Beleuchtung für die Patientenphotographie. Photomed 1991;4:21-34.

Williams AR, Nieuwenhuis G. Clinical and Operating Room Photography. In: Vetter, JP (Hrsg.): Biomedical Photography. Boston: Butterworth-.Heinemann 1992.

Woerrlein H, Neumann G. Perfekt präsentieren. München: Markt & Technik 1993.

Wolf H. Zwei Makroblitzgeräte im Test: Nikon Macro Speedlight SB-21 und Minolta Macro-Flash 1200 AF. Photomed 1988;1:111–124.

Index